OVERTOUN

VOLUME FOUR

OVERTOUN: KENTUCKY

Dr ALEX NIVEN

THANKS

Friend, talented novelist Jassy Mackenzie whose published works provide inspiration: *go Jade, go*, and advice. Check out her website at http://www.jassymackenzie.com. People of the towns and cities who set scenes including Dumbarton, Dumfries, and Johannesburg.

God, through The Lord Jesus Christ whose power to forgive, by continuously scalpels clean bring hope and promise.

Family, as always for providing the security of a loving nest in which to grow and express imagination. Melissa, Andrew, Christine, Holly, Callum, and Finley for their input.

CONTENTS

INTRODUCTION

Begin by stating, I accept mankind's role in life is imperfect. A fact which begins with me. In relation to our dealings with ourselves, and our fellow humans we act flawed, as warned by the theory of Original Sin.

While accepting it possible to control the devil inside and become the perfect human authored by the Supreme Being who made us Imago Dei, the image of God, appreciate most only attain that lofty state at or around their death... better described as a necessary, inevitable process allowing graduation to the next life.

This, as a well-recognised philosophy only takes on firm flesh as we mature and witness our own individual failings and those around us. Thus, as a veterinary surgeon working hard to attain mastery of animal behaviour and disease, contact with their owners, trainers, and caregivers, permitted insight into the darker side of relationships, the power of greed, and the difficult people face in forgiving others and especially important, themselves, did the notion of creating a novel develop.

Two incidents around the turn of the century, sparked action.

One was an actual human drama centred on the accidental... well neglectful mixing up of twins after birth in a maternity hospital.

The second related to how easily a Johannesburg horse trainer carried off multiple insurance frauds by falsifying documents and then killing the horses with insulin overdose.

While suspicion abounded, and fingers pointed, the lack of true evidence; although the local horse fraternity knew, allowed him to escape detection.

Why? How did these events push me into the novel Overtoun?

No answer! And then, as rhino poaching escalated, my active mind developed along Overtoun's conclusion in volume five. Daft, yes. But the ending needed a beginning.

Overtoun House in my hometown Dumbarton was the logical starting point.

Magnificent, please visit and gasp at the fabulous crafting of its ceilings. As the idea of swapping twins at birth commanded attention, so too did my profession offer the route map. So, here goes.

Alex Niven. Easter Sunday 2024

CHARACTERS

Angus Stewart Father of the swapped twins.

Margaret Stewart Twins mother.

Niall Cairns A Stewart twin swapped by Deirdre Cairns and raised by Fiona Cairns. As a researcher, develops with homoeopathy a cure for HIV.

Calder Stewart Fiona's true son by Henderson is tainted with his father's weak morals. Enters corrupt practices.

Alroy Stewart Niall's twin raised by Angus and Margaret Stewart. Police officer fighting fraud and corruption.

Wolf Alroy reports to him as Police Commissioner.

Alroy's team Henry, Pauline, Sophia, and others do outstanding work when combating fraud.

Flynn and Gordon Corrupt police officers.

Georgiou This bogus and corrupt vet encourages Calder Stewart into insurance fraud by killing healthy horses.

Sr Angela At Overtoun, her concerns over Deirdre's mental health, and management of nursing infants raises concern when revealed to Francesca.

Francesca Cormie Angus Stewart's illegitimate daughter. Engaged to Niall, who as Angus' son means disaster.

Sr Catherine Midwife at Overtoun, hospitalised and now recovering, as memory Corrupt US vets involved in dodgy European escapades to smuggle diamonds.

Patrick and Holly Overtoun's doctor, married to midwife and ICU specialist.

FBI Waterman and Blanchard are top field agents involved in taking down criminals in the US. They work alongside their GB counterparts. Designated to be the victim in an insurance fraud, his final whinny is loudest of all.

CATCH UP

With TOPSY TURVY; last chapter of Overtoun Volume Three.

TOPSY TURVY

Racing industry abounds with dodgy people.

Crime unfolds easier when large dollar signs flash.

While neither Yvette or Louis searched for cases, they found it easier when lukewarm enquiries enticed them to explore openings that burned with ambrosial aroma of easy dollars and attracted notice.

To be sure, when seriously searched, they appreciated pits of despair that dragged down disgruntled owners, realised just how ripe the field promised.

As a result of horses often disappointing owners, particularly well-bred and expensive individuals, situations abound where dissatisfied clients write off inferior charges.

Notwithstanding them still a loss, for major breeders and owners, those with vast sums to hand and hopeful replacements will fit the bill, laugh them off, mark them down as tax losses where creative accountants softened the blow.

For one thing, when they worked together, this vet couple followed the same path, knuckled down to building their relationship and veterinary practice and kept eyes open for lucrative, safe possibilities.

In Lionel Dixon, they soon lined up their foremost claim.

A general builder, astute Lionel, took cognisance of trend to mail order selling and with a junior partner, explored building warehouses.

Immediate success followed. Later he described success as unexpected, stupendous. Besides, as they embraced that initial successful streak with massive financial rewards, which allowed him to satisfy a life ambition of owning a racehorse.

To begin with, as a significant punter on ponies, one who kept meticulous records of investments, declared himself one of few professional gamblers who annually made money from betting. In contrast, having known hundreds of gamblers with fail proof systems, who lost fortunes, Louis tried it for one year.

Found it malodorous, never worked.

Forthwith, even with sound inside knowledge, he broke even after twenty-one betting; *cannot fail efforts*, and finding it not worth the emotional effort, appreciated pressure encouraged greed.

Excitement generated by a winning bet made him understand pitfalls, how easily addiction develops into flood of a monsoon.

Also, odd that we allow colossal amounts of betting marketing when knowing misery caused by addiction. Only greed allows the sporting industry to absorb gaps left after tobacco restrictions.

Mind you, still legal to sell cancer sticks.

For example, fascinated Louis to watch TV racing programs where palatable experts, often self-proclaimed, recommended punters where to place bets. Often shaking head, for he, knowing racing characters, reckoned only those earning delectable salaries from TV companies possessed more than three dollars to their name.

However, by establishing a system of setting a ceiling on how much to invest, and when to step back, reflect on how gamblers may indulge in crispy fun, and while never life-changing money, cavalcades of careful betters break even.

One nutty plan may burnish the wallet if content to place bets on the second favourite in a race. The casuistry of life ensures few possess required discipline. One misanthrope, after a dedicated season, complained he made only fifteen per cent profit.

Hang on... in that year the stock exchange only yielded seven!

Lionel's life reached a point where life flowed with enviable security and comfort. With basics of life fulfilled; family nestled in an exquisite home, and particulate, secured investments guaranteed financial security.

A residue of sufficient funds enabled him to realise dream of owning a racehorse. In fact, and without delay, Gertie, his statuesque wife, thrilled, when she announced her support. They gained unexpected rewards when acting together, their common interest in this fresh project found them regularly visiting racetracks.

Next, that fulfilled social implications necessary to satisfy his outgoing wife. Race meetings are often associated with lunch and smart dressing required for visits to parade ring.

Because she enjoyed the venture, they found entertaining friends a rung up on the wool-gathering one-upmanship that drives New York society, that ricocheted their social standing up the ladder.

An unexpected bonus supplanted earlier boredom when interacting with horses and racing meant they shared quality time together. Gertie thrilled at what she described as their Date Days, described how they regenerated earlier lively relationship that had with time stagnated. Thus, horse racing for them proved a win–win story.

So, they indulged in racing from the top side and having dealt profitably with Joao Gomes, a marketing man, took advice from Joao's sister, Sheila Ariadne, and bought a yearling.

The tough talking, hard drinking divorcé took no prisoners.

A hard, sober face adorned with excessive wrinkles generated by an all-weather outdoor lifestyle, meant she fitted mould of a professional, if unkempt horse lady, featured by long, straggling brown hair and chipped finger nails whose bright green covering while drawing attention to them, never hid defects.

Hence, when leading him by the... let us go with convention, say ear, she used him to make herself a fat commission.

Furthermore, surprised when a stroke of luck meant Topsy Turvy; now a three-year-old colt, won four races on the trot. Say surprised, because prospective owners disliked the horse, spun him because his heart produced an odd sound that suggested a defect.

The breeder conspired with Sheila, encouraged her to make Joao fork out one hundred and twenty thousand dollars for the horse, which enabled her to pocket a useful twenty thousand commission for the sneaky deal. In the meantime, the horse's early success, including a black-type feature race, meant his value soared, and rejecting big paydays to sell, aimed him for classic races.

On balance, Sheila, herself no tender bunch of violets, experienced in vagaries of horses, insisted, cajoled, or seduced him to give her an undervalued share,
They insured the horse for a vast sum.

Calamity that often dogs exercise physiology flared, because, after they rejected an offer to purchase of seven hundred and eighty thousand dollars. A simple respiratory virus that sneaked around stables changed aspirations. Regardless of TT experiencing clinical signs only after a gallop, the insidious virus strained, permanently so, an already genetically compromised heart.

Its associated weakened circulation reduced his twinkle toed efforts.

While the inherent anatomical heart murmur was of no clinical significance, when combined with viral induced carditis, that rendered Topsy Turvey's powertrain useless. Unable to run faster than the stable dogs, they termed him a useless hound.

Also, Lionel's business interests hit a sticky patch.

His minor partner made a significant, inappropriate investment without taking Lionel's opinion. An economic loss, it left them bogged down in an unsavoury mire patch that enforced them to tighten belts.

Lady Serendipity played her part with predictable coincidence when Yvette, as regular stable vet, gave Sheila unwelcome news.

With both in professional mode there was no need to euphemise or soft soap the problem so she dived straight in. 'The ECG evidence points to chronic, irreversible carditis.'

They stood inside the hospital barn, and as she fingered the collar of her sodden rain jacket, Sheila bemoaned poor decision making. 'Damn the thing. On the contrary, against better judgement, we turned down that great offer to sell. And now.' Stroked dirty fingers through equally untidy, rampant brown hair. 'If we give him a decent holiday, will that help?'

In adamant form, Yvette continued. 'As a handsome gelding, you might get eight grand as a jumper, and he may perform well even up to B-grade.'

'A disaster. There must be a solution. To think we insured him for a fortune, more than enough to restore our weak financial position.'

Sheila kicked off a life-changing career when staring at Yvette, she cocked her head and said, 'Now, honey child, if only he could die on us.'

Yvette and Louis put heads together and planned his execution.

Fast as that.

From unconsidered to complete planning, they uncovered a solution by the end of their second coffee. Yvette wagged a finger to foreboding strains of Handel's Messiah. Music appropriate for Holy Week before Easter.

In summary, if it took vets forty minutes to decide on the killing method.

Sheila's downright eagerness locked onto Yvette's eyes when she outlined the method. 'Agreed, so what next.'

First part settled on Sheila instructing head groom Miguel to restrict the horse's feed.

'No breakfast for TT, because we plan to treat him with specialised medicine this morning.'

When he and other grooms set off to feed the yard, she, employed best clandestine fashion of all sleuths, to slip two cupsful of the strongest coffee, mixed in banana essence, into the hungry horse's manger.

Watched as he gobbled this down then hung head over stable doors in harmony with compatriots while eagerly awaiting his five am, pre-exercise feed.

On an empty stomach, coffee soon triggered a period of intense excitement associated with palpitations and sweating. She called the pre-prepared Yvette; already dressed, about to exercise her horse, Sunshine.

She raced over and examined TT, diagnosed him affected by meningitis or encephalitis. 'A hangover from virus, could be a serious complication.'

Returned to car to fetch a dose of Domosedan to tranquilise horse, but on her return acted in a different manner. In a tight, tidy yard of only thirty horses, proved easy to overdose horse with a massive dose of insulin.

Thereafter, the animal experienced a dramatic lowering of blood glucose levels with concomitant severe neurological signs, including seizures. 'Sheila, we are too late. Also, ring owners, prepare them for the worst. Advise they seek a second opinion, for he may die.'

Sheila played her part, for as second owner, she at once called Francoise Cardin, senior vet in a rival practice to examine the horse.

Concurred with Yvette's opinion. 'Granted I, like you have experienced these sudden onset encephalitis cases before, and often in spring after fresh fly activity spreads viruses.'

Despite their detailed examination and administration of high doses of tranquilisers, when the horse collapsed, Francoise said, 'This horse will be dead in fifteen minutes.'

Not only did the horse die, but Yvette had an unexpected bonus when Francoise took on role of arranging postmortem and later certification. To emphasise usefulness of that move, he reduced any pressure Yvette may have experienced as stable vet.

'Sorry, Joao, while we did everything possible to save him, he died on us.'

Forthwith, it stunned Joao for they never discussed their plans with him, while the pragmatic Gertie, as she listened to the conversation, clapped hands. 'Magic. Stupid, useless creature has just earned us a big pay day.'

In time, with planned slaughter going off without a hitch, and paperwork easy to complete, Joao solved his financial snag.

Vets earned a fragrant forty thousand dollars from their first incursion into fraud.

And so, it continued.

Until greedy... vets stretched themselves.

People whispered.

Thereafter, as that whiff of suspicion became more than a soupcon of unpleasantness, they accepted it less than flavourful and took a positive stance. Cold facts allowed them to appreciate they acted blasé.

By managing their last case in careless fashion, which prompted them to take a preeminent decision.

Never trenchant, they sold off their expanding Florida business and relocated. Also, they swore their future professional must remain sacrosanct, no more indulging in mephitic fraud.

That said, the three hundred and twenty thousand dollars cash they had already earned worked wonders. For they judiciously used the clandestine cash netted from fourteen ventures in insurance fraud which, as it burned holes in pockets soon helped them found an equine practice in New York State.

Horse country of Newark embraced them, authorised them to take over an established, but ailing vet practice on Reynolds Road, close by a racing centre.

Renamed as HORSES 'R-U-S, ill-gotten gains helped them construct a well-equipped, custom-built practice.

Forthwith, registered in Yvette's name, they worked hard and earned well as practice boomed.

That changed for the better when propositioned by Chinese investors. This led to fresh, illegal gains earned in Europe, via an extraordinary novel approach.

Wealth multiplied at exponential rate.

1

WINE LUBRICATES

Racing industry abounds with fabulous people.

Those who work in the industry for love.

Horsey people share a fascination for everything connected with horses, from how they savour their wholesome, earthy smell to a remarkably sensual touch and primarily for their movement. And not necessarily or only the exquisite movement of Prix Saint George dressage, as even the plainest individual can produce extraordinary classic passes when on his own in a paddock and at that moment in time feels like showing-off by indulging in a series of bounces and flying changes.

Arguably Arabic poetry expresses this best and one of the better-known examples is the modern work of Saudi Arabia's Prince Khaled AlFaisal.

'From the daughters of the wind, I own a flighty chestnut mare.

When she flights, she's like a desert deer.

Any rider wishes a mare like her, as does all horse experts.

Her beauty is in her delicacy and majesty.'

Lee S, Dougherty[1] offers a poignant introduction to the involvement of the Bedouin people and horses. When she touches on how diverse people from artists to scholars symbolise the horse one feels the truth of where and the necessity for powerful partnerships arose and continue to develop man's awareness for the environment.

Gerda Stevenson offers a different route when she incorporates the human touch.

---

[1] Lee S. Dougherty. Arabian Horse World. Winter 2024.

Two horses against a hill,

shoulder to shoulder,

one faces East, the other West,

and I think of us –

how we can be,

sometimes, at our best:

opposites, yet close enough

to cradle each other's different worlds

in a wide arc of peripheral vision.

But when delicacy and majesty are insufficient for those connected with the animals, temptation strikes.

Other factors centred on money can come into play and may distastefully lead to greed and its buddy, crime.

Deceit, lies, and fraud unfold easier when dollar signs flash, as the carrot encouraged the horse to follow so does the prospect of easy money produce a flavoursome release of savoury factors which as they enter people's nostrils, attract, and excite.

This provides opportunity for lesser mortals; in terms of expected moral values, who as ears prick, search for bargains, and... well, yes, crime in all its manifestations rises to surface to detriment of not only horses but also, those associated with them.

While parttime criminals; astonishing numbers of them never actively search for cases but find them easier to stumble on when unexpected events raise sufficient interest. The ambrosial aroma of easy money, attract notice then maintains interest. There are others, those with an inherent tendency to easily commit crime and who diligently search for dodgy openings. They do so when fully aware of pitfalls of detection.

Yet, temptation to easy money may hold sway even when aware of potential disaster that follows capture as pits of despair swallow them when the judicial system metes out punishment.

All shady characters, cognisant of how poorly performing sport horses cause disappointment to identify disgruntled owners and persuade them to enter crime in hope of salvaging economic loss.

As a result of horses often disappointing owners, including well-bred and expensive individuals, situations abound where frustrated clients write-off inferior charges.

Notwithstanding, them still a loss, for major breeders and owners, those with vast sums to hand and aware of hopeful replacements growing back home in farm and stables, can afford to laugh them off, mark them down as tax losses where creative accountants soften the blow.

Partnerships do not always work.

But when effective, results can be spectacular.

More so when the parties work well together. Thus, consider how this vet couple entered into a solid romantic, professional and crime affiliation.

After surviving a near miss, they followed a fresh and declared mutual intention this should trace an honest open path. Knuckled down to building their relationship and using ill-gotten gains from clandestine practices equipped a finer equine veterinary hospital than most could ever manage from a basic start.

With enviable ambition they intended to create a five-star unit.

Until as expenses mounted.

Financial factors required to create their specialist facility soon ate into their capital and as they appreciated how reserves disappeared and convinced standard routes of obtaining capital unpleasant, scratched heads and looked around.

Inevitably, Louis looked back with longing. 'Dear one, almost there.'

Early evening, with glass of wine in hand, they prepared to stroll through hospital. When time allowed, this permitted a regular inspection of the inmates.

Different this time for it allowed them opportunity to consider final additions necessary to instruct builders and outfitters on the new theatre and investigation facility. 'Imagine with an additional three-hundred-thousands of ready cash we could cream this venture, set ourselves up forever.

'Yvette's push for supremacy in profession showed when as she stroked dated radiography equipment, she agreed. 'If only we could.'

Louis found it easy to agree, then introduced where he depressed over their latest financial projections outlined by accountant Mullins. 'Found Eddie's figures encouraging.' Stroked her arm. 'Decided we are on the right track, as with income increasing, we can employ a second assistant vet, and additional nurse, and still afford to pay off a reasonable loan.'

Yvette slugged down the remnants of her glass.

Studied his face, and uninvited took over his half full crystal. 'Love this chardonnay, but sense it not too your taste, so,' Brushed lips with tongue tip, 'let me pour you a glass of your favourite, rich merlot.

Before she reached their apartment, hesitated. 'Perhaps…'

He picked up a change in her tone and curious, said, 'Know that gleam, and as you spoil me, sense something big runs through that delightful mind?'

She held up a finger, winked, and said, 'Give me a minute,'

On her return, as she passed over his glass she returned to the subject. 'Well… While we agreed to keep business professional, straight down the line, wonder if we should keep eyes open for another lucrative, dead safe possibility or two.'

Yvette, without entering into reversion to unfold how their successful, fraudulent deals earned good money, waited, watched as he swirled a South African *Merlot* in a larger glass and inhaled its fragrance.

Remained patient as he admitted. 'This generous vintage shares a heavenly aroma.' Then, after a healthy, satisfying sip, mind harmonised with her opinion but expressed concern. 'Thanks, precious one, for while we did well, still shudder over how that case with *Flirting Surprise*, brought us close to disaster.'

Kissed top of her head. 'And thus, nervous to again involve ourselves in something tricky especially as we are already in a good spot.'

As they reached Sunshine's stable and still in thoughtful mode Yvette stroked the attentive horse's muzzle, and said, 'We were stupid, greedy with that case. With hindsight, avarice overruled brains for truly, neither of us felt it a safe scam worthy of our efforts.'

He sipped at wine as she offered a weak chortle. 'And appropriate, after we flirted with jail that time, decided enough, too dangerous.'

Encouraged one finger to match Yvette's rhythm on Sunshine's nose, and as empathy flowed, shared a more nervous chuckle at that difficult experience. 'Dead right girl, a near thing when that groom's curiosity almost spilled beans.'

Streak of her base toughness struck hard. 'Lucky, we found the halfwit easy to control.' As opinion firmed, Louis took discussion forward. 'Although when we consider earlier success, how easy it was to milk some cases, and if we do not look for cases, well… if the perfect one jumps out at us and screams dollars, agree we should consider opportunity.'

Next, as she warmed to memories where the chase thrilled, Yvette, nurtured greed and as she swirled wine in the manner of an official taster, without necessity of spitting sample out, admitted possibilities abounded.

After Louis nuzzled her neck below the left ear, she appreciated how he aroused flavours even more than the *Mcintyre Kimberly Vineyards Arroyo Seco*, bought before popular acclaim tripled the price, and allowed logic to have its way. 'Okay, but both must agree it a cast iron venture. Satisfied!'

2

A NEW VENTURE

Two men visited the hospital.

Insistent, charmed their way to an appointment with both vets.

When they dealt with practice manager Florence; despite her being regularly forewarned partners wished to interview only bona fide equine aficionados, by acting gentle, with heaps of flattery, their persuasive argument had its way.

Thereafter, as she offered Yvette an apology for arranging meeting with people her boss must decide not pucca horsey types, said, 'Both are so handsome, and dress and manners nutty, unfashionable for New York.' Pretended to swoon; said they caused quite a stir.

While Florence was clueless to former fraud, nervous anticipation made Louis at once en guard, suspicious them snooping FBI agents whose false names hid identities.

Inasmuch as Florence had arranged the meeting, discounted idea of cancelling for fear they raise red flags, also because they refused to leave their manager with contact details, met the two fashionably dressed men who arrived prompt, in reception area.

As the vet moved to greet, smaller of the two, he slipped off the hooded, snow flaked windproof while the other studied a series of smart, professionally produced photographs that accurately recorded a horse undergoing colic surgery in the clinic.

As Louis walked up, he emphatically endorsed the skill illustrations suggested. Most impressive. Makes me confident you are the right people to solve our conundrum.' Before he gave the vet time to form a decent impression, the visitors insisted Yvette join them. 'Her opinion is essential. Please. Guarantee she will find our meeting worthwhile.' Dived to point faster than a stooping peregrine.

In a strong voice made more attractive for her by its hint of an educated Eastern European accent, taller one said, 'We studied your interesting, adaptive their work in Florida.'

Both sets of eyes flared as vets looked at each other as he continued. 'Savoured your impressive resume and *reputation*.' When underscoring the word reputation, he set both pulses racing with remarkable harmony.

Raised eyebrows failed to settle as he dug into subject with mental agility of a horse on bovine somatotrophin, when he revealed results of their voracious research. 'Our posthumous investigations of insurance certification exposed your standing in the industry as professionals.'

Paused, studied vets' anxious faces with intensity of a forensic accountant. 'It came to our attention you are known to... be flexible with rules.'

Louis barely resisted a gulp, a remarkable sense of control not emulated by his partner, although their visitors never reacted to such overt distress. '

The shorter man smiled. 'Admired that, particularly your propensity for successfully making money by assisting deserving owners.'

Yvette's mind raced into depths that forecasted abyssal scenarios which included finding herself sealed under iron bars in a dank oubliette, with a myriad of black suited FBI special black ops agents.

It was how they pulled off toenails that induced another gulp from an already tight chest full of stale air. As she slapped a hand over her left breast, a second hideous thought dug into her brain where they tortured her with electric clips on nipples.

Furthermore, when Louis tried to interject, the smaller man, also touched with an Asian background; but not excessively so, expressed dominance when he reached out and placed a soft palm flat on Louis' chest.

In flawless English, used a gentle tone to bring calm. 'Please, do not insult our intelligence. Facts are facts and thus our industry, compared to attitude of standard legal opinion, awards you platitudes.'

As his partner issued a small chuckle he continued. 'We appreciate where you have been most helpful to distressed horse connections.'

As her pupils expanded, Yvette's eyes, while they by bathing her face in darkness created a stunning belladonna effect, confirmed secrets she hoped never to release while he went on. 'Those with significant, particular problems.'

Hesitant to apportion time for them to issue wasteful ancient statements declaring innocence, he, allowed that most powerful opening gambit, to sink in, while appreciating why neither of the professionals responded.

Gave another, advised them not to worry, for their outstanding history of gracious client support explained their desire to meet.

Even if his relaxed open statement never held tenor of suspicion or aggression, only a lamenting pibroch on a heather clad Scottish mountain top might have added to misery that perfused vets' psyche.

As Yvette released the final litres of trapped air that threatened to burst through her chest, she suddenly appreciated enormous relief. 'Wow! So, we are not off to jail. Magic.'

In time, the same man explained how they mesmerised over history.

Most impressive. (Heavy emphasis). With both vets still tongue tied, and as nails threatened to grow deep through the floor to create permanent anchors taller man emitted a hearty chuckle. 'Now, time to put you out of misery.'

With visitors, satisfied they had nicely softened Yvette and Louis they laughed again, and this time vet pulses dropped when they appreciated light-hearted tone of their banter.

As Yvette clung to Louis arm for support, he felt her tension drop as the leader of the two said, 'We need your help.' That short statement encouraged troubled brains to focus on what followed. 'For we have a difficult, but lucrative project in mind, and only you can solve our problem, bearing in mind it one that will prove of exceptional interest and be profitable.'

Distant from any of the normal health matters of veterinary practice, a remarkable conversation followed when, during a remarkable forty minutes, what proved the most absorbing meeting either vet experienced, unfolded.

Amid hurly-burly of expanding their new, well fitted veterinary hospital, they, satisfied they left a life of criminal fraudulent activities behind; these two fascinating men took them to areas never explored.

On balance, they presented two attractive prospects. First up, a well delivered, punchy argument struck home when they drew her attention to incredible; later, Yvette, mouth-watering, described them as obscene, profits.

Second, their ingrained approach to, and experience of international crime allowed vets to glimpse an unexplored vision of proper organised and efficient criminality in what smaller man named as real-world situations.

Clincher followed, one that harmonised with aspirations of the two competent, highly intelligent petty crooks, make them ask if corruption proved unbeatable, why not collaborate with experts in a safer environment and take a deserved share?

Then floored them when they claimed to be agents of a powerful, inordinately successful international smuggling ring. Granted that was now difficult, with traditional routes becoming increasingly better policed, they hoped vets could help them move contraband diamonds by developing innovative systems.

Tall man, all thoughts of soft approach gone, said, 'As you know the equine industry inside out, and benefit from a mutually dishonest partnership to encourage each other, which places you at an advantage over the two vets who are next line to approach, should your attitude... or efforts, discourage.

For fear, time must compromise their normal, slimy arrangements in harvesting dodgy diamonds; bloodstones from African continent through Asia and Russia to England and the US, their masters instructed them to open further new areas and routes to move an impressive collection of precious stones.

Altogether they displayed a sound knowledge of the industry, and centred debate on the booming international trade in elite sports horses.

With vets hooked, they suggested that meant a unique, potentially valuable opening for an exclusive sophisticated and mutually beneficial partnership in the smuggling trade. For, as proven smugglers, they desired skilled vets to assist by creating a novel method for trafficking already stockpiled diamonds.

Taller one gave vets a simple brief. 'We need you to put some effort into this project and research whether you can help us achieve our goals?'

A sweetener followed.

When, as evidence of faith in what seemed a system based as ludicrous as developing a breed of horse that required no feed, as visitors prepared to drift off into a cooling wintry evening, taller one as spokesperson, reiterated hopes they could produce a mutually valuable solution.

'One destined to be therapeutic to the financial status of professionals portaging through necessary financial minefields.'

Satisfied with their tour of hospital, they spotted possibilities for improvement, echoed Yvette's earlier comments. 'Love what you are doing with this place.'

Threw an arm around. 'Consider lady, what you might achieve with half a million dollars of safely laundered income. How that should support you to purchase the best of portable and fixed radiographic equipment'

When he noted how she caught bottom lip between teeth, he reinforced argument. 'Which must make this best private equine unit for miles around.'

Together with how he created a scene redolent in flamboyance of a classical conductor, he prolonged his control when he gestured at a smart paper bag emblazoned with the Chanel logo, his partner placed tantalisingly on a desk.

'Work with us and this, 'Fondled bag as though caressing a lady's thigh, 'is a mere fraction of what your efforts with us should accumulate.'

Louis walked them to their car, where they, despite suitably dressed to face windblown snow, shivered.

Vet watched as they left, active mind loaded with grey matter technobabble, too busy to consider steady drip of sleet as it dripped on head from the mature oak that dominated front car park.

3

GIRLS DESERVE CHANEL

Smugglers bid him goodbye.

Yvette remained leaning over counter.

Immobile, eyes fixed on that paper bag.

Impatient and as tongue sensuously licked lips, prayed they must soon disappear, get on with whatever they had next in mind.

On Louis return, silent and insistent, she dragged him off to their smart, two bedroomed apartment.

As Louis' confidence overflowed, mind solidly registered an outstanding financial future, he took the bag from her, bowed, and in humble mode, said, 'For you madame. As queen of Kentucky, you deserve honour of opening this mysterious gift.'

After he ceremoniously passed the bag to eager Yvette, she managed the structure with care usually only displayed when she operated on a horse's larynx, then, opened the carrier.

Withdrew a handbag protected by oodles of bubble wrapping.

Before she could speak, Louis smiled and said, 'That looks a fine bag.'

In full feminine mode, a million times more sensitive than her partners, Yvette gasped as she uncovered a fifteen thousand-dollar Chanel handbag.

In grey, quilted leather the caviar design left her speechless.

As he acceded to her superb taste in these things, and encouraged by her astonished gasp, even he gloried in the gift, imagined how it must suit his lady for smart functions. Considered this then switched focus as she opened watching focused attitude when opened bag to check out internal architecture.

Speechless, Yvette managed a brief. 'Gosh.'

For she ended the unwrapping ceremony with a heck of an inducement when she pulled out fifty thousand dollars in crisp new notes. Only as the dollar signs which clouded vision cleared, conversation escalated and magnified their interest in this incredible project to levels beyond stratospheric heights.

Although Yvette found it difficult to count money because she could not remove eyes from bag. Louis's basic and inherent greed summed things up when he declared. 'With this as a backhander, how much can we make from the real thing?'

Yvette, though she swithered between uncomfortable and ecstatic, remained intrigued at the project. 'Profitable... doubtless we must move forward... for this incentive makes their business proposition undeniably attractive.'

4

SENSIBLE SANDY

Niall needed a full three days to get his head right.

Because he and Francesca deserted the world.

Spent so much time enjoying each other with the egotistical passion which characterises fresh love. Selfish, this resulted in urgent truancy which although more than mutually satisfying threatened to derail medicine's urgent project.

Until as needs must, spent as any Atlantic hen salmon who, after laying eggs in redds of upper reaches of the Endrick River, drifts downstream. In a mostly haphazard, current controlled effort to return to Atlantic Ocean via Rivers Leven and Clyde.

Destined to be one of the few who recover after spawning to reach the ocean and continue to thrive, while her compatriots as they die and rot become part of the organic fabric of the river.

As Francesca drove, cabin reverberated to sound of *Alicia Keys* and *Fallin.* Which made conversation well-nigh impossible.

Niall, firmly stuck in decent music of eighties, never got head around how not only did Francesca indulge in modern strident music but also insisted on blasting it louder than he ever imagined a car sound system could produce.

Nor did he understand why she continuously repeated the same track. *Perhaps she is an unknown karaoke competitor, and I should consider this a serious rehearsal?*

Never realised her Golf had a custom-built system and might have choked at expense.

In carpark, he breathed silent, profound, as he said, 'My dearest, can we compromise on your various methods of aural torture.'

Concerns earned a slobbery kiss, as she ignored that comment.

After she negotiated a tricky corner at speed, waved off his concerns. 'Philistine.'

Then grabbed his hand and hurried them inside away from imminent threat of an onerous downpour. In time, with research project using homoeopathic remedies against HIV virus ready to move on, they extricated themselves from the super glue attachment which bound them together.

Guilty at neglecting work, Niall turned focus to consider team members and recognised with final tests now looming, back on track, then planned and savoured an extended meeting with Uncle Sandy.

Despite their improving success, one point still raised areas for concern. 'But Sandy, under pressure from team to add and change remedies.'

Wise man used right thumb and forefinger to squeeze lower lip into pouch while thinking, then offered advice. 'Cannot perceive us gaining anything hopeful by departing from the agreed plan.' Lip got another squeeze. 'No! For we burned gallons of midnight oil to create those formulations, so any ill-considered restructuring at this stage is inappropriate.'

Tenor of exchange rose for Sandy who had been around longer than Niall.

Anticipated disruption and half expected the Seekers; Niall's research team, for fear of missing something, to chop and change.

Took another moment to ponder his response then used wisdom to explain his projections. 'Experience leads me to understand that as we approach the conclusion of a project, must expect, and therefor anticipate unwarranted advice crops up.'

Happy that Niall followed his drift Sandy continued. 'Often, and without adding value, tension leads major players to be swayed by views of inexperienced and often tired, yet eager members.' Sandy, determined to make his point, offered a pertinent example.

***

'Often face similar difficulties with racehorse trainers.'

Niall chuckled, listened, and expected to gain a useful lesson from the hard field of the track.

'For example. Consider how a trainer and I, often with jockey input, plan a horse for a race until everyone agrees to follow a set exercise pattern.'

Niall held his tongue as Sandy went on. 'As human nerves twang, this causes niggling doubts, makes trainers contemporise and then often under an owner's opinion they deviate from the standard plan. A favoured comment, often if the owner has watched the final preparatory gallop, may go like this. *Unsure if colt needs to reduce last fast work, two or three days before race, by two hundred yards or must step it up by four hundred yards.*

Niall sympathised. 'This puts you under pressure. How do you cope?'

Sandy smiled. 'My job is to chat with her, hold hand and listen and then softly help to the trainer to appreciate the original exercise schedule was spot on. In the absence of any unexpected or unfamiliar problems, she should relax, make no changes.'

Highlighted how one trainer, with a superb horse, gave a harder than agreed gallop two days before a Group 1 race, when their charge was clear ante post favourite. 'Did so because, *they needed to be sure.*

As expected, the horse; *Change-a-Plenty,* put up a fabulous gallop, which satisfied connections.'

Niall noticed a frown trotted over Sandy's face as he said, 'Horse worked his heart out. Too much too close to the race.' Well in control, Sandy added. 'But then, noticed something. For the experienced Ferdie de Graaf, trainer of *Always Hope;* second favourite, watched that gallop. Saw him clap hands and pull out his phone to contact his owner.'

Sandy chuckled. 'Bear in mind that our tightly knitted training establishments allow efficient nosey parkers to watch everything. Because I lip read a bit, estimated he said something like, "Got them. Climb in now, hit bookies hard, for this morning they overworked their horse."'

Before the off, Ferdie's horse settled as clear favourite and during race as *Change-a-Plenty* felt effects of overwork he tired in final one hundred yards to finish a close run third.

Ferdie's owners made a killing at the bookies and sadly of lesser importance, collected a magnificent crystal trophy.

Sandy, pleased with how Niall accepted logic of that story, pushed shoulder with closed fist, three times at two second intervals. 'So, if your guts feel good, do not change course of this trial.'

Opinion satisfied Niall he made the correct decision and content with Sandy's assessment agreed it too late to add new remedies.

'Slow down, young man, take this steady.' Sandy held Niall's huge shoulders, forced him into a less than comfortable armchair. 'Recommend you stop your team searching outside project for additional holy grail remedies.' Sensible, offered a last piece of advice. 'But should this episode not go well, then we will be forced to backtrack, consider remedies earlier tried, and from there consider whether to make minor adjustments.'

Commonsense carried the day. Satisfied his team that while time might arrive when at a subsequent stage, as they reflect on results, then they may have to make potency adjustments.

Evan agreed. 'Ah! Got you now. You bolster confidence and perform as the visionary your team expect.' Of course. They continued to analyse, consider, debate, and as Niall displayed his normal enthusiasm and energy he prepared to close. 'So, we agree?'

Lack of contrary argument certified Sandy space to summarise. 'Yes. Only reservation relates to us discounting nosode Carcinosinum Burnett in the 30CH potency.'

At once, and irrespective of previous discussion, they changed minds, restored it for the test. 'Because of its link with chronic disease, especially for well-known association with weak immune systems and excellent therapeutic history in management of lung related conditions, consider it may be necessary.'

Niall also followed that route and expressed happiness, for Carc's regular employment in treatment of asthma and chronic bronchitis where patient coughs up a thick, often tacky gelatinous exudate is reminiscent of symptoms which plague patients with secondary TB infections.

'Indeed, that clinical picture fits as an unwelcome partner for so many AIDS sufferers, so, yes, must accept its powerful weighting.'

Prof clapped his shoulder and in a departure from normal invited. 'Business over. Time to visit my office for a celebratory nippy sweetie, a J&B.'

Hilda plugged on, reminded Niall of the French methodology. 'They produce and consume more homoeopathy than anyone else and prefer low potencies. So, am happy to increase numbers of nosodes by adding Carc to test number nine but let's be cautious and go with K12 potency.' Deal done. Evan laughed. 'Here we go, here we go.'

5

FINAL STRUCTURE

Breezed through the board meeting.

Successful, because everyone shared an air of optimism. Even obstreperous Carmichael surprised Francesca when he admitted to sharing their sense of profound optimism. *Niall has worked wonders there. Now keen.*

So, Niall sat back, basked in the cheerful assurance exuded by his team, as sudden rise in air temperature and its partner, a sneaky, fearful sun, made an appearance. So too, clouds of pessimism that had surrounded them like an intense Dumbarton fog dramatically revitalised them as it does over the estuary as nature steals it away from the River Clyde.

In harmony with improving weather, Niall embraced how air of growing confidence washed away negativity and lifted spirits in a cleansing wind of positive expectancy.

'No! Notwithstanding, this break finds my team rested, recognise they share eager eyes of the foraging Scottish Wild Cat once spotted on foothills of the Cairngorms.'

'So, ask again. Niall, are you ready for this?'

He started. 'Sorry Prof, wrapped up in the team's... well, youthful enthusiasm, ploughed through a sensitive, introverted moment.

'Prof, relaxed as anyone could remember, spilled his humane side. 'Well done, young man, and deservedly so. For we know how this project dragged you down, but now...' Gawked at everyone. 'let us kick hell out of it.'

Francesca added her report before they discussed makeup of final test. 'As a result of your increased confidence, introduced our exciting prospects with a potential investor.' Waved arms and in propitious yet encouraging manner. 'Subject to a further positive test, substantial funds are available.'

Keeping best for last, cheerful voice intimated that significant cash flow may allow for development of a new department focused on homoeopathy to develop new treatment protocols.'

That said, exercised firm self-control when not releasing how close the company was to signing a contract, for fear it might affect team, encourage negative anxiety during an emotionally charged time.

Especially, as they were keen on selecting Niall, despite relative inexperience, as Professor to run new department. Francesca chuckled inwardly at how that must deflate Carmichael's balloon for she retained intense, now ingrained dislike.

Straightaway, timing appropriate to discuss formulation for upcoming test twelve, Niall presented the following remedy selection as the team's best hope while she accented slight changes.

Test 12. Nosodes: Factor X, HIV, Herpvir, Tuberculinum and Carcinosinum. All at K12, and K30CH and K200CH.Remedies: Acidum phosphoricum, Baptisia tinctoria, Calcareum carbonicum, Cannabis sativa, Carcinosinum Burnett, Chininum arsenicosum, Echinacea angustifolia, Eleutherococcus senticosus, Thuja occidentalis. Potencies: K12X, K30CH, and K200CH.

Evan, aware of the formulation, surprised with his enthusiastic support, while Francesca, already his firm friend, smiled at hair dancing as flashing eyes expounded with confidence. 'Team. This it. About to hit crazy, extraordinary heights. Go for this.'

Besides, in an uncharacteristic move for a boardroom, slapped friend on arm. 'The time you spent discussing nosode, Carcinosinum in this potency with Sandy fits.'

Offered Niall a fist pump. 'Well done genius, glad this woman has not completely bonked out your brains.'

When someone laughed, Prof acted fast to suppress further ribald comments. 'Enough of unnecessary bawdy innuendo.' Eyes wandered room, then smiled, 'Although it looks like we develop a sound plan.' After he summarised their ponderous route to this point, he placed powerful emphasis on its magic.

As Niall drew together final threads, Prof asked the big question, one that stuck most lips together as fresh heather honey does when one appreciates exceptional sweetness.

Reluctant to spoil moment by swallowing it away to oblivion, asked. 'When?'

Eloise, who naturally fell into role of remedy quartermaster, accepted Niall's nod. 'Most remedies and labs are at our disposal.' Admitted only Cannabis sativa held them back. 'With world going *Tally Ho* over this remedy, have transposed normal restless energy into patience.'

Gave Francesca a thumbs up. 'As our super sleuth curbed enthusiasm, she demanded we wait until she sourced a long-term supply of best quality material from South Africa.' Evan interrupted. 'An astute move for when holidaying there on our friend Gugu's farm, half of the staff smoked it.' Made them laugh when he mimicked dreamy eyes. 'Of course, we use only modified, anti-inflammatory aspect and have refined out mood enhancing aspects.

'Niall agreed it appropriate they excluded THC, the mood enhancing portion of the cannabis, then, moved on in tangential route, again introduced how, in later work, hoped to lead them in a different direction. One in which they researched isolated CBD fragment of Cannabis to create novel products for treating people with CNS related problems including anxiety, depression, and epilepsy.

Which drew a chuckle from Prof, who then slapped hand on table, advised everyone knew Niall had an agenda of future products from arthritis to cancer and beyond, of where they intended experimenting in future. Laughed again, then clapped hands demanded. 'Focus, for I need my department to first crack this HIV story.' Only Eloise frowned, for she like Niall, shared healthy zest of a young Labrador during retrieval training. Already convinced. *Pray one day, world will open to hidden God-given gift homoeopathy presents.*

When they got back to work, a single, basic hiccough around quality assurance matters related to South African sourced Cannabis sativa by the meticulous Natura Company caused sensible delay.

6

GUGU DEBENZA

Scheduled test for thirteen days.

Only Eloise dreamed it the final one.

For confidence complete, she sensed they homed in on success.

Although further off than intended, Seekers gained an unexpected, much appreciated bonus. A necessary hiatus after energetic previous few months, in terms of an enforced holiday.

Astute, the Prof revealed his understanding of their efforts when he spread thick layers of intense appreciation. Surprised when ordering them to take a full ten days away from University. 'Can no longer watch you work like Clydesdale horses. Insist you take a break.'

Holiday proved propitious for Francesca, who, never one to waste time or opportunity, moved into Niall's apartment.

To begin with, interrupted intense, heady chatter that followed as Prof left the room. 'Brilliant, also, perfect time for us to invite team home for a full-blown Seekers housewarming function on Friday evening.'

Of course, never consulted Niall on either moving into his apartment, or to them hosting a party. He, in footsteps of successful husbands before, heard her out and issued the three magic words. *Yes, my dear.*

Because that simple answer saves so many problems for husbands and partners when they acknowledge their lady's superior knowledge, readily agree.

Sensible man happily fell into that group of men who perform best when organised by a confident and competent partner. In time, everyone learned description fitted Francesca to a tee.

Even, always the showman, arrived as was usual practice, last and caused a stir by bringing a partner. However, the lady on arm caused more than a touch of interest.

Not a partner in current sense, but a mutual friend to him and Niall.

Their initial meeting was an unlucky, yet fortunate encounter when all three were students at Glasgow University.

Niall, fresh from three days of dealing with a horrid tooth root abscess, was alone in the apartment shared with Evan.

Until disturbed at his nonappearance in Students Union where they planned to join a throbbing mob watching Scotland play England in quarter finals of the World Cup, Perplexed, Evan raced home to check on him. Found him asleep, as body washed out antibiotics and painkillers taken to control inflammation and infection after having abscess drained.

Accepting him a big soft lump, Evan removed bedclothes and shook him to life. 'Come on dunderhead, get yourself together for game is underway.'

Niall, improving after rest and treatment, thanked him for the reminder and, while stretching, peered around room, searching for clothes. But dissatisfied with progress, Evan, finding him slow and knowing desperately in need of cheer, urged speed. 'Come man. Run with me for we need to watch the game on the big screen. 'Come laddie, we can do this.'

Hoped to get there before end of the first half of a torrid match.

Scarce five minutes later, dragged Niall by hand, they headed off to University Avenue and arrived outside Union building. In time, both men pulled up by steps to Student's Union faced and faced an unusual sight. A delivery problem at normal door meant a man unloaded a load of large carboard cartons containing crisps on the pavement, which obstructed usual fluent access.

That said, a mere hiccup.

Until they jogged around the two-yard-tall pile of cartons, slammed into Gugu. She, only student in Glasgow with no interest in football, was leaving Union to search a quieter spot.

Whereas her diminutive figure, well-hidden by cardboard boxes full of chips meant containers disguised her diminutive frame from the boys.

When two big lads collided with her, both ended up on the pavement.

Five feet and two inches tall, six inches if we include a pair of her collection of four hundred sets of heels, Gugu Debeza's small frame caught them at chest height, the perfect elevation for the Zulu Pitbull of a lady to floor them.

Amid moaning and groaning... from boys, Gugu crossed arms over her plenteous bosom and watched, barely controlled herself from upsetting their dignity further by laughing.

Meanwhile, Evan held a hand over a red face, already busy producing an ugly black eye. Niall shocked, and concussed, slumped onto a step as blood flowed freely from a cut on cheek, induced when heel of Evans size eleven shoe caught him a glancing blow.

Morris Cumming, a fellow medical student, took pics of the accident, including a telling image of Gugu as she bent over the guys. As a prime piece of multicultural interaction, the student magazine published the pic. Notwithstanding masculine embarrassment, Morris agreed with editor's perfect title. *Tiny fourth-year medical Zulu Princess floors two giant Scotsmen.*

Gugu appreciated Niall's distress, and amid confusion, they clicked when in an extraordinary example of serendipity, procured instant and lifelong shine. To begin with, took control. 'No nonsense. Both! My apartment, on Great George Street, now.'

Furthermore, ten minutes later in the street's largest rooms which featured magnificent ceiling plasterwork, she acted firm, matronly and refused to allow them to watch the game live. Addressed injuries while recording game fort them on her giant TV.

No mother ever, flip no stepmother, exerted such control of second-year vet students; giant, handsome men as did that medical student, who after she patched them up, forced Niall to nap on her bed for an hour.

Despite trying, she never got chance to join him there... until much later.

With recovery, fed them and thus began a lifelong friendship, that Gugu, at once hooked on Niall, worked hard to partner him. Albeit a brilliant scholar, she walked her tiny, yet imposing frame, with confidence of a CFO walking into aboard room when in possession of files holding concrete evidence to unmask fraud.

Deserved, for as a bona fide Zulu princess, Gugu always commanded respect. Unusual for a Zulu, straight hair hung over shoulders, without treatment, she said.

***

As she walked into the apartment, Francesca spotted Gugu.

First thought reflected pleasure: *Evan has found a girl fit to introduce to the team.* Pleasure never lasted long, and smile disappeared when Gugu ran to Niall embraced, especially when she subjected him to an unsisterly display of lip locking.

Only a mother protecting infants could have matched Francesca's possessiveness as she complained. *No! Dislike this. Competition.*

Gugu's inherent, majestic presence ensured she commanded the room. Shared personality that only breeding and generations of culture can mould as she glided around to greet everyone and oozed natural grace unsurpassed by even an impala doe. Given that, naturalists describe that antelope as the perfect example of four-footed creatures.

Everyone else took an instant liking for Gugu at once captivated them. The lady whose disc-shaped, handsome face with well-formed lips oozed attractive kissability, and benefitted from complexion of a beautician who spent more time on her own skin than pound paying clients.

With glow of polished mahogany, she shone with health of carefully managed antique, French polished furniture. Not only Francesca noticed for Gugu attracted attention as ripe, juicy Pipkin apples demand sugar seeking bees.

In summary, jealous and as protective as Francesca, Eloise jabbed her man's ribs, gave him a sharp look while demanding he roll up his tongue and put it away.

Evan took over, introduced how their friendship started, and company appreciated this unexpected addition to their numbers. While one team member worked hard to make Gugu welcome, she and Francesca set to lock horns.

Instinctive, both ladies sensed aims and ambition and shared. *Niall is my man. Must claim him, protect against this ugly dwarf.*

At once, even before they met, Gugu's similar reaction must have stunned had Niall heard it expressed. *So that is the great fat cow that has my bull sniffing at her tail. Magic. For the way people talked, thought she was at least a little attractive.*

Followed that up with another tougher comment. *Suppose every man needs to drain his tubes, so, my gorgeous man, allow her to entertain your basic needs for now. But. Remember you will be mine*

But knowing life moves on, and as Eloise first turned towards them, and then stood with her back to window to emphasise role, and was awarded a sudden, dramatic congratulatory blessing from nature as a burst of sunshine bathed her in ethereal umbra of illuminated warmth.

Scene mirrored bird activity on the Antarctic seaboard where on an ice cliff, wings clashed, reluctant to be first to plunge into water for fear of predatory Leopard seals. Seekers and Board Members packed together, tight. Resembled Adelie penguins on Ross Island in Antarctica. On an ice cliff, wings clashed, reluctant to be first to plunge into water for fear of predatory Leopard seals.

Huddled collectively with a joining only mutual fear creates. Almost smiled at how boyfriend gasped as he watched, poured admiration.

Earlier, all acclaimed a thrilling end to football when Scotland lifted roof of the University Union when they scored winner against The Auld Enemy in extra time.

7

BIG RESULT

On the contrary, importance of their meeting nudged her along.

She played out her well-rehearsed report and provided she maintained stern fixed face, they followed delivery in a different, unexpected, and neutral manner.

Still, Seekers restricted breathing with synchronicity of penguins preparing to enter the ocean and scarcely moved while watching, nervous hopeful.

Three agonising days earlier, Niall and Eloise, when they strictly adhered to to same fixed protocol used in earlier rounds of testing, prepared petri dishes with their precious test samples.

Determined, used same reproducible methodology necessary to guarantee forthcoming results stood up to international, scientific scrutiny.

Overall, as Niall, satisfied group in harmony reiterated intentions as with previous range of tests but shared a note of apology.

'Know you have heard this before, however in anticipation of earth-shattering conclusions,' In danger of losing confidence, hesitated to grab air, 'we again apply our HIV1 culture as a monolayer cell to eighty-five identical vials. Next, grow them with live HIV virus samples at 37°C in a water bath.'

Niall's smile indicated relief nodding heads meant team in synch, everyone with him. 'Standard tissue culture methods confirm healthy virus growth. So, we monitor samples eight hourly until satisfied. For fear we miss anything, only when all eighty-five vials, following standard seventy-two-hour incubation process, exhibit uniform development, can we move on to phase two.'

Because of the excellence of their procedures, none doubted their well-tried setting up could fail.

Notwithstanding, they heard it all before; he continued and if a face could display a combination of confidence, anticipation, and fear, so describe such motions that flitting cross Niall's face.

Mirrored dancing moths flirting with a naked candle on a dark night. Besides, hoping for a kill result of over eighty per cent, everyone appreciated importance of what science prepared to unfold. Life changing, unforgettable hours stretched out as if months.

In a break from protocol, University's specialist photographer spent thirty minutes placing lighting strategically to record each step of the process.

By the time Eloise took centre stage, at most efficient, she impressed as she outlined their use of what they termed their three potentised big guns. These were test materials collected from patient X, and the CD4 and CCR5receptors.

For fear they miss anything, they had added these sequentially to cover all single and combinations of three antiviral agents. One sample dish held only live HIV virus colonies as control.

In contrast to vast accumulated specialist knowledge, common sense, often divorced from skill, declared these final set of dishes claimed their future.

Niall oversaw live HIV virus dishes containing chosen blend of homoeopathic remedies, and when setting up the others left platitudes behind. This live test must prove their results, the projects future.

***

Thirty-six hours later.

Time for the unveiling.

Francesca raised both arms above head, placed both palms on wall above viewing window, and with patience of a shrew watching an approaching grasshopper, never moved.

As her best male friend ever, Evan snuggled up behind and offered support, leaned chin on shoulder. But still a man, enjoyed delicious, sandalwood scent. *If not my type, this girl sure gets juices flowing.* In absentminded fashion reached down one hand, tousled hair then plonked it back into position.

Others assumed various positions as they desperately sought a comfortable, seconds eating stance as beggars any audience preparing for curtain rising at performance of a virgin Lloyd Webber musical. Eloise read samples, recorded findings, then stood back, gave no sign of findings.

Niall stepped forward, claimed her position, and methodically studied same recorded laboratory equipment and confirmed her findings.

Whereas watchers knew it essential to clarify and statistically confirm results, even if experience with previous tests meant them accurate.

Carmichael, acting as ever the pessimist, had planned to criticise, gasped. 'No!' Shoulders slumped with disappointment when neither of the two researchers in the testing chamber expressed news, nor declared joy.

A deathly silence gripped during thirty seconds required to record and compare notes. Then a screaming Eloise threw arms around Niall.

Still fully clothed in anti-infection outfits, both jumped up and down, shared their zesty excitement.

Test 12. Result: 96% kill rate.

8

DUMBARTON VISIT

A proud Niall took his lady to meet family.

He and Francesca stayed with mum Fiona and Aunt Deirdre.

A hectic, joyful weekend included Patrick and Holly hosting Clarice for the Saturday, and others joined when Holly presided over a delicious, evening dinner party that included Sandy.

For fear that plans go array, one always worries over family gatherings especially when introducing partners where those closest eagerly assess visitors as potential new relatives. They may be part of necessary, often complicated, often distressful vetting process. That said, love and lust may follow paths dissimilar to intentions and hopes of existing family structures.

Let us be honest in opinion of mum and concerned ladies, no girl could ever prove perfect match for our Niall! Holly confirmed this sentiment earlier when chatting with Patrick. 'Well husband, let's hope Niall found a good one.'

He shook head; confident sensible lad could never arrive with an unsuitable, waif-like model who tipped along on outlandish high heels in a clingfilm, silk dress marking her different to rest of family.

In any event, Holly appreciated Patrick's shared thoughts, laughed, asked if he remembered how sister Fiona in younger days, went through a similar, albeit fleeting phase.

Without delay, as a precursor to extending and continuing Cairns family into the future, Francesca need not have worried, for she proved an instant success. Besides, even Niall's sister Sara, always so protective over her big brother, delighted

Niall found a girl she considered fitted him as the complete partner. Also important, a girl can never own too many friends and as they hit it off made plans to get together. Clarice insisted she and Francesca attend Overtoun House.

Visit concluded with coffee on Saturday morning, a delectable pilgrimage for the girl, and let us be fair, as a journey along memory lane the place of one's birth stands up as unique occasion.

Before they entered Overtoun House she admired the splendid exterior and walked over distinctive, stone bridge that, unknown to them, featured in Cairns family history.

As Francesca snuggled her spine against the rough, stone parapet she ran a deferential finger over where the mason had expertly fashioned Lady Overtoun's name into stone. Never dreamed of two momentous events.

First, that spot marked exact point where Dierdre decided to swap infants which resulted in Niall's twin brother Alroy being reared at home in Dumfries by Margaret their birth mother who raised Fiona's son, now Calder Stewart, as her own.

Also, marked where Sister Catherine assaulted Midwife Celine, left her lying in a pool of bloody water.

Marvelled at unexpected opulence of the place.

Under expert guidance of its guardians, the house, with its role as a maternity home now in distant past, gained reputation as an international Christian centre for Hope and Healing.

Later, Angela joined them at Overtoun, first visit since retirement as matron nine years earlier when the Hospital closed, and took refreshments in elegant setting of Angel Room, where the fabulous, beautifully decorated ceiling was s a Dumbarton landmark.

Despite years passing since retirement, Angela's clever mind never dulled. Whereas memories often fade, others never develop even suspicion of a halo; the slight blurring round edges causing exaggerations and inaccuracies.

Doubtless, the fascinating story of Francesca's birth meant for both Angela and Clarice significant historical events connected with that birthing ensured their meeting progressed better than hoped. In the meantime, everything unfolded as expected with Clarice and Angela as comfortable with each as years earlier.

Until Angela, laughed at Clarice, said, 'Your confinement with us, its remarkable circumstances left an indelible mark.' Moreover, observed Clarice to make sure no negative signals came her way, and steered away from nitty-gritty.

Continued along a different route. 'But also, the Stewarts who had their twins at the same time, were also unforgettable.'

'The Stewarts! Who were they?'

Francesca, raised in the lie of her father as an unknown, untraceable AI donor, grew up in Dumfries and regularly picked up on the fact of the Stewart family in Lockerbie, because at least passing acquaintance with that prominent family was impossible to avoid.

Still, never knew Angela referred to them.

In a word, this caused Clarice's already heightened senses to further inflame. For instance, that unexpected change in direction introduced a rare occasion in life when hesitation reflected inner turmoil. Mention of the Stewarts raised warning flags flickering around hidden, unforgettable fact she with tasteless cunning, deliberately seduced Angus to fall pregnant by him, lifted pulse, made her catch breath.

Before she reacted, Angela continued. 'A lovely family; everyone's favourites.' Stopped to sip coffee as none dared disturb for fear of missing something important. In the meantime, with Clarice on high alert, Angela got back into story. 'Twin boys. How fortunate for everyone their birth and hospitalisation with us was a success, for those wee mites caused drama.'

Eyebrows raised towards dazzling ceiling. 'As indeed did Matron's own nephew. For Niall Henderson's bitter sickness at the same time created a charabanc of activity.' While grim to conceive, truth of matter testifies Angela never appreciated Francesca's connection with Niall's mother Fiona Cairns, whose sister Deirdre was Matron at Overtoun House in the days before Angela took over.

'Niall.' Francesca, while initially confused at naming of her partner, grabbed hold of unexpected mention to declare relationship with Cairn's family.

Angela entered that mental state where memories flooded back and relived that special time, most significant four days of health care ever experienced in career as midwife. Only days later, major factors associated with doubts and concerns about Deirdre's running of the hospital flared. Overall, unbelievable.

Needed time before circumstances of promotion to Matron and then separation from Overtoun regained their significance. In brief, concentrating on one aspect still alive from those days, said, 'No! It cannot be. Are you in a relationship with that same child?'

Next, amid excitement for Francesca, when updated about connection between Overtoun Hospital and Cairns family, who played an important part in Overtoun's history. As a result of Angela exposing facts around confinement of two of Overtoun's most significant mothers and children, Clarice, sensing she dug deeper into dangerous territory, worried, tried to escape. 'Indeed, fascinating times, and... time flies. We must get off and prepare for this evening.'

But others ignored, for with Angela and Francesca heavily into things, Angela deepened intrigue. 'Cannot forget how one of twins had loveliest pink birthmark high on inside of his thigh. Since it was the only one, I ever came across, so lovely.'
As a distraction she tried sipping from empty teacup, 'While birthmarks are rarer than most people imagine, that caught me out, for I assumed identical twins must share that feature.' Clapped hands. 'Wrong again.'

Thank heavens. Interruption for it saved Clarice from further awkward facts. Occurred when a group of noisy American tourists flooded room in a kafuffle which meant they lost Francesca's excited comment in the changing scene. 'Find this fascinating, or Niall also has a similar birthmark. How extraordinary.'

In like manner, Clarice, with no knowledge of them swapping infants, intuitively sensed a toe dipped into stagnant, murky waters.
Legal training added to basic maternal instincts flushed emails through brain. Even if messages were unclear, that line of enquiry proved out of order, irrelevant.
Satisfied they faced prospect of drowning in muddy waters Clarice terminated conversation before it escalated and soon, ladies took their leave of Overtoun.
Two drifted back to Dumbarton, to the Clyde Shore, where a fascinated Francesca at once checked out Niall's birthmark.

By the time they dressed for dinner, with house full of people, no appropriate moment cropped up for the girl to raise questions posed by Angela's revelation during their Overtoun visit. Clarice, mind troubled, added facts to an old, special mental folder. One crisp enough to never need dusting off. Labelled as Stewart.

The following morning after a farewell family breakfast, Francesca tried discussing her Overtoun birth with mum but disquieted over how subject caused Clarice to duck and dive like never before.

Late afternoon during a relaxed period with mum they headed home, men deserted them to fish for sea trout on River Leven.

A trip based on hope rather than opportunity, as low water made it unlikely fish ran in significant numbers.

Afternoon reiterated importance of fishing as companionship.

Francesca telephoned Angela, reported how their conversation raised interest. 'Could you find time to meet me again?'

9

DUMBARTON AGAIN

Three weeks slipped past.

At last, Angela and Francesca had their meeting.

Took tea in Balloch's Lomond Hotel. Remember that scene hosted Henderson and Fiona's first date when they met for coffee alongside bustling River Leven years before. Today's afternoon tea, taken outdoors under a thoughtful early summer's sun, although it lasted full forty minutes longer than allocated by Francesca, ended too soon.

Intense, discussion meant they ignored the fine river and assorted boats as they boiled in fast current, hoping for a swift journey to meet bigger River Clyde.

While pacing herself, aware time their enemy, she worked at Angela encouraged her to open with noteworthy facts. That included a detailed discussion on how Sister Grant deteriorated into mental illness. A briny, inexplicable subject, it held centre stage in Francesca's mind.

Accept proposed phenomenon of Morphic Resonance is uncertain, on occasions, even scientists cannot explain pathways which encourage searchers to trail wasteful routes.

So, it was with the girl when she displayed tenacity of limpets that hugged River Clyde's Red Rocks, when hanging on gamely to all aspects of Dumbarton, Cairns, and Overtoun history.

Furthermore, as the need to gain insight into family history raced through a prodigious brain, Francesca explored that situation in an atmosphere exuding comfort and support.

On balance, girl's paucity of family, accept that since meeting Niall and family, she also embraced Angela as part of her new, welcome extended family. Could not remember when last she savoured company of an older lady as the still dignified and elegant Angela.

It suddenly hit. *With Angela, see her as surrogate aunt, the one I always wanted, the one never owned.* As familiarity increased confidence, she investigated. 'Sister Grant, although fondly remembered sounds a fascinating lady.'

In synch, Francesca pleasured in the girl's company and opened. 'Odd. For she developed an unhealthy dislike that degenerated from dislike into frank hatred for Cairns family. Surfaced when she emphasised the Cairns name every time it came up during conservations.'

Shuddered, held Francesca's arm, then whispered. 'Other staff members reported she talked to herself...' Mouthed the last part, to walls. Now, as she almost forgot Francesca, Angela slipped into a disconsolate place, that while never fearful, introduced best forgotten memory, one she could not yet share. 'Then one day glimpsed her banging head against corridor wall and grunting something I took to mean: *Cairns... Cairns... and now I get them. Pay them back.*'

Francesca watched, staggered as older lady half closed eyes and relived what must have been an unpleasant experience, drifted away. *Remembers something, and big, not ready to share it with me. Must concern Aunt Deirdre, or even Niall as an infant, or does she lead into other sensitive areas?*

'Nothing explained such animosity.' By then, aware, threw arms around, then leaned forward as though launching into something tasty. 'In fact.' Spoke softly as if afraid of information overload. 'When she degenerated into mental ill health, staff concerned about possible madness.'

That said, Francesca's eyebrows reached for stars while she gripped Angela's arm. 'My oh my, a terrible day.' By then, Angela had no choice, and when attempting to draw Francesca away from infants, as part of her escape strategy she felt comfortable to release other secrets best kept hidden. 'Attacked Nurse Celine, beat up the poor girl, a shocking day.'

Francesca's mouth opened wider with each revelation. *Sense something odd around that time. My, but these are strange stories.*

Still, with the speed of the Overtoun burn in spate, Angela held nothing back. 'And then, worse followed when I witnessed her terrible accident. A road accident when she almost died, added another awful day to Overtoun history.'

With information overload speeding up Francesca's breathing, she probed. 'Was Sister Grant badly hurt? What happened to her?'

'She had, and still has several problems, although as we speak, thank God I can report she improves, but...' And here took a break. 'Silly me. And sure, if you wish to catch up on that story, speak to Holly. Yes! She knows her better than anyone, still visits her in the nursing home.'

'Holly, do you mean Niall's aunt?'

'Yes, my dear. Same one, and Sister Grant's own niece, Eileen Fraser, now Sister Eileen and married to a doctor, although I cannot remember her married name. For sure, they should be happy to add background to capture family's fascinating history for posterity.'

Then Angela described how Deirdre's state raised suspicions around odd, unusual, and even unprofessional activity. 'Because something untoward happened with those infants, including your...'

Inappropriate information release hit so fast and hard, excitement caused carelessness resulting in overbalancing when trying to rise.

As Francesca caught her, that prevented a fall, but to girl's dismay, also gave Angela opportunity to appreciate she went too far and thus closed that part of conversation.

Careful. For it was suspicion and intrigue around, infant care led to Angela's promotion. But with Francesca in danger of running late for an early evening meeting with the Prof, she closed; and hating doing so, conversation. 'Sorry Angela but I really must rush. Got to go.'

Not to worry my dear.' As they kissed goodbye, Angela continued. 'Enjoy your company; we must do this again.'

'For sure, my friend, for sure. See ya later.'

'

10

WE DO THIS

The smuggling subject perplexed vets.

Insistent, filled waking minds.

Not merely a distraction which governed minds, even nagged during intricate cases with demanding horses and ever increasing managemental factors related to an enlarging staff and ancillary needs that form part of a busy hospital's day.

Not only financial reward occupied minds, because, as scientists, enquiring minds accepted challenge of the unknown. For always reaching out to improve already excellent techniques, developing this unique concept caught brain's processing powers centred on imagination.

Chinese approach encouraged a glorious, enviable harmony whose shared, restless desire meant the couple inspired each other and encouraged them to develop a fresh slant to ingenuity with unexpected urgency.

Brains demanded inspiration, but by gnawing at edges of brilliance they searched for that single flash of inventiveness to bring a solution.

Over weeks, both vets considered their involvement, debated, and discussed historical methods used for transporting diamonds, while striving to hit on an effective program. If they never adopted same mindset as Ian Fleming's characters in *The Diamond Smugglers*, although one readily imagines how that thriller triggered similar neural pathways, while practical approaches led to them discounting systems as fast as they materialised.

May surprise reader to reflect on how, after those first heady and intriguing days, notion of financial reward while it never disappeared sneaked into a cupboard, as with remarkable focus, they disciplined themselves to concentrate on solutions.

At once, discarded equipment and personnel as obvious, too dangerous.

Neither did lack of success bring frustration, for by exercising patience, they developed an orderly, structured system of reasoning that guaranteed, in their eyes, a successful setup.

Time disappeared, and as logic declared novel arrangements around certain equipment routes impossible, narrowed down scenarios to those that directly involved horses. Each time they declined to accept evidence produced after investigating one route, the next appeared.

Combined and considerable brain power kept them hopeful, never despaired when forced to discard embryonic avenues.

Considered their involvement purely as them developing a solution for a client. Prospect of them physically doing the job never emerged.

Nor did guilt enter minds for excitement caused by skirting law raised fascinating queries.

Never bothered with people, cast doubt on best route of smuggling via diplomatic pouches as out of the question. Already so packed with rhino horn that limited space.

HORSES-R-US thrived.

Their business, mainly because financial oil from earlier payouts in fraudulent equine insurance industry, lubricated purchase of an existing tired practice for a reasonable sum.

Delectable ill-gotten dollars funded and equipped their specialist equine veterinary practice.

No fools.

Aware of prying eyes and professional jealousy generated by extraordinary investment, which ensured they borrowed, took sufficient loans to satisfy those who watched, even snooped around their extraordinary development.

Windfalls from deceased family estates carried insufficient weight, logic demanded they follow those standard financing channels.

Easier to pay off huge loans when they minimised non-taxable and personal financial drawings by using hidden cash reserves.

Business grew exponentially because both were top clinicians and surgeons, and better placed than most owners of fresh practices, their modernised hospital staffed with keen fresh minds attracted attention.

Inasmuch as Louis earned Master's in Equine Surgery, that touch of one-upmanship lifted him a rung, attracted respect, for theoretical and solid practical approach ensured he advised on cases from colleagues.

Although not as professionally qualified on paper, sensitive fingers endorsed Yvette to gain a sound local, and spreading reputation for managing surgical approach to throat conditions in racehorses.

These include palate disease and particularly LSRH; the left sided recurrent hemiplegia that causes partial collapse of larynx, proved her forte.

Her approach to Tie-Back surgery garnered notice. By suturing nerve induced weak cartilage into place, which, by opening larynx, improves inspiratory phase of breathing in damaged horses.

A tricky procedure. In Yvette's hands, hopeless racers returned to the track and achieved their potential. *Achieved their potential* is a fair term. For, and in contrast to shenanigans of former days, when trainers tried everything from cortisone and adrenaline to elephant juice, extra improvement hoped for by trainers and owners follows standard medical processes.

One memorable event occurred when Melanie Tinder, a trainer, hopeful of pulling off a betting coup on a four-year-old called Del Monte, pleaded. 'If only I could give him the same boost I get from a snort of cocaine.'

Doubtless, Louis, safely burying early adventures with white powder understood how that heightened her manner and energy after a sneaky sniff.

But with experience ensuring modern racing industry could never condone drugs, nor hide them, wished to move on.

Melanie, sharp asked about using cocaine in homoeopathic form as reports indicated various derivatives of the Coca plant rather than the opium poppy benefit individuals by improving red cell and haemoglobin management.

While Louis, stroked brain around that possibility, he accepted major differences between opium poppy produced cocaine and the *Divine plant of the Inca*, barely missed her disappear for two minutes.

Hair stood on end when on return, she handed Louis a see-through packet of the white stuff. Life never ceases to amaze, especially when he imagined a number of negative scenarios, paramount those relating to ending in jail, struck from Veterinary Register, so much so and to Melanie's amusement, Louis ran away, changed clothes.

Ability of specialist equine vets to stretch knowledge of exercise physiology and circulation to work on and facilitate performance of weaker individuals reflects pursuit of excellence.

Experts who can manipulate those factors, correctly diagnose then remove pain induced by exercise induced strains, often encourage disappointing horses to race better, to achieve maximum use of inherent ability.

Besides, in the modern day, where swab testing to detect illegal, better termed prohibited substances, in horse's system is so efficient, only stupid trainers' resort to administering inappropriate chemicals.

Louis remembered how one researcher claimed testing so smart, they detected illicit anti-inflammatorys days after use and in remarkably lower concentration. One report claimed by testing sewer systems, researchers could backtrack through sewage flow and reach original source where the guilty flushed drugs down toilet.

Their practice, supported by skill and efficiency grew until they employed six veterinary colleagues to help service stables. That plus when winter's icy claws gripped and caused the racing season to dip offered them a discrete degree of freedom to concentrate on their Chinese project. In time, hint of success exposed itself during a case of colic.

Problem of colic in horses presents as a recurrent, often urgent, potentially fatal condition. On balance, argue this increased in significance because people changed shape of the animal from original, tougher, smaller versions of Przewalski types originating in Steppes of Central Asia. For instance, during fascinating process of selective breeding, when humans selectively breeding animals, stretched horses, various parts never developed as well as others.

Some anatomical structures reacted less well to change than others, and, for example, intestinal tract did not evolve as fast as increased height and weight. LSLH mentioned earlier is commoner in bigger horses, as are colic and lameness conditions. As a result of them regularly managing colic cases by hospitalisation, they gained experience treating medically and occasionally surgically.

A field where colleagues noticed Louis' mastery.

To emphasise, when we have stressed exceptional skill of both vets as surgeons, their sound professional base, and financial success, it leaves us entitled to wonder at them finding it necessary to bend rules, and eagerly so. Greed played a part.

The case of *Maryland Grandmaster* caused excitement. The tall, bay three-year-old was not the most attractive horse in New York State, but he could run a bit, as older type trainers often remarked.

Fast. Raced three times at end of the two-year-old season, recording blistering pace over fourteen hundred and then a sixteen-hundred-yard feature race. Success ensured Bob Righton, his trainer whose Flying Paddocks racing yard abutted on vet hospital, nominated for major three-year old classics.

Three-thirty am, and a diligent night-watchman groom found him upside down and rolling in pain from colic.

Panic set in and, requiring urgent treatment, Aidan Murphy, practice's senior assistant examined the horse. Clinical signs (signs in animals, symptoms in people), including sensitive palpation of posterior bowel via a rectal examination, diagnosed mild nephron-splenic entrapment.

After treating with anti-inflammatory Flunixin, admitted to hospital. One of the beauties of working in a hospital environment, with like-minded and sympathetic colleagues, is ready availability of extra hands and brains.

On balance, under Aiden's, then with Louis input, horse improved enough for Aiden to comment. 'Better. Seems flunixin, combined with delectable colocynthis and other complementary homoeopathic remedies for gut pain, avoids him presenting as a surgical candidate.'

Superb news brought Bob relief. 'While I have experienced your excellent success with surgery, pleases me to find it unnecessary. So, well done guys.'

'Let me keep him overnight, for not yet passing proper droppings, so will wean off strong drugs. Later, will administer further doses of homoeopathy, lubrication, and electrolytes.'

After dinner, both Louis and Yvette strolled around their hospital.

Although well-wrapped against cold evening, both sensed mercury rising, thought of spring bouncing steps. She chatted to her two riding horses, bid them goodnight with same honest open-hearted approach Louis sensed must use with their children. A happy thought already hopefully expressed by her, while Louis deferred pregnancy for two years.

Maryland Grandmaster settled into an improving state, but Louis, disappointed he never drank enough, administered four litres of a warm electrolyte solution orally. In the meantime, when withdrawing the transparent plastic tube from MG's nose, turned to duty groom. 'Thanks Miguel should relax now. Will monitor him from inside the flat but please check in three hours. You may get off now.'

They stabled the horse in a purpose-built recovery box, as a virtual padded cell, which permitted space and a secure environment for horse to lie down and roll around. With heavily bandaged legs that protected him from further self-inflicted damage.

An idea hit. *Wonder if we could transport diamonds inside a horse's gut.*

Forthwith, excited at prospect, he jogged up to stable number twelve and reached it as Yvette closed door after kissing Sunshine goodnight. With bristly excitement, picked her up, twirled around.

'To clarify my reasoning, hug you, not because of any sudden interest in your magnificent body.' Hugged hard and long.

'Because this genius may have cracked our transport conundrum.'

She slapped a shoulder. 'Genius indeed. Knew a good reason encouraged me to love you.' Besides his news, sudden generous attention warmed her in other ways, and after treating to a swift snogging session loaded with promise, invited an explanation. Suggested transporting diamonds inside the horse. A well-tried route in people, modern radiography at airports reduced chances of that system's success.

Yvette, shared his aspirations, said, 'This genius,' Pointed both thumbs at size thirty-six boobs, 'now adds to your brilliance by declaring us ready to test your theory.'

Straightaway, never surprised, for as one of best lateral thinkers ever, she regularly found solutions. 'In fact,' Now sharing excitement, and on a roll by then, said, 'we put six or seven sparklers into a plastic tube and slip them inside horse while tubing with usual pre-travel electrolytes.'

Excitement meant her unable to sit still, so pointed at beloved Sunshine's face, mimed tubing process and while declaring that simple solution, then comically posed as someone taking a dump. 'Moreover, two days later, we wash droppings and collect sparklers.'

Gave her a smacker on lips, suggested he never deserved such a brilliant, fantastic partner.

11

NOVEL DELIVERY

Enamoured by innovative possibility, they practised.

With secrecy important, at first, hid actions from clinic personnel.

To begin with, sneaked around hospital in evenings, which proved a difficult exercise, for as well as vets, grooms and nurses abounded.

Overall, following another clandestine ten pm session, Yvette called a halt, demanded they formulate a sensible excuse, a lie to defray concerns.

Louis, whose mind raced along a similar track, agreed. 'If we oversee this well, opposite is also possible. May get a sympathetic approach from staff, even encourage them to take a hearty interest in a velvety, new project.'

With Yvette, spending two full ways in hospital, not visiting stables, which permitted her to take on a positive role in their investigation, she began by updating staff. By managing this well, using a matter-of-fact manner when telling them a pharmaceutical company commissioned them in the development of a new delivery method for bypassing stomach and small intestine with a different, potentially dangerous drug.

A sensitive relaxed manner ensured staff, familiar with secretive nature of drug company's development strategy, keen to assist. Need not have worried over possible negative reactions, for they by understanding how everything around competitive drug development is associated with secrecy, accepted that explanation and moved on.

Meanwhile, found Yvette and Aiden at a propitious time when they discussed modern rock music over coffee, Louis made a clever move. In reasonable frame, mentioned broad outline of their research.

Aiden, finding Yvette's interest contagious, rose to bait as expected by Louis, satisfied the practical man must prove keen.

Even offered to chew over methodology with them. 'Anything to help.'

Besides, Aiden, and here we blame Irish parents, matched Yvette's voracity.

Perfect time for Louis, a firm fan of softer melodic music of the seventies, to leave them immersed in discordant, metallic sounds of screeching rock music.

Never one to rush, Aiden considered their plan and came back two days later with a positive suggestion.

Aiden conducted the anaesthesia while Louis endoscopically removed a carpal chip in a three-year-old's joint.

In left field mode, offered a suggestion. 'Chewed over that interesting question of yours on delivering drug. Should consider coating capsules with a membrane, something that will protect the product. Until, four to six hours later, as digestive juices exert normal actions, which will soften and disintegrate the shell.'

Because normal processes of food breakdown must then release product for lower, less acid bowel to absorb active ingredient.

By the time Aiden and other vets took an interest during their discussions, they impressed Louis how easily staff absorbed and considered the idea for Aidan's developing suggestion, offered a workable but embryonic plan for success.

'What we need is a cellulose membrane, one easy to shrink wrap, and when moulding around capsules containing active ingredient, its natural form must not affect gut motility.'

Aiden's idea open doors to them developing an exceptional technique. Years later he developed it into a commercial success with Glaxo for delivering anthelmintics.

In contrast to other vets who may have had to establish a source of horses outside practice buildings, because their hospital always housed horses as patients that gave them an on-tap source of guinea pigs.

In addition, as Yvette rode daily, they initially focused on her well-mannered riding horses as consummate test subjects. Albeit their idea showed promise, needed refinement before guaranteeing fit to service diamonds worth a fortune. Aware of colossal value of pretty stones, everyone agreed it of paramount importance their system prove safe and effective.

The inside of the horse must inevitably be worth more than the vehicle; the horse, which carried them.

Five weeks later, after routinely examining Sunshine's droppings, they congratulated themselves on perfecting the method.

The striking thoroughbred gelding, Sunshine, after ten similar treatments, delivered package timeously without anticipated problems, including colic. Sunshine, alongside four similar grain fed horses, accepted, and safely transported plastic tubes through gut.

Of course, only they handled final product, indestructible, malleable tubes, while reinforcing lie they developed Aiden's idea of sing tubes formed of readily absorbable cellulose membrane.

Research established gut transit varied according to tube size; the smaller ones moved faster through gut.

In time, established a consistent product, one that reliably satisfied requirements, stablishing materials travelled safe through gut without causing any discomfort and ended up in faeces, perfectly timed after forty to fifty hours. Important for that fitted with transport arrangements, allowing horses to travel to selected destinations with a safe period after arriving before delivering goods with efficiency of DHL.

Finally, they settled on three-inch tubes, containing six glass balls of a size that matched six to eight carat diamonds. Discounted larger stones because when tested they delayed gut travel times, as did heavier steel ball bearings. Twice, using steel marbles in six-inch tubes, two subjects developed mild impaction colic.

On balance, even when a colic case proved mild, they worried those hoping to travel horses knowing that hours of transit must exacerbate the condition.

Without delay, continued and after successfully trialling fifty-five separate treatments, Louis concurred with Yvette. 'Time to invite Chinese back here and demonstrate our system with Sunny.'

Yvette, now in monetary mode conjectured how much they might earn for developing the plan.

12

FRANCESCA GRILLS FIONA

Francesca's met with Angela during their Dumbarton visit.

Left Niall snoring, akimbo as any purring fireside cat.

The big lad stretched out, flattened after another exhausting session with his lady, enjoyed a nap in the bedroom.

Francesca, savouring peaceful atmosphere left him to a deserved slumber, wandered downstairs, and joining Fiona in lounge, offered to make tea.

'You are a sweet girl, for offering, and Deirdre will also take, for here she comes.'

Forthwith, they sat in lounge and engaged in a comfortable chat. Francesca pleased how easily she fitted into Niall's family was eager to build on Angela's revelations, and hoping timing good, explored. 'Niall's birthing was, according to Matron Angela, an intense time at Overtoun.'

Remarkable, as without a word, Deirdre rose with speed of a startled partridge, spilling drops of tea, then muttering incomprehensible somethings under breath, ran off to her bedroom.

That said, she alarmed Francesca who stared open-mouthed.

Fiona's voice dropped into a sad phase when tutting. 'Touched on a tricky subject. Altogether gruelling, for my sister barely survived an incredibly strained time, and besides, her relationship with Niall's father stretched already squishy, mental faculties.'

Stared after her as though watching Deirdre through walls of bedroom and fearful her state must set into a tearful, phase, Fiona's eyes moistened in harmony. 'A dreadful time.' Rose and poured tea, and inclining chin to Francesca, said, 'No! We ever talk about it.'

Inasmuch as Francesca, was fully into the story and with tension mounting could not hang back, revealed brutal persistence of a lawn burrowing mole after information. 'Niall does not talk about father and without seeming rude, what happened?'

Fiona sat upright, stretched finger towards her and through a series of short, deep sighs, stumbled beginnings of an explanation. 'Notwithstanding, that a challenging time. I, well, none of us, like talking. No!' Despite increasing tension thickening atmosphere with viscosity of glycerine, Francesca could not let go. 'Now that I am family, surely that entitles me to know full story. Deserve to understand everything and then fully armed, can support Niall as he deserves.'

Whereas Fiona, now animated, reacted positively, exhibited a moment of tenderness when taking both hands, pulled Francesca to feet, and hugged. 'Do not think so. Not yet. Hard, sad.' Sipped at tea. 'Niall remains unaware of details around my marriage to his father... No! Too hard.'

Aware she wandered too far, Francesca picked up a steely glint and sensing pain, closed off discussion.

13

PAULINE'S DELAY

Six thirty am.

Pauline dressed for exercise.

Normal thirty minute, never classified as jogging, fast run.

Smooth tarmac took her along Tufnell Road, into and around park of same name. Shared an interest in environment with Henry, particularly trees, where the areas mature Limes, Pin oaks and Horse chestnuts were favourites.

Dedicated one wall of bedroom and study, to an impressive display of photographic series of one massive Horse chestnut, collected on a bimonthly basis throughout a year. Entitled as *My Guardian*, acknowledged tree's worth for dominating road on opposite pavement of her home.

From the roof terrace, accessed by a cute spiral staircase, head almost reached tree's uppermost branches.

Financial stability permitted by inheriting property rather than having to pay outright for dwelling helped. For instance, which permitted her to take out a reasonable mortgage to refurbish unit into an exquisitely modern, home. In 2018, a local agent valued her home at seven hundred and twenty thousand pounds.

Dressed for her run in a luminescent multicoloured track suit, on opening front door, to descend steps toward road, plans changed. During the previous evening, an ugly but not desperate electrical storm associated with seventy mile per hour winds caused local damage.

Common during May, it never bothered her until she appreciated devastation which embraced the road in front of her dwelling and both pavements.

The fact My Guardian braced himself against wind never fazed for during its sixty-five-year reign, had coped with worse.

But when a single spike of lightning ran through trunk from underground, iron rich sedimentary rocks that tipped balance against him, issued his execution order. That bolt of lightning travelled so fast, only a specialised camera set to record at one hundred thousand frames per second could trap the perfect discharge that ended MG's life.

Unbelievable power ripped through nutrient rich, softer layers of cambium layers, splitting tree vertically into three pieces.

The part opposite Pauline'sproperty, heavier fragment, headed for car, which because of a late evening she left, with others on street. A row of younger Linden trees on pavement closer to home saved car from extensive damage after storm also pounded the thirty-year-old fine specimens. They, after a severe winter pruning never withstood power of MG's redundant carcase hammering into two, although when lodging there, delayed his earthbound journey.

Amid a scene of distress, barely reacted before efficient local council authorities arrived to unblock road. While we often criticise, this team, on top form, set about dealing with obstruction, after a resident raised alarm.

'Good morning, Bernard and sorry, for in a fix, cannot make meeting.'

He, with an important subject for debate, understood and scheduled a video conference via TeamViewer for ten am. Such was proficiency and adaptability of Alroy's excellent team their meeting began on schedule.

On balance, Pauline's glitch took centre stage, and using Apple phone, illustrated calamity by relaying a video of scene outside her door. After expected series of oohs and aahs, got down to business.

Earlier, Anderson and Bernard, in Pauline's absence enjoyed a useful meeting to reflect on information gleaned during her talk with Flowers. In the meantime, Inspector Flowers' information rang bells with a remarkably composed Pauline, and chewing over notes, bigger the bell got.

Until, when they latched onto the Houdalakis name, it took on sombre, powerful resonance of famous one ringing over Thames. To clarify her hunch, advised Bernard to conduct investigations via his powerful computer setup.

Altogether careful, only when satisfied computer probing secure, he dug into police, insurance, and Jockey Club files while Pauline and Anderson explored tangential avenues. Grimaced as nasty story of Heraldon, the other horses and Shawn's deaths unfolded in more detail than originally noted. When he released information to others, everyone whistled with harmony of courting wrens at size of insurance pay-out.

Admirable records allowed them to list personnel involved in the insurance investigation, including vets, while Pauline, walking to window to assess tree fellers in action, alarmed at them working close to car.

'Have something fresh for us to ponder. This Greek vet called Houdalakis!'

Despite his name being on the board, and although Alroy mentioned how Fortsy passed it on during his first conference, but thus far no one chased the trail. She said, 'I wonder. This, particularly, may be a part of what we are after, so keep digging.'

Bernard's magic fingers danced over keyboards as Pauline left him to chat to Anderson.

14

CASANOVA

Bernard begged thirty minutes to update Pauline.

Touched sides only during lunch the following day.

With road open, car barely scratched, the loss of her guardian angel left Pauline disappointed. Although she never slipped into the intense sense of loss which some feel after unexpected family bereavement, disappointment had her vacillate on edge of loneliness and anger.

Had it not been for growing dependence on her police family, she for the first time since taking a knock from unrequited love as a seventeen-year-old might have taken to her bed for two days.

Brave; *resist temptation to suggest it's only a tree*; she got back to work where life reclaimed her shape.

Acted back to best, listened, attentive as Bernard said, 'Should like this, for have uncovered an interesting snippet.' Unintentionally flashed the smile that increasingly made her weak knees wobble. Despite best intentions and obvious mismatch in terms of age, personalities, and habits, she continued to experience an unexpected, stonker of attraction.

'That vet Houdalakis is overall worth following up.'

Pauline stood behind, overlooked his shoulder to study one of five screens. Moreover, he tried to ignore how she stroked his bare shoulder, although as any male must, eased into her intimate touch. As it continued, inhaled pungent, not overpowering rose fragrance, and an unidentifiable something else she exuded, her personal odour.

A poor libido, and an enviable ability to focus on work, meant him backward and a rigid sense of application excluded all efforts he may have in that arena.

She sensed his negative reaction, backed off, aware they must focus on an interesting twist to earlier investigations.

Bernard patted his own back, awarded a healthy round of congratulations for uncovering that excellent lead. 'Preeminent, consider this brilliant work when a lesser mortal than me might have dropped this line of enquiry.'

'My but you are now quite the super sleuth, not merely an information cruncher.'

Laughed as he reached out and stroked one of his huge desktop screens. 'My girls.'

'Smile got her, and while determined not to push onwards with flirting, said, 'Now then, Casanova, what else have you uncovered?'

'Casanova. Why that name? Odd!' Besides, never adept in the sex game or much interested at present, still never suspected her crush.

Pauline's self-control held up admirably when she declared it related to something elsewhere on her mind. 'So, forget it and tell me the story.'

Since she left him curious, he studied her face as any analyst does when they look for clues might and continued. 'Tracked down that vet Houdalakis who acts as stable vet at the Saunders yard.' Cocked his head, 'Mean the vet who does most work there.'

Instructed him to proceed, Did that with an unintentional tap on that shoulder.

'Although actual brief investigation involved usual people; veterinary experts, pathologists, trainer, and grooms.'

Pauline's active nose flickered at prospect of active information.

'Accept that as standard approach, but' Scratched cute nose, 'have you found something to suggest Houdalakis influenced their decision?'

As he turned towards her, Bernard unconsciously flourished that same smile, which forced her to clear her throat and use her best formal voice. 'You may have uncovered a valuable point.'

He said, 'It gets better, for investigators never questioned Houdalakis. Although it was a detailed, around the table discussion, only his boss, senior partner in the firm assisted the investigative team.'

A puzzled expression drenched face when describing how superficially they closed the case. 'At any rate, decided deaths as accidentally induced by severe thunderstorms damaging electrical cables.

Dug into a pile of notes and after an intense fifteen seconds, held up a finger, and spoke. 'One person's report caught my eye. An electrical engineer, Dr Thomas

O'Brien, commented negatively about electrical wiring to one block of stables in the yard.'

Here, when Bernard sensed a track, forgot himself, and as he mouthed a pinkie, dug deeper. 'Now, odd.' Drew attention to how they discounted the engineer's testimony.

Pauline insinuated herself into his narrative. 'Never! In my experience, such technical experts always command attention. Odd.'

He enjoyed her interest. 'Strange. One wonders why they ignored what appears to me, at any rate as valuable evidence of preexisting faulty workmanship capable of contributing to disaster.'

'Was there a history of electrical snags in stable or general area?'

She ignored hormones as he bobbed head and said, 'Failed to uncover anything yet. Besides, await an official council report on an electrical compliance investigation conducted three years before.'

In restless, ferret mode, she dipped her chin and hunted that point. 'To begin with, could be significant. For researchers regularly blame arson attacks on faulty wiring, so that should have raised warning flags. Will read through that report for you when it arrives but now let's take a coffee break.'

Henry joined them, Bernard filled him in on discussions with Pauline and Anderson. Likewise, after answering questions, added a different slant, for something bugged with vet Houdalakis. 'On the whole, after digging deeper into background, he pricked my ears.'

Touched one earlobe, pulled hard. 'Because, as Pauline already noted, Houdalakis works in that practice.'

Henry picked up how Bernard concentrated as he said, 'My nose,' Tapped ear again, 'Well, still uncomfortable with this chap, can I dig deeper?'

'Nice one, Bernard. Could be something there.' Pauline agreed, that fitted earlier thoughts. 'Detectives hate word coincidence, so, yes, interesting.'

As they continued to discuss the investigation, watched close, wrapped themselves up in Bernard's boiling excitement when he slapped desk. 'In short, gets better.' Rubbed hands. 'Searched database for Houdalakis... and bingo! Name arose in an insurance case involving sudden death of a second horse...' Glanced at notes. 'One called Craggy Moor.'

Hands still washed together as Pauline enjoyed how his youthful enthusiasm poured over them as he said, 'Now dead!' Slapped desk again. 'As well, that resulted in a significant, easily processed claim.'

Henry took command. In formal mode said, 'No coincidence, so get Alroy and rest of team together.' Henry thumped hands. 'Great work, you two. Fabulous.'

Before they moved on, Bernard added information. 'Hence Morag, sorry! Meant Sergeant Anderson,' Henry laughed as Bernard slapped own wrist, 'is busy collecting original files from local nicks and the insurance company. Incidentally, the same company, *EquiLife Incorporated*, took both hits.'

Held hands up. For fear they suggest he spread information too wide, said, 'She understands how sensitive this investigation is, and am confident will take care when collecting required data.'

Issued an even bigger smile, raised eyebrows. 'Surreptitious was her word. Nice one!'

15

WHO IS THIS VET?

A busy morning.

Henry stressed the possibility someone had them under surveillance.

Now, suspicious an internal spy unit may have started to unofficially investigate them in serious vein. Altogether, tenor of meeting changed as they shared his sense of urgency and caused debate to flow.

Of paramount significance they considered how best to work around this irritating but valuable evidence and at the same time researched how best to implement evidence from earlier discussions.

Anderson, set up and decorated an impressive incident room.

No matter boards barely half complete, Alroy studied their effort with deserved diligence. In time, underscored how well they emphasised pieces, including closely typed script, copies of false certificates, and photographs.

Spent time on descriptions of diamond classifications, where they came from, including known routes describing circulation. But consequences of one colourful report in red and marked as *Blood Diamonds*, caught everyone's eyes and imagination when it cropped up for the first time.

As chart illustrated actual diamonds related to prices, Alroy harrumphed. 'If I were of that notion, how much must a decent engagement ring set me back? Incredible.'

Pauline's artistic flair ensured they displayed reports in garish format, enough evidence to catch attention of eyes of any nosey parkers who might pop in.

Boss chuckled, pointed out a trail related to diamond theft and smuggling. 'Fascinated at this business.' Tapped the board. 'Of diamonds and drug shipments.'

Traced a finger between three reports and back again. 'How you stress actual docks, could fool me. Why, these customs certificates should demand I accept them as accurate.'

Smug, Pauline advised with shipping schedules readily available on internet, Anderson updated them daily.

After Alroy absorbed much of those statistics, Pauline took things further. 'Because of our intention to leak information, here are transcript of calls placed this morning.' illustrated how most were accurate but innocuous. 'Something for vinegary sniffers to experiment with.'

That said, continued by asking for help. 'Hit on an incredible piece of luck, for this transcript covers a real time fraud. Relates to a load scheduled to arrive in Dover tomorrow.'

Allowed a moment for that to sink in then outlined how he got it from one of his safe drug sources. 'This has to excite any listeners, because and serendipitous, if you place this call at four pm tomorrow to the drugs squad, a genuine arrest will by then be underway.'

Explained it best if he placed call, so with an air of excitement, asked him to mention two names. 'Need your help, so request you to follow this up for us by placing that call,' Repeated. 'must be exactly at four pm.' Because by then, my man, who is expecting your call, will collaborate your insightful tip off, and when he spreads the word to his squad it can do no harm.'

When Alroy placed that call on the compromised telephone line, they hooked a massive fish. After a touch of expert fiddling and fine tuning, he reported. 'To emphasise necessary value of us taking care, Sgt Anderson confirmed a spy logged onto your call.'

A still youthful face hardened when he outlined how solid evidence traced it originated from inside the Met. 'Although left it there, fearful their sensitive tracking systems might ping our interest.'

Gained Brownie points for being on their toes for the bust's success gave them increased credibility with Met's spies, who impressed, quietly congratulated them on busting that smuggling ring.

Overall, twice happy. For, having no direct connection with that crime, basked in the assurance threat of Alroy's unit as an undercover unit researching officers never posed a threat.

In addition, confirmed evidence from Commissioner's office that neither did PA Inspector Parker, find suspicious activity around Alroy. Given that Alroy read transcripts and studied corroborating evidence attached to the wall mounted boards, he impressed at their efforts.

Soon, shook head in disbelief at the same time, as on one false report signed off as his, read where his unnamed snitch deserved a congratulatory bonus. The man, or was it a woman, deserved top pay for providing name and eta of equine transporters bringing in a shipment of horses into Dover. 'So believable. Also, far away from our working areas, chances of anyone accurately checking this pathway are remote.'

'Wonder.' Henry, in processing mode wished to take this further. 'Yes Alroy. True, although so important, suggest when we get the second team set up, they should believe truth of these reports.'

Pauline clapped hands. 'Fool proof detective work.' On reflection, continued by outlining how, as Bernard helped create these false reports, they accidentally stumbled on dodgy areas.

Chinese smugglers were busy with select shipments from Africa through Russia. Mused this, originally seen as background effort, not only added credibility to their efforts, but may itself, with effort, expose useful information on existing, yet unexplored, areas.

'Hmm!' Pauline's revelation got Alroy going. 'Will four additional team members be enough? Hope, Henry, when you flesh out diamond story with your new team, we may gain considerable credibility and even find something.'

He smiled at her. 'Which, backing up your hunch, may lead to successful closure in areas not initially deemed of interest.' Instructed Pauline. 'You and Bernard continue. Dig deeper. Since with this, Houdalakis name cropping up here and in Athens, fascinates. Find family connections or history between these vets here or overseas. Start with Kentucky.'

Pauline rubbed hands together and suggested a tangential drift. 'Besides that, important search, can I now also dig deeper into Inspector Pastor?'

Alroy, while ready to agree, apologised. 'Mea culpa. Also, had to drag you away from Houdalakis while setting up this diamond story cover. Now, with timing suitable, go for it.'

Final briefing illustrated track for them to follow. 'Time for me and Sophia, with a touch of Bernard's expertise, when Pauline can spare him, to dig into Met's top ranks. With only a handful of players, we begin by first investigating Superintendent Flynn and his connections.'

Given that Alroy's personal investigations dragged grey marks, still nowhere sufficient to initiate proper investigations, over three top-ranking officers. But Flynn's name cropped up most often.

DS Anderson chimed in. 'Must continue to research bloodlines, breeders, and farms. Imagine we will nail down a connection between vets and trainers here and in US.'

Hence, while they planned campaigns, Bernard joined them as Pauline said, 'Know we go softly on this, but as you hinted... please consider adding officers to our team. Besides, as we face increasing levels of standard police legwork, suggest we need help now.'

Alroy gave others a moment to add comments for as he and Henry had revisited this subject again, invited opinions. 'What do you think?' Henry nodded. 'Doubtless, with timing right, so let us ask Pauline to bring all four officers, earlier identified into scene now.'

One negative point flared when Bernard worried over how physically to manage increased labour force to their already implemented excellent standards divulged concern. 'Not crying foul over overworking, but to set them up as we manage our existing team. A huge task and ask if we may get too big.'

In the meantime, Henry pointed at Alroy's chest to indicate he should continue by introducing their theory around man management.

Alroy moved to the paper board. 'We discussed this and now offer a solution.' Drew circles to indicate code names of existing five members and duties inside circles, outlined how he interlocked them like Olympic Games logo.

Next, drew bigger circle at side, then added four names of new officers he wished to join them. 'Now, please note how their circle does not, at this stage, divulge any relationship with this team.'

'Like it. A team within a team reporting indirectly, yet autonomous.'

As an adamant Pauline declared agreement, she satisfied Alroy to move on. 'When Henry and I considered this earlier decided it workable. In fact, now officially second in command, only he will collaborate with them. They will report directly and will be issued with secure mobiles-without realising top-class safety features. They will, however, use standard equipment, and pool cars.'

Pauline summarised how as they swung into his system it must help relax noisy parkers. 'As far as outsiders are concerned, they are normal police officers investigating diamond smuggling rackets. A solid idea.'

Henry continued. 'Our object is still to keep tight, although that new team will operate from empty offices next door.' He smiled. 'Once again, admirable forward planning, Pauline.'

They chewed this over until Henry said, 'Repeat. To begin with, carefully keep both squads apart. Furthermore, insist on us maintain this level of secrecy. But if a bad big boy upstairs sniffs around too much... then he can feed off my team, leave this main unit in peace.'

After coffee, Alroy continued. 'Walked around station, snooped. Amid energy generated by busy officers thronging these corridors the place resembles a rabbit warren. So, no one will ever notice an additional officer here and there.'

Anderson said, 'I can assist CI Henry by doing admin for both groups, although envisage us keeping them mobile.' Bernard said, 'Although Pauline vetted their records, only Henry interviewed them, and you do not wish any of us to mix with them, anyway.'

After a chorus of agreement, Alroy concluding their briefing. 'But enough for today. By ten am two days from now, Henry, after briefing his team, will fill us in with their working details.'

Henry added comment, one at first sight loaded with potential difficulties. 'In view of them taking on our diamond story. Say we transfer that dodgy telephone line to them. They could easily do this without alerting sniffers to main operation.'

As others accepted logic of that system, concluded. 'That should, by offering a diversion, keep prowlers away from us.'

16

FEED HORSES DIAMONDS

Louis phoned potential partners.

Chinese agents reacted well.

Yvette's tone convinced them of a solution and wishing to proceed, arranged a meeting. Not only that but also, they guessed at where some new and ingenuous method must add an additional notch to how they conducted their smuggling enterprise, which buoyed their already high confidence.

They met in the hospital.

This time, to impress professionalism and lead into an explanation of how they investigated their research project, arranged for fraudsters to attend on a peaceful Sunday afternoon.

Besides, that freed up time to treat Chinese to a more in-depth tour of hospital's premises and facilities than previously experienced.

For starters, outlined how their purchase of the original hospital buildings proved successful. With land a premium in the state, fact of them squeezing into a three-acre site jammed tight between existing racing yards meant they used land deemed unsuitable for anything other than horses.

With that significant step complete, and the vets still having cash secreted away from earlier fraud, they restructured rather than refurbished.

To their surprise, surveyor indicated while the existing barn and offices were rundown, shabby, found them structurally sound. Encouraged by that report they built on and doubled the unit's size.

A touch of luck followed when Lionel Dixon, TT's owner, thrilled at how his share of insurance payback on TT amounted to four hundred and thirty thousand dollars, bent over backwards to help.

For instance, using company's specialised workforce, they completed work to an exemplary standard, at discounted cost, and absorbed dodgy cash.

Of course, Lionel knew nothing of their complicity, nor payback on horse's death. Yet, a clever man, accepted something which may have been untoward had nevertheless got him out of a jam.

The building project's main feature involved doubling size of original horse barn into a sixteen yards wide and thirty-six yards long structure. North side included twelve stables and two functional rooms for miscellaneous items of horse equipment. A clammy, building on north side, distant to stables, although adjoining via a weatherproof walkway, formerly housed bedding, and feed supplies.

While it impressed new clients, Yvette explained their updated design minimised dust associated with straw and grass circulating into work areas as horses even more so than most horsey people imagine, are allergic to musty moulds transmitted by grasses.

Notwithstanding that side of the new facility progressed well, they added a new wing on south side for reception, offices, an operating theatre, treatment room, and knockdown box.

Chinese marvelled at the structure and how professionally they developed their operating facility.

One, known to them as Chao, hoped they might attend during a working day. Because he especially wished to witness complex process of horse anaesthesia, process by which they took a live, standing horse and safely rendered unconscious by drugs, fascinates those unfamiliar with the effort.

'You appreciate we deal with valuable animals.' Louis extended arm. 'Thus, note sophistication of our new close circuit tv system.'

Chinese marvelled at vet's care and Louis raised eyebrows when he indicated where a bank of monitors allowed them to oversee every horse inside the stables and throughout the hospital. 'We also installed a similar, smaller system inside our home apartment to satisfy constant observation valuable charges deserve.'

'Given these well-placed cameras, take it these feeds mean, besides horses, you fitted a bank of sophisticated security cameras.'

'In contrast to local racing stables you smartened the exterior.' The second man, now identified by unlikely name of Gregor, displayed a sensitive approach to architecture.

Yvette, who shared his design empathy explained how the builder, with a significant amount of recycled *Connecticut Brownstone* available, clad the main, public walls. As that part of the building attracted most people's attention, every visitor appreciated that exuded an air of professionalism.

That said, as vets hinted at their solution, others shared mounting enthusiasm and excitement.

Next step fell into order when Yvette handed them samples of tubing, they decided appropriate. As with any type of experiment, opportunity to oversee and visualise process firsthand impressed and made Gregor ask. 'Understand how you, by experimenting with these glass balls to represent stones, created a workable system. But how will you use them, conceal them in equipment to avoid detection? Need you to offer me a foolproof solution around that critical point.'

'Inside the horse.'

Faces went blank.

Yvette continued discussion by taking them into areas never fantasised.'

While the two men scrutinised each other, they remained so quiet, Louis perceived they must communicate on a level of unknown telepathy or the mind synching processes loved by science fiction novels.

Gregor again. 'But if you implant them surgically, surely that by creating wounds, must result in obvious scars?'

'Also, what risks does that entail?' Chao's mind also buzzed with novelty of concept.

In contrast to their concerned approach, Yvette calmed by declaring they established a simple, safe, effective process. 'Foolproof. A touch of genius. Although, for you to be cognisant of process, wish to demonstrate our unique, first ever technique.'

Prepared for such an intervention, as they walked towards Sunshine's stable, Louis picked up a standard stomach tube and a two-litre jug and matching, funnel.

Chao, most affected by entire process, lost his jolly, energetic mien. On the contrary, unable to speak fixed eyes on the eight-foot, clear tube.

Stopped outside stable number eleven, further designated by the stainless-steel name tag *Sunshine*, directly screwed into wooden door.

Yvette slipped the bolt and without fitting a head collar stroked horse's head. On balance, with content creature understanding the process, he nuzzled her arm as Louis joined them inside stable.

Yvette stood on horse's left side, slipped right arm under and then around his muzzle, encircled it to ensure stability.

Unlike anything fraudsters ever witnessed, Louis, stood by the horse's neck on right side, half-filled jug with water from the automatic drinker, then asked Gregor, who demonstrated no fear of approaching the horse, to hold that and funnel.

Next, without fuss, inserted tip of the tube into Sunshine's right nostril. With hardly any effort from him and no fuss from horse, he slid tube inside horse's head until four feet disappeared.

'Now, during this part of the exercise, we demonstrate a routine process, one we undertake daily.'

To prevent the tube slipping, Louis held it firm against horse's nostril with one finger. He collected the funnel from Gregor with the other hand and asked him to help attach this to end of the tube. 'And now, for something we believe unique.'

After collecting the insignificant plastic tube Yvette passed, dropped it into funnel. 'Now Gregor, pour half of the water from jug into funnel... and watch.'

Louis held funnel up higher than his head and without fuss, eyes fixated on plastic, watched as tube disappeared inside horse.

Neither Gregor nor Chao moved or spoke as Louis with one smooth effort, withdrew tube, and walked out of stable.

Yvette stroked the horse's nose and then, on impulse, caught Chao's hand, encouraged him forward and invited to stroke the horse.

To begin with, hesitant, allowed fingers to brush horse's muzzle on sensitive skin at a point where a generous pink snip of unpigmented skin drifted into left nostril.

Gregor soon joined in the exercise and much to Sunshine's pleasure enjoyed touching the horse. First experience of being that close to one, they relished velvet like skin which made Chao say, 'Skin feels even softer than inside of a boy's thigh.'

Unable to comment on the implications of that statement, both vets stared at each other as Chao, now he understood the process changed tack. 'You mean for horses to carry our precious diamonds inside their stomach. Remarkable.'

Quicker on uptake than Chao, Gregor anticipated a delivery method that involved a horse able to carry eight of these insignificant tubes with a maximum payload of forty-eight, ten-carat diamonds at a time. 'Yes?' Ran one empty tube through fingers.

Nevertheless, fearful how flighty he got when racing onwards, Yvette's practical side encouraged necessary reality. Explained where during rigorous testing, when they experimented with numbers, sizes, and weights, such a substantial number was impractical.

After she invited Louis' support, he insisted. 'Our studies indicate with care, and by sticking to our now well-established method, we envisage a horse will carry five tubes. By adding four to six stones of around the six-carat mark into each tube, which should allow your overseas vets to meet requirements.'

Gregor, aware vets never knew plans for them, ignored his comment around *your vets*, as he clapped hands and predicted their system, while a malodorous, even nauseating method for handling product, should prove effective.

In contrast to earlier reticence and doubt, capable vets infected them with deserved confidence.

Moreover, as Yvette had diligently researched the diamond market, confidence oozed. 'Besides, with average value of top-quality stones around twelve to twenty thousand dollars per carat.' Allowed a ripe pause, then decided this method offered a valuable consignment.

Henceforth, as Louis studied faces, greed in their eyes stunned, then flared when he recognised Yvette shared their avarice.

Taller of the two agreed those figures correct with reasonable stones, although, and now he treated her childlike, described they intended using only their rarest, most valuable products.

Chao's excitement mounted. 'Our Zhāng brother's friends.' Held up hand in horror. 'Sorry, my fault.' Cringed as the clearly dominant Gregor stared. 'No names. Sorry.'

'Although you are now our business *partners*.' Gregor stopped scowling at Chao and attempted to defuse situation with a tight, forced laugh. Emphasised word partners and, as he glowered at Chao, described how they stockpiled impeccable stones from corrupt African countries.

Made Yvette's eyes dilate when informed each had a value closer to thirty thousand dollars per carat.' Rubbed hands together. 'And so, one tube with five stones at six carats each...' Calculated that fortune. In contrast to her valuation, which figure astonished Yvette.

She, especially after giving one of her spectacular gasps, played with intended load of twenty diamonds. 'Each horse could transport up to three-quarters of a million dollars' worth of your precious stones.'

Furthermore, they added to her surprise, when even more hopeful than she, declared plan even better than their rampant imagination ever envisaged.

'Wonderful.'

When Chao received a nod of affirmation from Gregor, fingers dragged a pouch from trouser pocket and without giving Yvette time to gasp, with a magician's flamboyance, spread twelve sparkling diamonds of matched sizes over her palm.

Yvette's jaw slackened, as she gazed, dumfounded, at nonchalance when he ran stones through fingers, better suited to a crop dealer demonstrating yield of harvested wheat to prospective purchasers in Dumbarton's vintage Corn Exchange.

On balance, unable to talk, revealed avarice of a Verreaux eagle chick who, when fighting for strips of dassie flesh, barges into its smaller, doomed sibling.

Gregor guessed her hooked and sneaked a thin smile as he watched tender fingers that graced the operating theatre, fondle stones, then advised they needed the vets to repeat the test. 'Now.'

Forthwith, Louis allowed a reluctant note to thread through his voice, for as they reached crunch time, stone's value encouraged anxiety, asked them to confirm. 'You wish me to demonstrate our technique... now!'

Emphatic, Gregor declared only then could they understand their confidence. Still nervous, Louis worried what happen if something went wrong. 'What if Murphy himself creates havoc with our effort?'

Chao stepped back, confused at him for mentioning this Murphy person, worried they brought in a partner. Calmed when Yvette reported Murphy a slang term for things going unexpectedly wrong.

They bid Sunshine goodbye, then moved back to their compact laboratory adjacent to the office.

In time, Yvette prepared three tubes to carry eleven diamonds. Matched stones to tube's internal diameter, and after squeezing four stones into one, cut off tube's end, leaving a one cm stalk.

With aid of a Bunsen burner, melted plastic ends to seal the tube. Next, dropped that on a stainless-steel tray to cool, and repeated the process with other two tubes and the remaining seven diamonds.

Suddenly, with confidence overpouring, Gregor marched them back into the yard.

Albeit Yvette decided her second horse, Brightman, a handsome bay with a plain head should take this load.

Again, proved a perfect gentleman, never moved as he received the stomach tube.

The horse never knew value of his participation, as inaugural subject in the experiment. Abdomen now contained its valuable load of three diamond packed tubes slipped inside his nose enroute to stomach, and fame.

Gregor admitted it a rank, uncomfortable experience, yet... simple.

Yvette reiterated they often tubed horses, found it a straightforward technique.

Final effort centred on explaining how she recovered stones. 'And then, I monitor droppings, every single dump he produces.' Chaos eyes widened as she explained the process, how she washed and sieved faeces to recover the tubes.

'This never happens before twenty-four hours, often between thirty and forty hours after insertion.'

'Only after collecting all three tubes, shall we arrange a meeting.' Yvette expressed her worry. 'While unlikely, how to tackle an incident if a packet lodges inside and cannot pass?'

To show their complete disregard for animals, which matched Georgiou Houdalakis, Chao stroked Brightman's face. 'No problem. Kill. Cut him up, remove stones. No setback.' Smiled while tickling Brightman's nose. 'Yes. Solved.'

Yvette experienced a night of restless terror as she pictured some callous vet killing her friend Sunshine to find diamonds.

17

DIAMONDS TO HAND

Three nights later.

Vets and Chinese business partners met in a busy car park.

One that served a sprawling but vibrant *All Star* supermarket.

Chao's idea. He advised they rarely used same venue than twice, seldom met partners more than five times.

To begin with, Yvette barely snuggled into leather seats of Mercedes SUV before she pulled a plain paper bag from inside her anorak. As Gregor held out his palm, she counted while pouring diamonds. 'And you must agree sir...we introduce a world first.'

Chao expressed an outpouring of intense emotion which threatened tears, mumbled, *perfect, perfect.*

Gregor and Chao studied stones.

Demonstrated professionalism when he fished out a 10X magnification jewellers' lens and examined each diamond.

When satisfied, he returned eyes to her. 'In our business, having dealt with crooks...' Laughed. 'Rather than bona fide, proficient professional manipulators of law, we check every detail.'

With vets slow to comment, continued. 'That said, having checked stones handed to me and as I declare them correct, that covers you.'

Chao echoed that theme. 'Besides, your exemplary handling of the process satisfies us your expertise will deliver our stones and cannot cheat.'

Still vets, although they displayed mounting curiosity, and remember, were still convinced their role was as purely to develop a workable pattern for smuggling, never dreamed them directly involved.

Comfortable with that scenario assumed a further healthy researcher's fee must wing their way as Yvette's ambition considered they must earn commission as diamonds moved.

In conclusion, satisfied they solved how to transport diamonds inside horses, Yvette and Louis assiduously discussed and researched how partners intended sourcing suitable horses. Asked where they intended moving horses from and their destinations.

But also, Yvette in cautious mode apologised. 'Sorry. Have no right to ask questions. Indeed.' Hesitated. 'Despite our curiosity, probably best we remain ignorant around delivery mechanics.' Although this problem remained that having spent endless hours investigating, curiosity ate them alive.

Of course, Chao and Gregor had solved what the perceived as glitches and began with a fascinating introduction which illuminated the extent of their organisation for it included specialised partners knowledgeable about European horse breeding, and how they sourced quality, sound horses of first-rate breeding.

'Thorough research and mindfulness meant they began laying foundation for this project eighteen months ago when they bought yearlings throughout Europe, including Poland, Belgium, and France.' Enjoyed how that opened Yvette's eyes. 'Understand why you astonish at our professionalism.' Chuckled. 'Found other, more fashionable countries expensive.'

Yvette picked up on the emphasis, while both listened spellbound as they explained they used expert horse vets and breeders to purchase young horses, with id documents.

Albeit that brought hesitation from vets, which permitted them to continue and did so to outline how they arranged, via an intricate process to collect eight horses bred by AI from top bloodlines. 'These, normally prohibitively expensive animals are impossible to source, but by making use of a tedious bribing process we collected them for the US market at sixty percent of their true value. Again, with traceable passports.'

'A labour intensive, expensive business. How will you proceed? What are your main routes?' Louis, enthralled at operation's sheer complexity, needed information. 'Main routes are from Belgium, France, and Holland. Two loads via cross-channel ferries to Dover. Others via KLM to the US.'

Notwithstanding their interest, Gregor hit them with the big one. 'After the horses arrive at holding stables before overseas transport only you two will manage and treat them for export.'

Besides unable to reply, with clueless Yvette wishing for time to chat to already suspicious Louis, remained still, soundless as Gregor continued.

Yvette, staggered at effort already worked into this project, sat open-mouthed as Chao reiterated. 'Repeat. Since we have already sourced pristine horses, and pre-booked facilities in Europe for you to prepare them. Trust only you to supervise travel and stone collection.'

Raced on. 'You will receive animals in batches of three to five at a time. Close to airports and docks, you treat them in overnight rest stops in Calais, then travel with them.'

Gregor smiled at their consternation. 'We envisage one acts as the vet,' Here he smiled, 'while the second plays role of groom.'

Despite Yvette's intense and incredulous expression, Louis smiled, imagined how much more experienced in the horse world they were than he imagined. Also chuckled at prospect of himself as a highly paid groom.

Yvette stared at Louis, wondered at his thoughts, although the crinkles that surrounded her eyes predicted where her mind raced in parallel with hers.

Although experienced in killing horses criminally and fraudulently, this lifted involvement in crime to unimagined levels.

Louis, noted Yvette's concern, said, 'If we decide not to continue?'

Gregor laughed. 'You will not disappear... nor will we involve authorities.' Slipped into a silent phase, then gave each a heavily weighted stare. 'Forget old Mafia stories. Things are different these days.'

Tapped Louis's shoulder. 'You require no threats. Greed for money, our promise to find you oodles of it is sufficient incentive. Money, easy money, more than you can earn in a lifetime of sticking plastic tubes up horse's noses.'

As he paused. Chao took a turn. 'For developing the theme, you deserve a bonus.' Passed Yvette a bag, a supermarket marked shopping carrier, miles distant from her much-prized handbag. 'Now, time for you to take a short break, then we shall contact you again as final plans fall into place.'

Brains danced as vets headed across carpark and home.

18

DIAMOND SMUGGLING

Neither spoke as they headed for home.

Tongues thicker than a horse's when entrapped by an elastic band.

With business quiet, unnoticed, they slipped in rear entrance to their flat.

Louis, if he never slammed the door, made it shudder to a stop. 'All of a sudden, am at a loss to establish what comes next?

'In a remarkable state of either self-control or numbness, she moved into the kitchen, poured coffee. His white, hers black with a teaspoonful of thick, natural honey.

Snuggled up beside him, they sipped, staring at the money bag.

Part of her brain that earlier detached, firmed, and gaining substance, reached for the bag, opened it, and poured notes over the occasional table.

When counted, he said, 'Two hundred thousand dollars.'

Yvette dug fingers into the pile and turned over neatly stacked piles together, without a trace of excitement repeated. 'Two hundred thousand dollars.'

Fingered new burner phone that travelled with money. 'That makes a quarter of a million dollars already earned for uncovering a solution.'

With both mesmerised, they took a brief time out.

Sufficient for Yvette to scrutinise the side table against the wall on which she proudly displayed her handbag. 'And my bag.' Still thrilled, had not yet found a suitable occasion to introduce it to usual contents, never dared take it out with her.

He pulled her to feet, led her to bedroom and after an hour doing things big boys and girls do, showered together, and returned to lounge.

With pressure released, and now comfortably engaged in preparing a simple dinner of lamb chops and oven fried chips with garden peas, they stretched active brains.

Yvette, thrilled at money, anticipated how much still to come, said, 'Impossible not to join them.'

'Hear you, although best think this through because I envisage five trips, each including travelling time of around seven to ten days if jetting back and forth.'

'Suppose they will set everything up.' When halfway through pouring rich coffee, held her eyes. 'They fund all expenses.'

'In that case, plan for a month, say six weeks. Notwithstanding preparations take time, with business steady, we can disappear to continent, conduct local trips, and when done...'

She threw arms and legs around him and launched another belter of an idea. 'First. We can have a quickie wedding. Our excuse for a continental honeymoon. Yes! Perfect.'

Amid excitement, he overjoyed, delighted how she changed mind about marriage; *will never marry,* and encouraged him into another celebratory bedroom trip.

19

FLOWERS FAMILY

Team considered the Flowers information.

Alroy added fresh facts.

Considered them alongside Bernard's gripping information and interest in both Houdalakis leads and took a positive step. 'But Sophia, while these are positive facts, I need you to make a trip.'

She, understanding the importance of his interest, appreciated concerns, and readily agreed to travel to York and nail down Faith Flower's evidence.

Alroy said, 'Convinced the girl holds information, and as an intelligent person, may have sifted out facts at first marked down as unimportant.'

In contrast to Alroy's earlier gentle efforts with facts and staff, others realised how depth and power of his investigative brain worked when he said, 'Remain convinced that you as a mature lady, can grill her in obscure fashion.'

She almost wilted as eyes sunk into her, held her gaze with a soul probing effort. 'Find missing data for she must possess material evidence, snippets to help.'

Appreciated how Sophia's recent York visit to attend the annual Trainer's Dinner brought success.

After hours of tasteless, often tart chit-chat around increasing expenses horse functions demanded, when others deciding her effort fruitless, Sophia's sensitive snooping brought results.

To emphasise importance of constant probing, she uncovered useful information around trainer Saunders.

Repeated how, by uncovering solid evidence of marked financial improvement after Heraldon's death and link with Paolo Grizelli in Kentucky which prepared ground for promising research.

To protect her mission from both her targets and their local spying eyes, instructed her to drive. 'First, contact a friend or family member via your safe phone and prepare ground. Then, from our compromised phone, declare your eagerness to visit them for a weekend.'

Suggested she then detour from York and share R&R with that friend on homeward journey to stamp the visit. Sophia agreed to that basic logic. 'Shall visit my friend Melissa in East Retford, just off the A1, sound thinking.'

Thus, her visit to York should leave no obvious trail, decided it unlikely snoopers were ready to dig into vast amounts of CCC cameras along the motorway.

Pauline, enthusiasm for this trail obvious, offered to go with Sophia, and, while the latter agreed, Henry interjected. 'Yes, and no. For that means Pauline loses two or three days from her investigation into Pastor and Flynn.' Eyebrows danced. 'Too much at this critical stage.'

Pauline at once agreed to that logic and withdrew offer.

In synch with Alroy's opinion, which closed the debate, Sophia said, 'In that case, let me get myself and Felicity into gear.'

Called Jermaine Flowers, and as she found him at home and available, he agreed to meet her that afternoon. The perfect coincidence meant Faith was also at home for the weekend.

Overall, unsure time needed for interview, never booked overnight accommodation in York which freed her to stop off with Melissa that night or, if late, to book into a hotel. Sophia immersed herself into the 220-mile trip to York.

Felicity: her ostentatious, red Ford CMax drove like a dream. Indeed, with only 1800 miles on the clock, she instructed her to toddle along at sixty-mph. While a tough, fearless detective, well-seasoned in hunting criminals, she never stressed family members.

Sophia rarely stretched her fine machine.

Throw in a couple of light classical discs, which as they played in the background so as not to disturb the regular one-way conversation between Felicity and her mother, the officer enjoyed her most perfectly relaxing day experienced for months. Left the A1/M1 for the A1036, found Tadcaster Road sign well-marked and pleased, said, 'Sooper Felicity, like it when they clearly mark road signs. Good.'

The notice she paid to the gleaming dashboard suggested her a woman deserving of an intimate friend, a companion who could talk back to her. That said, a fair assessment.

'Now. Yes, indeed. DI Flowers seems a charming man. Accepted my suggestion of our double telephonic conversations as though an everyday occurrence in his business.' Paid attention to dashboard. 'Doubtless, a police officer.'

St Helens Road junction with Thanet road swam into view, then Eason Road and Eason View, a mile from York racecourse. Number 147 sported a smart brass number, as expected of a classy area.

Relished their easy journey, how simply they found destination. SatNav helped.

'Why Felicity, we face a fine property. Not only that but also twice as big, and only half price of our London residence.' A detached four-bedroom dwelling, less than five years old, Sophia admired place's clean lines.

Light coloured face brick walls matched deep brown tiles. Also, generous, modern moulded composite windows added to home's unsullied attractiveness as tarred driveway, encouraged her to proceed to the main door, near double garage.

'Sorry my darling, shall not stretch our relationship by making your wait overlong.' Sophia, although eagerly anticipating the interviews, seemed to a passing observer reluctant to leave her vehicle.

A two-yard-wide path; unusually laid out in same face brick as house, led to a double sized bright red wooden door.

When he opened the door before belling, Sophia, settled, instantly at ease with the man who greeted her, relaxed into a firm, confident handshake that matched hers.

At around retirement age, late fifties, for a lifetime officer in Special Investigations Branch of defence force, fitted her earlier description of Major DI Flowers. A finger width short of six feet, slim, fit with upright bearing of an officer, correct with a capital 'C,' astonished herself by being at once attracted to him.

The interesting man earned a degree in law from York University before he enlisted in force after graduation. In the meantime, a lucky man, also work hobby, authored his thesis on development of criminology in the British Army police force.

Sophia with iron clad homework under her belt since she checked him out after their first interaction, appreciated sharp, clipped accent, almost minimalistic word usage.

One of the few she experienced who articulated intentions concisely yet left nothing out. Besides, an introductory comment typified that approach. 'Faith is intelligent and sensible, facts which declare we must investigate her experience.'

Employed his shy smile, broad as his daughters, less often than she.

Intuitive, sensitive Sophia appreciated lingering presence of his long-departed wife, Sophia's mother.

She found the attractive, outward going Faith relaxed, absorbed in their discussion, and with enthusiasm of all youngsters in pursuing justice raring to go. As Sophia examined her, appreciated excitement that mounted in her own breast. 'Good. Sense this fine girl may own valuable information.'

Besides, gaining confidence, Faith, and Flowers had as requested kept mum on the story, so promised regular updates as case progressed.

Took tea together when the absence of gossip or idle chit chat encouraged business. When set up with notebook and recorder, Sophia asked. 'Please take your time but need your complete story from beginning.'

Chuckled her high-pitched, charming trill, a cultivated, successful effort that disarmed and eased people into interviews. 'And! Indulge me with the girly version, not the one I expect from the seasoned Major.'

Both ladies enjoyed that, the soldier less so.

As information chugged along, Sophia interrupted Faith. 'Prior to this event. What impression had you formed of the trainer? Attitude and dealings with people and horses.'

Before answering, a five second break meant Faith organising opinion. 'Seemed hard, but fair... usually.' The girl took another, shorter pause as though fearful of breaking a confidence, or nervous about rendering judgement, rather than facts.

Sophia acted like any seasoned investigator when she sensed they were on cusp of a breakthrough, so to reduce tension, shifted gaze to window and remained still. Doubtless a learned, oft practiced ploy designed to give nervous people space by reducing pressure.

Of course, it worked again, gave Faith confidence to renew conversation, and then started to bring out deeper, concealed facts. 'What I never appreciated was his poor relationship with horses.'

After she considered her dad, threw a hand in front of face, and apologised. 'Never found him cruel or mean, but disappointed to understand he had no real interest in them as... well, animals.'

'Did he not pat noses or stroke necks? things normal animal lovers engage in?'

'No! Although that changed whenever an owner or agent visited. Then he acted touchy-feely, but afterwards I reflected on how he evaluated them as... just racing machines. Money earners.'

'Ah! Interesting.' Investigative rules exist to bring results, but Sophia eased accepted standards. 'While not at liberty to divulge our interest, can outline where suspicious circumstances existing around those horse deaths have commandeered notice.'

'Agree with your thinking.' At that point Sophia observed where the girl shifted in her seat, upright and animated then led her through events earlier outlined.

'What made you approach him about the incident?'

Although she often pondered that question, Faith never discussed the depth of emotional strain Saunders caused with her father. But with Sophia, the police officer's expert skilled, velvet touch encouraged her to open heart. 'Suppose confront sits as an accurate expression for how I raised the subject. Yes, *confront* fits. Because...'

Following that highlight, Faith sipped tea. 'Father brought me up well, and much as I love him to bits and back,' Stroked his arm. 'Well, he is male, a soldier, and having no mum or sisters, and...'

Sophia savoured how as Faith stroked, disarmed dad with best flashy smile, he relaxed, increasing attractiveness for a man to a level absent for a decade.

'Perhaps I act tougher than most girls.'

He smiled when she described how she reached salient facts faster than her peers.

'Nice, one young lady. Know where you come from.'

After a second-round tea, and this time in a convivial manner, Sophia never resisted the cream scone with jam foisted on her by the major... now Jermaine. 'Can you describe his reaction, especially here? Ask you to be accurate, leave out nothing.'

Because Faith prepared for that question, she issued her answer with aplomb. 'Saunders rocked back on heels, blushed furious from what I sensed as fear, shame, or embarrassment. Then...'

After a sip of tea Faith rose from a comfortable leather armchair in regulation brown, walked to window and back. As though acting, smoothed down one leg of smart spotted slacks, took a deep breath, and surprised herself when she accurately described Saunders' reaction. 'Shocked me,'

Stroked his arm again. 'and I apologise, dad, for not disclosing severe verbal abuse, or how he,' Ran a hand through hair, 'raised a hand to me.'

For fear that her father might react negatively, she spluttered.

Faced a turning point where she prepared to water down her testimony, until and in extraordinarily brave mode, while she admitted he never touched her. 'But dad, that threat most fearful ever experienced mollified my approach.'

That said, Flowers, who remained serene, supportive throughout the session, changed his attitude in a way that marked up another gold star for Sophia's escalating feelings for him, when rising to kiss, commented for first time during the interview.

Gazed at daughter, touched her tender on cheek, and directed a firm, yet compassionate and knowing stare at Sophia, said, 'Glad you open up dearest one, for doubtless, only guilt makes criminals take that stance.'

Sophia harmonised with the family and flabbergasted herself at the empathy that flowed among all three of them. *Now Girl, careful, for this fine man envelops me in an air of quite unexpected, but delicious empathy and humanity.*

Then and to accord with his view, gave him a knowing nod and a personal, almost intimate smile, which as it was instantly shared, raised Faith's eyebrows.

To summarise her thoroughness, they chatted on for fifty minutes, rehashed and merged facts before Sophia reluctantly said, 'Thank you both for giving me useful material to chew on, although, please, may we chat again?'

After them replying in affirmative, examined her watch. 'Probably best I dodge into traffic now, before it...'

Faith jumped to her feet. 'No!'

And before she could continue, Jermaine prompted her offer. 'In fact, Sophia, in the hope this meeting went well we prepared a bed for you in the spare room. Dislike notion of a lady taking another long drive as traffic builds, so will not take no for an answer. Final.'

Without delay, Sophia accepted their hospitality invited them to dinner. 'This special unit I work for has a lavish entertainment facility. So, allow me to treat you to a swish meal.'

20

ROMANCE?

Albeit a Thursday evening the City lay undisturbed.

Sophia relished taking them out for dinner.

Rare chance to flash her expense account credit card, she thrilled at the idea of dinner.

Faith suggested if they hurried, they might claim a well-positioned table at the often-busy York Marriott Hotel that abuts onto York Racecourse.

Despite their arrival coinciding with the closure of the late afternoon meeting at five thirty commandeered a decent window seat, only one available because its lunch occupants rushed off early.

As Sophia's eyes, and ears never closed, overheard a woman muttering to husband to control gambling, berating him for losing too much money.

As their table overlooked the track, even before they relished a glass of wine, their party shared excitement of fellow diners as they watched powerful thoroughbreds flash by on the left-handed track, bursting hearts out in the penultimate event.

Sophia admitted while involved in a specialist police unit that focused on racing, her involvement with and knowledge of tracks and racehorses was minimal. 'Encouraged by family, rode competitively up to intermediate level dressage, but never discussed thoroughbred racing,' Issued a soft chuckle which Flowers found endearing. 'except compulsory Derby and Grand National.'

Faith took that as her cue for she, also with a solid basis in riding, filled Sophia in on inside information around the industry touching her as a student.

York Racecourse is financially the third biggest in Britain in terms of stakes and attracts three-hundred-and-fifty thousand racegoers annually. Holds three of the countries thirty-six Group 1 races, including Yorkshire Oaks, with Ebor Handicap meeting its main draw card.

Still known locally as The Knavesmire from Anglo-Saxon *knave* for man and *mire* for boggy land, the City records horse racing events from as far back as early sixteenth century. Back then, in significantly colder days, they ice raced on the frozen River Ouse. York was the second course after Newmarket to structure meetings.

If the Ebor festival in August stands up as most attractive and while horses claim significant attendances, none matched visitor numbers when on 31st May 1982, Pope John Paul's visit attracted one hundred and eighty thousand.

In time, Faith, illustrated a knowledge of racing and betting that alarmed father, when she outlined the influence gambling has on racing. 'To begin with, betting methods changed with the digital era. On course wagering, I mean by those attending tracks, continues to drop as people throw away their money using online methods.'

Now Jermaine, having often witnessed human misery after lifestyle changes due to how people frittered away savings on horse and dog racing, listened with intensity, and with paternal unease as daughter disclosed strong interest in gambling. Changed tack when she criticised the habit, and softened, he gave Sophia a raised eyebrow and a *phew* comment. 'Pleases me to find while you understand the system, you find money too precious to indulge in gambling.'

As a result of them sharing a rare sense of and increasing camaraderie akin to the family group Faith already aspired to, she chuckled.

Next, enlightened Sophia with basic rooted decency, again gave her father that favoured shoulder attention. Then, with a warm touch of affection appreciated by the others, reached over and held Sophia's hand. 'In the first place, appreciate sacrifices dad makes to support and educate me.'

Sophia, distracted by glorious familiarity appreciated her single, unattached life deserved rashers of similar affection.

When she returned to him, Faith's eyes flushed with glow only unconditional love offers. 'So, how could I ever dream of wasting your money on gambling?'

The detective, united with their wholesomeness sat back and watched them share a special, silent exchange. Despite herself, tinged those thoughts with a hint of jealousy. Granted, they assigned to each depth of sentiment never owned as a youngster. While never wanting for anything financial, with divorced parents passing her between them and lavishing expensive presents not hugs, she, well, you know the story!

Faith jolted her back to reality after a delicious curry when she continued to underscore where thoroughbred racing, despite its international size, exists because of gambling. 'Thus, if betting were eradicated, while the toll of human misery could be reduced,' Threw arms and heart wide open, 'population of racing thoroughbreds must dwindle.'

On balance, indicated how it must then become again the sport of Kings. 'Fun for the fabulously wealthy, with money to burn.'

Shocked Sophia and father when she declared to keep a horse in a decent training yard cost basic fees of around twenty-five-thousand pounds per year. That simple expose on the value of gambling reinforced the education Alroy's team gained from Bernard's research.

Peace embalmed Sophia in the rest of the just, snug in a large, comfortable bedroom decorated in girly mellifluous pinks and apple tinted cream. In keeping with most officers, despite heady thoughts on romance, relished all rest as available, could sleep anywhere.

Notwithstanding their fruitful relationship, a disappointed Sophia relished Flowers' warm hug and soft, overlong cheek kiss as he got off soldiering after breakfast.

With Faith and Sophia settled into a final chat, besides, now on their own, Sophia, as she sensed information that still remained hidden, grasped this period as opportune to go over old ground. 'Now with your gorgeous father off working, good to share a final coffee and enjoy a girly chat between friends before I hit the road?'

Faith, perceptive as any woman, picked up on her special send off with father and her use of the word *gorgeous* but sensibly and not to risk putting her off, kept potent mental meanderings safe. *Exciting. Because you are the woman my father has shown interest in since mum passed on. Now, Sophia does this hold something promising for the future?*

Overall, dumfounded, took them fifteen minutes to discount minor flirtations around that subject for Sophia had steeled herself to drop interest in men since being disappointed ten years earlier by a man who floated her boat. Now, and unbelievably, she mentally agreed with Faith, and opportunities of a relationship flooded her mind with unexpected possibilities.

21

DISCLOSURE

In time, discussed official business.

Detective matters ensured further probing.

'Wonder if anything else about that night, a discarded point heightened by yesterday's discussions is now ready to surface? Anything at all?'

She discarded thoughts of romance for the moment, reinvented herself as an experienced detective, one whose sixth sense nagged, advised Faith was in possession of information that could contribute to the story.

Something which made the girl unsure to share in front of her father.

'Wish you could help me with a positive id for the third character.

Faith mused. A although convinced one was vet Houdalakis, the Greek,' Head stuffed full of romance, declared. 'Gosh! So handsome, and well...' Blushed.

After a pause, introduced a point around how the unknown man deferred to the vet, that the character depended on him, followed instructions.'

As Faith revisited that terrible night, asked her brain to evaluate sightings, confirmed initial findings the men worked together as though in harmony. Animated, clapped hands. 'That's it Sophia, now certain they worked as a team. In synch.'

Sophia concerned she allowed enthusiasm to run amok asked. 'You feel they may have implemented a well-constructed plan.'

But also, if wrong, this could make my visit worthwhile. Sophia raised a finger in air and while she pointed it at ceiling encouraged the left digit to move back and forwards at two second intervals while she made notes with right hand.

Repeat. 'So, you remain positive the Greek vet and him functioned as one, that the third character was not linked to Saunders?'

Adamant and confident, Faith's opinion strengthened. 'No chance the trainer directly influenced him. No chance.'

Sophia was no ordinary detective, for years of experience in wide ranging fields honed her investigative technique and, despite impression those who never knew her gained from their meetings, intellect worked with restless inquisitiveness of a basketful of six-week-old Labrador puppies.

Now, fresh on a new trail, gentle as a Black-browed albatross skims waves, probed. 'In the meantime, while understanding and appreciating your position, accept the weather was horrid. And as you were fifty feet away, upstairs. Are you sure?'

Unexpected, she triggered off a sudden burst of emotion, for Faith frowned, then burst into tears and launched into Sophia's arms, and as she wept in torrents, hugged hard.

Besides, she admitted their new and exciting friendship, the promise it might develop into special scenarios, made her ready to confide in Sophia as a sister, even a substitute mother.

'Sorry but am ready to share a touchy spot.' Hesitant cheeks blanched at what she considered a shameful act. 'One I could not disclose to my father, for my actions, even if useful, must have caused upset.'

Big, beautiful eyes reddened by the minute.

After blowing nose on tissues Sophia proffered as though by magic, she continued but took a wavy road to get there. 'Enjoy birding, something dad and I often do together.'

After another reluctant ten seconds, Faith went on. 'There is a wetland close by the stables, one I was able to study from the vantage point offered by my upstairs room.'

Sophia, basked in girl's company as more than a witness, remained patient until she recovered. With Faith quiet, she guessed. 'Binoculars. You tuned into them, studied unfolding events?'

Amid a scene restored to a healthy discussion, Faith admitted exceptional quality Schwarzkopf binoculars, even under bad lighting conditions, made her confident she positively identified Georgiou. 'And, because of a series of illuminating flashes of lightning, caught the mysterious man's features.'

'You may not have recognised him? But believe if I tie him down, find pics, that may allow for a positive ID?'

'Confident, so yes.'

Satisfied she had collected all evidence, Sophia took Faith into her confidence, advised of her nervousness they had a spy in the force. 'Must warn you may be contacted by a police officer, one who claims to follow up on your father's earlier report.'

Given these points, Sophia advised Faith none of her fellow officers would contact her. Furthermore, should anyone attempt to reach out to her, Faith must play an Oscar winning actress. 'As we fear this fraud case may develop into something more substantial, need you to convince them the police closed the investigation as fruitless.' With she and Faith in synch, the girl chuckled. 'So, for you my dear, I must lie.'

Flowers interrupted them when he rang Faith and made Sophia laugh as he began with his normal opening. 'Hello, my favourite daughter, has Sophia left yet?'

'No darling father and here she is.' In her own girly fashion, probed. 'Of course, She is keen to talk with you.' Handed Sophia the phone, made a smooching sound, winked, and left them to chat.

Jermaine thanked her for visiting them, admitted with bashful hesitation he enjoyed her company, and revealed he planned to visit London next week. Embarrassment showed as he stammered through the call. Hoped to return the favour, invited her to dinner.

Couched it in terms suggesting opportunity to tidy loose ends, never formally suggesting their meeting a date.

Of course, that information left Faith in a spin.

Sophia and filly hit the road.

Appreciated their trip headed to Retford and a relaxed catch-up weekend with a friend, smug in knowledge Faith's questioning convinced her of illegal activity around Shaun's death in Saunders's yard that evening.

Spent twenty minutes on catchup calls with Henry and Alroy and constantly thanked Bernard for his expertise in providing them with secure lines of contact.

Moreover, just before she exited A1 for Retford, a phone call from Faith reinforced that thought. 'You impress me, DI Sophia.'

'Nice one friend. But what warms up that magnificent brain?'

Girl's voice bubbled with excitement, trickled along internet with emotion of a happy trout stream. 'Because, I have this minute received a call from a lady who intimated she was a police officer with an administrative position. No name. A mature, polite, correct lady. Apologised for the interruption, explained her call was a final check to ensure there were no developments on the case.'

'Lovely, lovely. Of course, you played her. Led her along with our well-rehearsed plan... to a tee?'

'A capital T, my dear. And I deserve that Oscar for leaving her content. That call satisfied me you are on to something.'

'Must bid you goodbye but let us get together soon. Will keep you posted.'

That said, when she turned into her friend's driveway, she brought Alroy up to date on that final, confirmatory note.

'Brilliant work, Sophia, we get closer.'

22

FRANCESCA AND ANGELA

Two weeks flew past for Francesca.

When they again met, she hugged Angela hard.

In tell-tale manner of ladies destined to be fast friends, not only did arms express happiness but also voice quivered with emotion. 'So nice to meet you again. How does life treat you?'

This girl, who stood up for herself in board meetings, held own against likes of the repulsive Carmichael, never displayed similar resilience during meetings or conversations which hinted at family matters.

In sync, understanding natural depth of girl's greeting, returned kiss with genuine warmth. To begin with, preliminaries scarcely drifted, when, with speed and energy of fast-flowing River Leven bordering terrace where they settled for coffee, Angela reverted to their earlier conversation.

'Have constantly reflected on our chat. Because, having no proper family, you triggered off vulnerable emotions never experienced.'

Spontaneous nature meant she reached over, held Angela's arm, and begged for relevant facts. 'So yes. Has meeting me triggered off memories?' Hoped former discussions activated curious, remarkable items from Niall's family history.

Francesca deserved historical facts to help her become a complete part of the Cairns' family. Continued to stroke Angela's arm with tender fingers, which as it sparked imagination hauled her into confidences. 'Love Niall. Share an unusually strong bond, which convinces me we face a life of intense togetherness few are fortunate to enjoy.'

Angela held tongue for a moment while she drank in the girl's passion.

Patience permitted Francesca's joy and aspirations to overflow.

This uncovered personal disappointment in relationships, which made Angela again regret she never claimed a partner, the spouse with whom to share life and family. Allowed her mind to play over Patrick's friend Sandy, reflected on how despite never having shared a date, they might have made a decent couple.

'Of course, any information you deem fit to share helps build trust.' Increased pressure of fingers on Angela's arm. 'Niall never talks of his past, beyond Uncle Patrick's family, Deirdre and Sandy.'

Repeated her need to research, enquire, emphasised how a clearer knowledge of Niall's childhood must help reinforce their relationship. Hesitated as though either nervous or unsure if she used the right words.

That pause; often an efficient lawyer's trick worked like a charm when used by Francesca, but not now.

Different this time, for it happened naturally and unintentional, allowed Angela space to take over. 'To understand, to support him. Do you have something like that in mind?'

'Perceptive of you, but yes, for life is harder than imagined. Couples need to draw strength when and wherever they find it. So yes.'

In a complete reversal, asked Angela why never married, did she enjoy being on her own, was there ever a special one?

Despite being famous in her own circles for that direct approach, her blunderbuss tactic shook Angela. But where it often caused resentment, this time it had the opposite effect and for the first time, Angela opened to the man she thought of minutes earlier.

'Notwithstanding two hopeless boyfriends set me back for years, often had illusory notions of Niall's Uncle Sandy as a husband. Well, if not true uncle, they embrace the special man as family.'

Francesca, her romantic heart already overflowing, found space to squeeze in an additional gap for what intuition hinted might make a spectacular love story. 'You missed out with Sandy. A fine man loved by everyone, one who needs the perfect partner.'

Aghast at how Angela might react to her next thought, Francesca plunged in. 'When you hit on him, what happened when explaining your feelings?'

As a result of her direct attack, when she stabbed Angela sharp as finest stiletto heels on a dance partner's toe, she flared into embarrassment, admitted she never explored a relationship, never dated. 'And yet.' Drifted off for a minute. 'Odd, because when together we enjoy each other's company, so yes, you may be right.'

Angela gripped Francesca's arm, firm enough for strong fingers to threaten a bruise. 'Anyway, doubtless with limited time, allow me to explore your needs. Begin with Sister Grant's story, for her part holds a certain, relevant depth.'

Furthermore,' Francesca held herself in check as Angela continued. 'Underestimated how much she disliked Dr Patrick's family. Of course, your own family now.' Bit off a sizeable piece of apple tart, munched it as a squirrel does after finding nuts hidden nut hoard.

In time, she wiped her mouth with a napkin, folded it, continued. 'Considered taking you to visit her in the nursing home, although on reflection decided no.'

'You intimated to that possibility before but left me believing her hopelessly out of things.' Surprise in voice was genuine. 'Is she now active?'

'Recovery is slow, intermittent. Occasionally coherent, understands our discussions while at others drifts into past mysteries, loses the plot.'

Francesca's horse grabbed the bit, took free rein proffered by a hyper imaginative brain. 'Why did she reveal such a strong dislike for my people, my Cairns family?'

Angela, although prepared to talk, worked to control herself. *Besides, best to hide unpleasantness for the present.*

Still, allowed bits and pieces to reveal themselves, teased out snippets by reminding, or convincing herself they touched on medical ethics. On balance, a reasonable excuse for not yet betraying family confidences.

But ladies, being of that sharing ilk, snippets slipped.

Francesca eagerly seized on a singular interesting comment. One where Angela returned to babies and birth marks. Spluttered. 'Babies. Birth marks you say. One marks my Niall, so, could another child own something similar?'

'Well... My dear, impossible. Chances of two boys bearing identical marks unlikely unless them twins.' Eyebrows slid gently to reach hair line, while she slowly shook locks. 'None of us, staff of the day, admitted to noticing birthmarks.'

Took a steady sip of coffee. 'Let's not waste time on that, for she is still obviously confused.' Held Francesca's elbow. 'No worries on that score. Nothing my dear.'

In another example of her readiness to dive in the girl jumped off deep end. 'What was the problem with Niall's father?'

'Jings!' Angela sat upright. 'My young lady, but you are straightforward.'

The tough girl blew out a big bag of warm air, and as she stretched arms upwards in characteristic fashion, apologised. 'True enough. While directness proves a useful trait in business.' Explained she often found it counterproductive in family and social matters.

That said, she smiled, strengthened apology, and released history of her background. 'Since I never knew my father.' Ran a palm over face as if washing herself. 'Because mum's pregnancy, well...mine as well, resulted from artificial insemination. While it worked out, still left a vacant space, and a chronic emptiness.'

Overall, surprised herself, especially at how Angela provoked in her an extraordinary depth of sensitivity. 'Mum and I share a fabulous relationship. Often, act like sisters. Although a gap exists. Every girl deserves a loving dad.'

Two lazy tears slipped down face, forcing her to dive into handbag for a tissue.

Angela rose, went to her, embraced the taller girl, and after twenty seconds whispered. 'Yes, yes, my dear, poor girl, with that harsh upbringing, share your sense of loss, abandonment.'

Francesca picked up on the word abandonment, admitted she never imagined that option possible. 'You touch on points never considered. Although mum worked extraordinary hard to heal the gap, I sense how my father by relinquishing his responsibility, deserted me after supplying sperm, left with a sense of rejection.'

In contrast to hopes for their meeting, Francesca gained valuable insight into deep seated, embryonic feelings. Overall, Angela unexpectedly drew out undiscovered reactions to Overtoun's past, knew to improve stability, even if never travelling the route, expected their chat to follow.

Although disappointed how fast time drifted on, when their meeting ended, Angela's parting thought offered something for the future. 'When next we, and soon, may visit Sister Catherine and discuss Niall's father and Deirdre.'

Suggested they kick off that meeting at the Gossip Shop coffeehouse on Dumbarton's High Street. A place holding special memories for Angela, because from there she witnessed accident that almost ended Sister Catherine's life.

23

GOSSIP SHOP

Niall loved Dumbarton.

So, he encouraged Francesca to explore his hometown.

Desirous of her experiencing the sense of history, geographical beauty, and strategic positioning as gateway to the rugged, yet still magnificent highlands of Scotland he taught her to explore the region.

Thus, after three visits, she travelled comfortably through the town, already feeling a part of it, accepting the embrace of ancient Lennox wisdom.

On her way to keep her appointment with Angela, she drove to the quayside and parked behind the Harp Social Club, itself a sign of the times where ancient Christian sacred wine now replaced by modern beverages, entertained rather than spiritually supported congregations.

In suitable time for her appointment, Francesca leaned over the railings that protected people from falling into water.

On a relaxed morning, studied sluggish River Leven roll past. Big near its junction with the River Clyde, a substantial body of water swollen by tide and recent rains followed its ponderous path, with heavy waters as the turn of the tide mandated Highland water to accept their inexorable journey towards Firth and Atlantic Ocean.

Their drift part of the resolute progress of nature.

As eyes chased swans as they worked against the current, observed how they took in every pedestrian in hope of inappropriate food.

Stopped short at magnificent sight of Dumbarton Rock.

And why not?

For the ancient indomitable volcanic plug hosts Dumbarton Castle.

This featured extensively in Scotland's famous, usually troubled history with notable characters spending time there including Sir William Wallace and King Robert the Bruce.

Most famous for the hapless Mary Queen of Scots.

From Dumbarton Castle as a girl, Mary, future rightful Queen of Scots embarked with an escort of six thousand Scottish soldiers for France to supplement their battle against the English.

Strategically placed at the confluence of the two rivers, Dumbarton Castle defended the West of Scotland for centuries for the River Clyde was, at one time a powerful shipping route for travel between Scotland and Europe.

A swift glance at her watch suggested it time for Francesca to head for the meeting.

But a child's wayward, multi-coloured balloon, low on life-giving nitrogen, danced as its bouncy momentum fled from the distraught owner into her arms. As she caught it two five-year-old girls arrived to claim their property.

Long black hair streamed behind twins as they rushed towards her.

The children's young mother, a replica of girls, who in Francesca's mind, hardly seemed old enough to be their mother, thanked Francesca for trapping the balloon.

Exchanged happy smiles all around and then she encouraged her babies to follow her along the quayside.

Those attractive twins, as they bubbled with carefree, infectious enthusiasm of childhood, induced in Francesca a poignant, unforeseen moment. *And yes, with my man Niall as the perfect husband, as early as next year, we must consider embracing a happy event.*

Angela arrived at upstairs Gossip Shop before Francesca where her friend, and owner Mary Jo, welcomed. 'Come my dear, have reserved your favourite table.' That site commanded a window offering an excellent view of Dumbarton High Street.

Years earlier, from that lofty eyrie spotted Sister Catherine as she walked Dumbarton's High Street to meet when she witnessed the horrifying accident that hospitalised Catherine.

After greetings and first sips of fragrant refreshment, Angela suggested. 'Now, knowing you are free from strict time constraints that normally limit our meetings, decided best we met here before moving on to Lochside.'

She gazed out of the window, lost in her own deep thoughts for twenty seconds and then extended her hand towards the town.

More than a hint of disappointment and regret suffused her voice as she said, 'For it was from this spot I witnessed Catherine's accident.'

In halting, often painful yet enthusiastic terms, repeated, as though only yesterday, Catherine's stumbling, careless progress along High Street until, falling off pavement, she met a car.

Voice struggled, for irrespective of how often she reflected on the incident, its drama, pain, always brought a tear. Francesca passed her older friend a tissue to mop sorry moisture off cheeks.

24

SISTER CATHERINE

They, having survived that experience, moved on.

With necessity insisting they both drive, they arrived together.

Although Angela still gave Francesca a cheery wave when they met in the car park. Francesca's vivid red VW GTI sparkled in late morning sunshine as Angela greeted as though this was their meeting in weeks.

Effusive as always, their joining took place on the lawn area designated for parking at Everglades Nursing Home. Angela took her hand, led over manicured grass to pebbled beach of Loch Lomond. Eager and expectant, watched, curious to study Francesca's reaction.

Girl played her part as most people do when she paused, breathed deep of clean fresh air encouraged by a recent rain shower. After a moment, smiled and said, 'Sometimes words are unnecessary. This Loch is a special place. Sense it steeped in an environment of health and wellbeing, banishing tension and anticipation threatening to envelop me when journeying to meet Sister Catherine.'

'Guessed, hoped our meeting here should encourage, for in an area remarkable for beauty, this exceptional spot offers insight into Scotland's grandeur.'

Hung in situ; arms locked as minutes slipped past. Until Angela shook both, and said, 'Enough dreaming.'

Giggled like nervous teenagers. 'Wait here. Drink in tranquillity only sublime nature of Loch Lomond offers while I fetch Catherine.' Pointed to a prominent wicker container on covered veranda. 'Please collect armfuls of cushions and take them over to those benches.'

A finger indicated where two double seaters facing each other, closer to the loch.

'Enjoy the benevolent protection of our mighty but generous beech tree. 'Make yourself comfortable. We will join you shortly.'

Francesca watched her walk away then collected a bundle of soft, well-maintained cushions, arranged them on benches, then strolled along the water's edge. Enticed by shimmering vastness of a loch set in one of most picturesque places in the world, appreciated Loch Lomond's subliminal support and encouragement.

Those who appreciate ability of, and desperate urgency of, natural things pulling and pushing strings of life in positive directions will offer a knowing chin dip, having experienced similar moments.

Despite being unsure what to expect, anticipate today will uncover important, facts useful even helpful. But also, notion of something sinister frozen in mists of time that awaits thawing prods me to take care.

Negative emotions, placed out of kilter with that backdrop, caused her to reflect on previous touristy drives escorted by Niall.

She drank in the loch's beauty, orientated herself. 'So, Auchenheglish Lodges lie there, to my left. Around corner from here Duck Bay Marina and Cameron House.' Well into swing of things, conducted tour as though guiding a group of visitors.

'Out, over the water sits, serene as any duck comfortable in-home waters, the big island of Inchmurrin. Straight across is interesting Ross Priory where Niall took me to visit last month.'

Shimmer of ancient beech trees, and susurration caused by leaves as they gently caressed each other added to heady atmosphere. Smiled, shared same notions that affect millions of visitors seduced by the area's beauty. In contrast to an agitated world, this place settles troubled minds.

That said, a banging door introduced reality.

Even from thirty yards away, appreciated the patient's frailty. Grimaced as Catherine took tentative steps of a foal when it first finds its feet. Supported on Angela's arm, she walked slow over lawn towards her.

Francesca closed distance between them, held out hand as Angela introduced. 'Now, Catherine, this is special treat. Brought along Francesca, the lovely girl I told you is to marry Fiona's son, Niall.'

Catherine reached out with both hands. When they met, grip seemed remarkable strong. Until Francesca realised it did not clasp as a greeting but was a request for further support needed by elderly, frail lady.

Put on her best smile, and despite inexplicable and growing trepidation, forced a note of ringing cheer. 'Lovely to meet you. Let me help you to this comfortable seat.'

Catherine flopped heavy down and, grunted as she took two full minutes to fit skinny bum into a comfortable state.

That accomplished, reached out, and took the still standing Francesca's arm. Eyeballed her, then cast gaze up and down and, while again peering into Francesca's face, said, 'My Elaine, but you present yourself different today, are you pregnant, for you have put on weight.'

Thirty minutes later, interview over, Angela, disappointed at their tiring, unfruitful meeting, consoled Francesca. 'Sorry, my dear. Guessed at a strained meeting, but not this bad. A disaster, complete waste of time. Can only hope your next attempt will go better.'

'What a sad lady, indeed. Anyway, time for tea and a chat.' As cars conveyed them up driveway, away from the home, neither noticed a thin, tight face fix its gaze on the departing Golf from an upstairs room. Her state, emphasising fluctuating nature of recovery from brain injuries exposed change.

Catherine's demeanour lifted by the minute.

Stretched a hand towards the disappearing car, then slapped it onto glass while she whispered a single word three times at four second intervals. 'Cairns... Cairns... Cairns.' When she escalated her call and associated it with rhythmic slaps against glass, a high-pitched ringing rang out with final repeat loud, it brought an attendant rushing to assist.

***

Confidants settled into a smart tearoom in Balloch.

Ordered tea and an open, rare Angus beef sandwich for lunch.

Francesca's mind whirred, unable to clasp import of that meeting, she sighed Albeit she sensed Catherine had at one point noted her presence, connected it with the Cairns name.

'Yes. A sad meeting, although wayward behaviour convinces me her merely having a dreadful day.'

'Indeed, also share your thoughts.' It was often Angela's way to make a statement then sip tea with delicacy of a songbird. While repeating that habit, she alerted the smart Francesca to sense it a ploy to grasp space, so, remained tranquil as Angela recovered and continued. 'In truth, although regularly incoherent, often physically stronger than we found her today.'

Sip of tea slipped down as though she sat alone. 'Occasionally engage in a reasonable conversation, thrilled at demeanour during my last visit. Overall, that gave me confidence to invite you to attend.'

Francesca sighed in harmony with friend's disappointment. 'Nevertheless, I shall continue to explore. In a firmer tone, growing in confidence, explored. 'Cannot forget our meeting when you alluded to difficulties in my Cairns family history.'

Angela offered a sweet smile, moved squeaky chair closer, looked around as if searching for spies, a furtive move Francesca took as a hopeful sign. 'So, are you up to me unfolding information about Niall's father, or' Deliberately forced a dejected note into voice, 'shall we leave it for another time?'

She smiled and stroked Francesca's arm. 'No. You and I share a sense of closeness, rare in non-family members. Reflected on our discussion, and as you graciously opened to me, agree it important you know his situation. Although I do not know the complete story, be patient. Permit me to outline pertinent points.'

Over twenty-five minutes, Angela, if at first hesitant, filled the sponge of a girl with sufficient information to swamp a lesser person. As a result of his relationship with Fiona and her siblings taking centre stage, she soaked up every word and soon appreciated how the man's enormous influence on Deirdre pressured her already strained mental health.

Francesca breathed fast when she assimilated information about how Henderson's lack of attention made Fiona's life miserable. 'No, my dear. Miserable is not the correct phrase. Since we, as staff, remain convinced cruelty to Fiona and reaction to Deirdre, forced her into early retirement.'

As the conversation deepened, she appreciated, then accepted, how intensely Angela had disliked her late father-in-law. Odd, but as Francesca soon accepted him ugly, found describing him as family distasteful. While exploring Henderson's darkness, Angela, even after years slipped past, outlined experiences in an air of palpable drama.

In the meantime, as Francesca reacted to horrid news of Niall's father, she released involuntary shivers until as Angela responded to the girl reactions and suspecting her chilling, asked should she fetch a scarf or heavier pashmina.

Emotions flared as Angela psyched herself to release a potent fact which must signal the endgame. One, stored inside for so long it deserved to flood restraining banks, knowing she must also gain from uncovering distasteful facts and inferences, which poisoned insides with sneaky, insidious, cancer-like growth of all progressive mental diseases.

As facts and half facts tumbled, Angela, nearing end of her expose, said, 'And rumours fed by staff unused too much personal excitement in our parochial hospital, went wild.'

Threw out questions, suspecting they might never find answers. 'Why did Deirdre decide to visit his home that day? What happened to him? Was it merely a propitious visit that caused her to arrive as the man lay dying? Did Deirdre do enough to help the man,' Eyes flared into a bottomless pit of suspicion, 'to save his life.'

Sustained a prolonged pause, then said, 'Some asserted she could have done more.'

Because Francesca enjoyed her share of TV soapies as much as anyone, and here, faced with an episode of raw life, she gasped at thought of a terrible, terrifying ending. 'No! Deirdre. Did she kill him?'

25

HENRY'S TEAM

Henry summoned his team.

The four socialised over coffee; intrigued and excited.

First to arrive, Abisade walked along the corridor and bumped into Mohammed a colleague from ten years earlier. Because he already understood need for exceptional secrecy around new position, merely touched sides, promised to get together, then moved on.

As he entered the Ops room, Mandy greeted with a swift nod.

Then, greeted by DS Anderson, in usual immaculate uniform, she indicated they help themselves to decent coffee while they waited for rest of the team to assemble.

Abisade's eyes lit up when he spotted modern coffee percolators, and smart new, hand painted coffee mugs depicting indigenous duck species. In plain clothes, knew nothing of rank, but suspected them part of Henry's new team.

Frank and Mamad walked through front door of Shoreditch Police Station together in association with three permanent staff, including Bernard. In the throb of the than 120 regular officers calling station their base, ignored each other.

Henry joined them from inner Ops Room, greeted them, and as he poured coffee instructed them to join them into their Incident / Ops room, under supervision of DS Anderson.

Soon, down to business, and departing from informality of Alroy's group, introduced himself as the CI to whom they would report. While outlining history, asked they not discuss name of reporting superintendent.

Before he asked them to introduce themselves, added to information received earlier during interviews, advising them specially selected for a new and undercover drug team, with an interest in diamond smuggling from Europe to South of England.

Then introduced Mandy as second in command, asked her and then others to give a resume of careers and family backgrounds. Unique for the force, explained their role brand-new. 'Our task to consider if smugglers use now extensive movement of sporting horses throughout Europe as a cover for diamond smuggling crimes supported by huge wealth generated by sale of so-called blood diamonds from Africa via China and Russia.

Information pricked ears, raised interest levels to fascination particularly at mention of an unknown, horse connection. News of them breaking fresh ground brought smiles all around, particularly from DS Abisade Kasir; a 32-year-old British born Nigerian, who after recent promotion to DS and being invited to join drug squad, disappointed when they tore him away.

A significant part he played in breaking down a money laundering scheme through Greece proved a pointer drawing notice to marked ability.

Not always appreciated, as typified by one commanding officer in charge of that investigation, who and in loud-mouthed fashion, declared. 'Not only does he own a big, axe-like nose, but uses it effectively for sniffing out unsavoury connections.' Did not go down well.

While Alroy never approved of officer's tone or attitude, such loose talk during an advanced course on communications in detection alerted him to the man's skill.

DI Mandy McDonald imposed when she held the floor.

Six-feet-tall, thirteen stone of solid muscle, this West Indian Oxford graduate claimed respect throughout the departments. Efforts in various fraud investigations pushed her to inspector status over male colleagues, as the force began to recognise the diligence and leadership qualities that made her an obvious choice to advance role of women in hierarchy.

A natural commander, this forty-two-year-old mother of ten-year-old twin girls, was an expert at balancing work and family life. Afrikaner husband Hendrik, naturalised Brit of eight years, was a medical GP who ran their home base, surgery he shared with four colleagues, two nurses, a physiotherapist, and a psychologist.

Notwithstanding this a successful business, he understood Mandy's role in the force and displayed rare appreciation for her profession. Thus, eased back on his own medical career to embrace role of family man which allowed her leeway to manage extraordinary working hours more demanding than most GPs expected.

Henry, having touched sides with her professionally, and aware of that harmonious background, decided her textbook in the role and enjoyed when a sense of humour made her interject. 'Wonder if them having four legs makes them twice as hard to catch as normal villains?'

Mamad liked her approach. 'Nice one, DI, but suspect combination of two legs for rider, and four for horse means... them three times as slippery.'

They selected DS Mamad Aswat; a Scots born Algerian, for his flair for African languages. The 36-year-old established a superb reputation in the drug squad. Ambitious, already passed DI examinations and hoped for a promotion.

His short; at five feet six inches, and plain appearance belied fact he held a black belt in judo. Also dabbled in competition chess and attained respect as London Police champion.

Unmarried, slowly recovering from a six-year relationship that ended because partner Chantelle, demanding more companionship than force allowed, dropped him for a schoolteacher.

Three months on, dependence on her softened, although found their separation tough.

DS Frank Brooke hung back, kept to himself, for the remarkably peaceful; unflappable character was naturally shy for a true Cockney. Included him in team for excellent reputation in social media and electronics. Henry decided him perfect to work with and learn from Bernard.

Twenty-eight with in Lisa, a steady girlfriend of four months. Lisa, deciding he needed a makeover, encouraged him to grow a mass of dense, chestnut hair.

Later, Pauline agreed, described him to Sophia as graced with the touch of Brad Pitt.

Earlier, having planned on recruiting Mandy for team, Henry asked her to interview Frank. Report included. 'Find him quiet, but intelligent, honest, and resolute. To me, ideal background expert to complement ever-increasing need for technical expertise, although may have limited effect in the field.'

Henry thought. *Bingo, a Bernard clone, should complement our expert, hopefully in time will reduce how we pressurise him.*

Henry subjected them to two days of formal briefing, more intense than any ever underwent. As a result of the time and effort Alroy's team conducted when preparing the field, he desired to share that, where expedience and secrecy allowed, Frank should get them up and flying, fast. Although it followed the already established routes, Henry led team along standard lines where dressing casual along usual plain clothes dress, enforced rank.

He and Alroy established they manage this group as a standard police task force unit, explored and confirmed this important from view of how they use the group to, and without them being aware, leak false information to remove pressure from main team.

Received their cell phones and laptops; pre-programmed to Bernard's specs who anonymously provided detailed written information on software. Without delay, this surprised and delighted Frank, who after working through Bernard's systems caught on to their unit being more important than Henry led them to believe. That and constantly reinforced emphasis on secrecy, particularly from family and colleagues, heightened sense of adventure and intrigue. Kept this to himself.

Henry instructed them to concentrate their research on trafficking in diamonds, and to establish routes hinting suspicion of horse involvement. 'In brief, where any unit mentions horse trade never ignore as irrelevant, mark each finding down as potentially significant worth sharing with team.'

Advised that included any cases alerting them to, even when stumbling across information hinting at insurance fraud involving horses. Important, avoided any suspicion of where their future, and key role was the investigation of corrupt colleagues.

The fact their offices barely positioned ten yards from Alroy's team never mattered. For the station throbbed with different, overworked task forces who rarely interacted or even greeted each other.

Both task forces used same DS Anderson and with offices permanently locked; buzzed in visitors, including members of Henry's team. Only she, Alroy, and Henry carried office keys. Amid hubbub of controlling two related yet dissimilar teams, her laudable competence ensured they never mixed.

DS Anderson, via Henry, was their only link with Alroy.

26

EUROPE AND DIAMONDS

Henry linked the two Ms.

Confident in their ability to work unaided.

Demonstrated experience when appreciating they needed more time to prepare groundwork than most new units, determined before calibrating future intensive investigations, issued guidelines, asking them to always report via DI Mandy.

The four had individual desks in one sizeable room suitable for eight officers.

After moving her up the chain of command her work thrilled Henry.

Started off only four days after releasing them from starting stalls, Mamad approached Mandy. 'DI McDonald, may I interrupt? For preliminary work already sources enough tantalising evidence to take forward. An interesting point around diamond movements catches my eye.'

'Fire away Sgt, what you got?'

To begin with, waved a sheaf of notes, moved towards a still virgin board as Mandy rose from desk to attend. Others were out of office, on the road, following up early leads.

Loomed over as he used magnetic plugs to pin up basic notes. 'Early days but may have uncovered an interesting lead on diamonds. As you know, Antwerp World Diamond Centre was traditional leader in diamonds, but now the Russians, who produce more than three billion dollars' worth annually, consider Europe inodorous because of sanctions.'

She, already tracing parallel Russian involvement, nodded at confirmatory evidence as he described how, and overtly when compared to usual, Russians attempted to strengthen what was originally a tentative base in Zimbabwe and South Africa. 'Good work. Thanks for that, for regardless of me also coming across matching information and linking this to Southern African countries still wooing communist politicians.'

He stepped back, illustrated slight nervousness. 'Not only that but also, picked up how favourable tax incentives in Dubai and Hong Kong now confuse the issue as well.'

She tapped his lineup of four A3 notes. 'Also, like your layout. Helps to keep things neat and ordered.'

'So, we agree on those basic points.' With little groundbreaking evidence, he, happy them running in parallel lines, added fresh information. 'But then, and I should have missed this had our DCI not stressed the horse slant, since by adding these factors that introduces a different and stimulating complexity that needs more work.'

With Mandy remaining quiet her bowed head, encouraged him onward, with confidence restored, stabbed an index finger against a series of photographs of horse's professionally crated for transport overseas including channel ferries and planes and beside them a colourful, heavily annotated in three colours of magic marker picked out routes used by professional horse transporters.

'Impressive.'

'Thanks DCI, and here it gets even more striking.'

Changed the subject, asked her to contemplate how as international horse movement exploded, figures involved raised eyebrows.' When appending more work sheets, Illustrated how industry peaked at over seven million dollars' worth of travel expenses from Belgium alone during 2012... and still increasing. Indicated two graphs for her, to demonstrate sport horse movement from four mainland European countries to England.

'That I did not know. Do those individual horses originate from Belgium itself? No, sorry.' Traced a tight report in plain black, 8-point print. 'Sorry, note where you present different figures for France, Germany.'

DI Mandy developed a remarkable habit when fully focused. Left foot sneaked forward to end up almost two feet in front of its mate. But also, by rocking backward and forward as though trying to unknot kinks in calf muscles tight after a bout of overexercise, produced a remarkable series of movements. Her thing.

Fellow officers she worked with spent time developing a monicker for that movement, settling on describing that pose as an involuntary, but bravura stylised version of a Jamaican rumba. One that intensified when she concentrated hard.

Of course, none dared designate that to her face! Also, found it odd such a fierce investigative mind never cottoned on to them taking the mickey.

Mamad, unused to her rumba, while he tried not to smile at such obvious idiosyncrasy, said, 'Still more, for now it becomes thought provoking, although early days.'

While he traced journeys made by bigger players, noted where Russian horse dealers, whose bona fide reasons for involvement with horses never gelled with him as logically founded. 'Why are these Russians horse trading with Chinese dealers when I trace no direct equestrian activity.

'While distributing horses throughout usual channels, those already known, when researching horses' final destinations, they rarely turn up at major show jumping, dressage, or racing events.'

Mandy empathised with his quandary. For yet, neither could she explain why these horses, at considerable expense, made repeat journeys.

'Nor do they move on through usual sales channels.' Mamad placed two further evidence markers on board. 'And now! These same characters orchestrate movement of horses. Showjumpers, to be specific, throughout Europe to Belgium, and from there... they face the world. Undoubtedly, recognise these horses as international superstars, regularly competing up to Olympic games standards.'

He continued to reveal a remarkable aptitude for active and divergent thought processes and work rate when admitting occasional horses disappeared from the limelight, became irrelevant. 'Only reasonable conclusion is they must be moving contraband using horse transport as...and no pun intended, the vehicle.'

'Good. Like this Chinese involvement, and following your theme, confirm worth continuing to search for evidence of smuggling.'

Mamad held up a lone finger and begged a moment. Moved back to his desk, stroked his keyboard, led her into initial stages of study on four people, three Chinese and one Russian. 'Now, having traced these, find them disgustingly wealthy oligarch Russians drowning in money from oil and gas. Enormous wealth.'

Mandy presented a prime example of her rumba when agreeing them new moneyed people of Europe and added a valuable point. 'People who accumulate this wealth are desperate to put it to work, launder in other, savoury areas. You will stagger at the amount of property and businesses falling into their hands.'

Led him on, described how he and others should take this forward.

By Monday, after drawing together preliminary reports, he intended to instruct team members to change direction and follow his lead, to dig into drugs and whatever. 'Something important, even vast, may come up in that direction.'

As Mamad, delighted in that response he found it easy to agree with logic, noted her intention they circulate a draft report for CI and then, subject to his okay, the others. 'But mam, If you agree, give me four days to put flesh on some of these points, and then you can help me focus on how best to present for DCI Henry.'

'Yes, sergeant. Interested in you finding how they fund these showjumpers. For this international show jumping is big business, involving top people.'

Scanned London's traffic from window for five minutes, while thinking. Only when that bout of Jamaican rumba ended, she came back to him. 'Cannot understand how people justify enormous expenses involved in cross-border transport of horses that seem to disappear. They invest staggering sums yet in real terms, prize money... a pittance. So, money comes from somewhere. But why, what do they get from this?'

As Mamad held his council she added. 'Yes! That is a route to follow, so research background of these competitors, home bases, how they earn a living.'

Now, Mamad added a useful point. 'Also, worth monitoring overt sponsors, establish how upfront sources provide funding. Agree important to uncover any deficits in balance sheets by comparing expenses against income. They do not do this for the joy of collecting flowery rosettes.'

27

PING

Alroy and Henry plotted.

Amid one of their regular, twice weekly meetings.

Assessed what information they collected on Houdalakis families. 'Almost time to start digging into this vet's financial matters.'

Henry, while keen to plug on, expressed opinion with enough doubt in voice to make Alroy agree. 'Close, but not quite enough.' Wished to defer detailed investigation as risky, for collecting bank records involved them approaching other departmental units, an association fraught with danger, as it increased possibility of opening enquiries to prying eyes.

They decided that risk of blowing cover, especially as the bank investigators gossiped most, so not yet worth taking chances. 'Small fry in relation to our top targets and cannot rule out possibility of them leading to a substantial big fish.'

Henry, alerted by phone flashing apologised to answer. As Bernard rarely interrupted, it usually meant important business.

Bang on the money, the call hit a sweet spot.

Bernard's strained voice on speaker mode alerted both senior officers to a crucial development. 'Hi Henry, we have just been pinged.' Without delay, or any of unnecessary whitewashing Henry painstakingly dissuaded, their tech wizard Bernard released not totally unexpected news how a warning ping from Henry's car reached him.

'Instrumentation alerted me to where a boffin actively tampered with your car downstairs in the police garage, as we speak.'

Henry was undecided whether to be sad or glad. 'Barely five minutes after locking it and climbing stairs to the office.'

'If Pauline has returned, shall I join you now?' Bernard was anxious to dig into this cheeky development.

'Not yet... although here she comes.' Henry swung head up as Pauline, unaware of the poser, walked into the office.

Sophia was on the road, dead ending a trail after a top showjumper involved in minor fraud, whose case she passed on to the local police unit.

Ten minutes later, the four sat down to discuss the matter, and quickly decided not to draw notice to the insult, Henry should function as though nothing happened. Agreed it a reminder for everyone to ensure they maintained their usual security practices.

Moreover, when Pauline's car got the same double ping two days later, Alroy changed his mind and decided time to investigate. Instructed Pauline and Bernard to meet at Henry's home where his roomy garage possessed the wherewithal and security to allow Bernard to conduct an intensive search.

Pauline and Bernard use time consuming, separate clandestine public transport and taxis to get there. While a nuisance, Alroy insisted, worried that two pings suggested someone on to them. After a careful search, Bernard found no evidence of how or who entered the vehicle. Each time warnings sounded they activated after someone opened driver's door with a copy key and during the incursion, Bernard received the second ping after intruder breached engine compartments.

Later, back in the office, Bernard emphasised findings that revealed how during both invasions, his sophisticated monitoring system declared perpetrators remained unaware of an erudite detection technique related to specialised keying methods Bernard placed.

Chuffed, reported how he investigated the trail following them searching the engine compartment. 'As they did not take that further, by tracking bar codes back to the website, seems uncovering nothing of interest backed off.'

At this point, what had seemed a useless exercise, but insisted on by Alroy, Pauline's snoop phone played its part. Because of heightened awareness after Henry's first insult, it was her way to hide a second, burner mobile between two front seats as if accidentally dropped.

'Bingo.' Bernard, using sophisticated equipment, detected where an investigator downloaded information from her snoop phone. Harmless SMSs' and short, coded but pointless messages false contacts, also using additional untraceable burner phones in their possession. If used irregularly, they added to intrigue by incorporating secretive undercover work, as officers did when communicating with snitches, leaving leads on the phone's sim card.

Pauline smiled at Alroy, congratulated him on thoughtful planning when he instructed her to act in careless fashion. The extent of Bernard's security measures impressed everyone and allowed Alroy to comment. 'So, we now know a department scrutinises our efforts. While they found nothing of value, this means we continue by being more vigilant than ever.'

Henry said, 'Even in the two years I spent with internal security we never had expertise, need or authorisation to search officer's cars without them being present.'

Pleased Pauline to note efforts she made when painstakingly laying down false trails proved fruitful. 'This contains faithful records which mark me as I used my phone, the tampered one on fourteen occasions. Every snitch call is traceable if they can breakthrough what Bernard's impressive levels of security.'

Patient, Henry asked her to restate each call she made on that burner phone contained trackable but misleading facts which must lead people away from team's proper work, before returning to the vehicle to collect the phone.

'Give them time to download the sim card.'

After replying in a positive manner, she returned to the car and when she reached it, issued a flustered impression. Tried to appear concerned, while muttering aloud *how stupid I was to leave that phone in my car.*

On return to office, admitted that while not deliberately checking, surreptitious searches from corners of eyes and via compact mirror uncovered no suspicious activity. 'A girl regularly checks her makeup.' Showed her girly side.

With Sophia called back to join the meeting, she congratulated Pauline on that correct response and expressed concern. 'Dislike this, especially as such detailed examination could only have been conducted under authority of a high-ranking officer above DCI level.'

Alroy brushed off her concerns. 'Dead right to be bothered, Sophia, although,' Face firmed, took on sheen of glistening quartzite, 'take a realistic position.'

Accepted Henry's nod meant him comfortable with his drift, approving reasoning. 'No matter our concerns, understand and accept this invasion of our cars as a positive reaction to our efforts. Overall, we home in on something big.'

Although he never shared disappointment of his junior officers, Alroy announced time to revisit their most recent lines of enquiry. 'In brief, this suggests one of our freshest enquiry lines hotter than imagined. So, backtrack, identify that line of sensitive investigation concerning our wraiths. Then probe it thoroughly.'

As an afterthought swung eyes Henry's way he said, 'Also, possible one of your team has already struck a nerve. Could be them we track and as you link with this team, they are so nervous they widen their search.'

'Gosh boss,' In partnership with the others even experienced Sophia never had an inkling of backtracking with Alroy's intensity. 'but only now do I get an impression of the investigative nous of your fine brain.'

Henry had initially accepted that as unlikely and soon shared Sophia's concerns, that Alroy may have played a masterstroke. 'With this a sound plan of attack from some clever, but bent officer, have we anything to lose by bringing both teams together earlier than envisaged?'

Pauline added a useful point. 'May even worthwhile dropping a line to our personnel department that after completing their basic training with Henry, now time to amalgamate our task force.'

Albeit less worried that before, Pauline congratulated Bernard. 'Nice work. Because I thought you over the top when delving into these fancy toys. And now apologise, for in the wrong, once again acknowledge your brilliance.' Genuflected as though she visited her confessor.

28

CHINA AND USA

Two sergeants collaborated with DCI Henry.

Henry often collaborated with would-be soloists during his career.

Found their approach unsuccessful, so enjoyed his miniature team. Sure, individuals often surprised with flaring brilliance, but inability to share and learn from fellow officers, often emphasised deficiencies. But harmony already expressed by his team's ability to accept Alroy harnessing them together, moved them with concert of harmony of electroplating electrons.

After Mamad and DI Mandy outlined preliminary findings for the others, he encouraged 'While you uncover several worthwhile avenues surrounding horse movement, the who and what around funding huge expenses involved in international competition, transport and so forth...'

Held their attention. 'Background that for the moment. With my investigations underscoring heroin-based drugs, that field must now be your focus.'

Watched how Mamad who initially frowned at losing his horse investigation, then brightened when instructed to get back into drugs. 'Your job is now to uncover routes brokered by the Chinese, irrespective of where they originate from.

Stepped away from the board and sat beside them. 'Overall, be different, innovative. For now, discount how main players in Britain deal in drugs.'

Tapped a finger against a desk and continued in a peppery tone. 'Force has a comprehensive drug squad focusing on internal problems, so need you to take this further. From poppy farms through European countries and Russia at this stage, experience shows powerful Chinese cartels control these routes. With their ancient history of learning art of growing poppies and refining techniques from India, and increasing use of neat heroine, we know during the diaspora of that nation they took it throughout the world.'

When taking queries, DS Brooke asked. 'Sir. Any objections if, and discretely, I seek help from a sound connection in the drug squad?'

A lack of response meant he accepted that as a positive and Henry indicated Mamad's history with drug squad jumped him to front of the cue for selection to this team, then approved his request.

'That was my suggestion. Please get them on board.'

'Now you excite me sir. For with my background and experience at street level the human misery caused by drugs shocked, which has built me up with a pathological hatred for the traffic.'

The DCI, while he outwardly applauded Mamad's zeal, appreciated he needed control to help stretch mind in a practical sense along traffic with a capital *T* as the sergeant continued. 'Alongside another officer, we initiated investigations into Chinese involvement, and although they gave us a bare two months, immensity of the trade surprised.'

Surveyed the others. 'Simple techniques stunned us when we realised the blasé attitude, or naivety of some enormous shipments and just as we touched on a route from Russia into Britain, got excited at a possible big breakthrough, our DCI announced a dramatic shift, moved us back into the basic areas of drug usage.'

Henry's ears pricked at evidence of senior command interfering, that someone had directed officers away from what they deemed dangerous material likely to point at internal corruption.

Now, as he responded to that observation Henry scented a pot of gold as Mamad continued. 'While I tried hard to control feelings that DCI's dissatisfaction was obvious, for earlier he rejoiced with us over how we sniffed an extraordinary, basic connection between Britain and the US. While we tried hard, time never permitted us to expose anything concrete, nothing we could then tie down.'

The DS punched one hand into the palm of the other. 'Sir, I believe being so close to this in the past, a free hand will produce evidence. Besides, always hoped for an opportunity to dig into that side of things, convinced those good leads may have allowed us name big players.'

Took a breath then said, 'On a deeper note, what if we skirted with internal corruption in the force. What might we have uncovered should we have followed that slippery path?'

At once, two points stood out as flawless. *This team needed less than one month before they are ready to integrate with team one. Also, if Mamad finds his contact useful, we may bring him over.*

Henry reverted to another consideration of Alroy's brilliance when he confirmed it likely his car was pinged because of Mamad's work.

Henry exercised a special ability, one necessary for a commanding officer, when he revealed an ability to extend people's opinions and views into tangible, worthwhile plans while they spoke. That showed, especially intrigued by fresh, relevant information new team brought to the party, but hid enthusiasm. 'Yes... and no! Suggest we split this in two for the present.'

Nodded at them. 'DS Brookee, concentrate on basic Europe and the Russians. DS Kasir can investigate Chinese drug trail into and out of the US.' Decided on that route for Alroy's team needed commensal support to deepen and merge their investigations. Delighted in their enthusiasm, Henry pushed them harder. 'Allow you one week. In the meantime, my job, alongside DI Mandy, is to pick brains of friendly, but dedicated senior personnel who we already understand are knowledgeable in this field.'

Winced at Mandy's thoughtful expression. Already sniffing our corruption theme, must dangle a carrot. 'May uncover sensitive, under wraps information.' Inhaled the air of syrupy insight the perceptive Mandy blew his way.

29

TWO SERGEANTS

The two sergeants as team members worked apart.

Heads down for five days, never managed a coffee together.

DS Brooke caught up with DS Kasir on the phone. 'Jings Abisade, but time fly's past.'

'Sure, does man. And, to coagulate my running points need you, for we must report in two days.'

To begin with, Brooke, introduced the subject by admitting nervousness around their project. 'That's why I phoned. Can we get together, compare notes and act in harmony.'

Two seconds hesitation forced a different drift. 'Or go on our own?'

'No!' Abisade was firm. 'Besides, talked to an old friend who was on the CI's team at one time, thought it useful to sound him out.' Reported the CI big on teamwork and then officers worked together, preferred them to report as one. 'So, we get together.'

Brooke, happy his information matched Abisade's, responded in cheerful mode. 'On balance, you supply me with relevant info and suits me to join you. Can you do 8 o'clock tomorrow morning in the office?'

'Dead right man, dead right.' Chortled with a bizarre ringing tone down one nostril. An injury during a motor vehicle accident left the right side permanently occluded. 'Do not know how DS Anderson swings it, but a pleasure to work with, especially as she brews best coffee in town.'

They compared the shared information.

When into second coffee refills, Abisade said, 'Time to condense our verbal report.'

Brooke touched his elbow. 'Agree as we think this down, better for us both to look at it for then we may conglomerate prose into detailed information.' Waved three pages in front of Abisade. 'On the whole, lets knuckle down and get this ready this for the boss, am sure that approach will suit.'

'Solid man. Simple, direct, and straightforward.' Brooke agreed. 'Despite warnings to that effect, it was always my predicament at school.' Chuckled fast. 'Too many frills.'

Spent afternoon getting their report together. Notwithstanding their efforts, Henry brought Alroy's team up to date. 'We move faster than either of us dreamed.' Even Henry, after his years in the force, thrilled at how evidence from diverse sources came together and probing, rejoiced at their positive track.

With Alroy sharing their enthusiasm, he added to his mood. 'We consider bringing both teams together faster than earlier imagined.' With piles of hot evidence mounting, their information boards developed a necessary ergonomic outline, bathing in urgency final stages of chases always engender.

Alroy, sensed their investigation upgraded from a charabanc of loosestrife odds to a limousine of fact, confirmed they raced towards their goal. 'Not only that but also, worrying over security, sense a moving keystone. A DS somewhere, using gingery senses, hoping to infiltrate us.'

'Despite agreeing with you, let me take my meeting with two of my sergeants next door. And then if they add significant research, talk again.'

As Henry left, Alroy's thoughts turned to Wolf. Torn over when to bring him up to date. But not yet.

30

TROUBLED SERGEANTS

'Great. Like this. Perfect.'

Henry spent fifteen minutes reading.

Then, pondered their report and only after he grasped jist of their evidence, asked for a verbal report.

Pleased to find they worked well together.

In synch, DI Mandy's advice proved invaluable; they presented useful evidence in a professional manner.

Positive response made Abisade wink at Brookee. *Told you so.*

'Now, dissect this properly, fill me in on how and what real police work behind this summary offers.'

Brooke moved to wall boards and said, 'Here we list routes and main players as we... sorry boss, your info helped.' For Henry's contacts added much to their good, solid police work. 'Zhāng twins are up to something...and oddly enough, although their loose approach, one officer described them nonchalant, we hit an impasse.

Abisade added his observations. 'Find no evidence of anyone hunting them.'

When Mamad took his turn, a hesitant approach made Henry take a closer look. 'Find this surprising, sir. Besides, contacts assure me circumstances around where Zhāng wins unfold into multiple trails of destruction and crime. Odd, for like restless teenagers, they in profligate fashion are careless. Contacts assure me while senior officers reported their concerns, yet...'

Mamad's ongoing hesitancy caused Henry to get tough and bark. 'Come on man, stop pussyfooting around for noting your concern, tell me what causes your diffident approach?'

Abisade, naturally a tougher character helped him out. 'If we may be frank, sir?'

As he continued to exercise natural authority, Henry, convinced men performed better under pressure, pushed. 'Yes. Go ahead, men. What makes you indecisive?

When Brooke took over, he went to the board and pinned up a sheet titled, inside job, said, 'several officers are concerned over a sensitive area.' Cocked head to side as though seeking permission to continue. With nothing to dissuade his disinclination to uncovering sensitive opinion, said, 'A worry exists. A rumour circulates around casuistry, that one of our top brass sits on this.'

Pointed at the board, tapped where they accented the Zhāng twins' names. 'While it forms part of our police nature to be suspicious, but to act on facts, we may be mistaken.'

Abisade decided Brookee's alarmed facial expression meant he needed support and taking over admitted. 'Of course, we may be wrong. Since as a superintendent, if he, understanding bigger picture, illustrates brinkmanship of command.'

A lone finger instructed hunters to remain calm and after four poignant seconds Henry developed that theme. 'Do we face a criminal mind tucked inside a carapace of deceit, or a mastermind collating reports from field workers?'

Said that to cover up what was on both sergeant's minds. 'Albeit, when timing ripe, we will then act and make arrests.'

At first, Henry maintained his inflexible approach but then in paternal mode softened. 'Although my growing suspicions suggest my team hides critical information from me.'

'Well sir,' Mamad intervened. 'our idea does not bear thinking about...'

'Now then, sergeant. Out with it.'

Mamad took an abysmally profound breath, fully aware of entering dangerous waters. 'As sergeant Brooke said, confirmed for me from a different source. Talk, sir. Rumours here and there,' Paused and when Henry deigned to comment, pushed on, 'conjecture a senior officer may attempt to delay or even squash this investigation. Sir.'

At last outlined suspicions of corruption involving at least one Met officer. Henry slapped palm on desk, insulted wood hard enough to enjoy how both of men jumped. 'Now you give me something substantial to discuss.'

Moved to the window and after two minutes spent watching flow of London's snarled traffic came back to his men. 'A serious allegation. Are you aware how, if this proves unfounded, it may macerate careers?'

With both sets of eyes marking concern, Mamad took a brave position. 'Only bring this to you with great care, Sir. We, however, do our duty. Besides, cannot hide facts.

Brooke blurted out their conclusion. 'Early evidence,' Looked at boards, flashed ten fingers with artistry of a musicologist, 'convinced us of serious skulduggery. In time, we may diagnose profound, cancerous, and evil infiltration in a seriously fraudulent department.'

Henry's attitude changed, softened as he congratulated them. 'Well done, men. Your excellent work surprises, for you had already began uncovering concerns of my own.

Well done. Superb police work.' Paused. Then again, voice hinted at intrigue. 'And of course, none of you, or us, know who or why or what the hell goes on. Right!'

Henry, pierced by this news of information that collaborated lines of investigation undergoing research by Alroy's team made known concerns while repeatedly palm lapping desk, then sat and set all finger's a-tapping.

Eventually, he began to reveal true nature of their investigation. 'Agree with where the fruit of your investigation smells out corruption and confirms we face something dodgy in the offing.'

Both sergeants offered synchronous sighs of relief, and then Abisade said, 'Thanks for hearing us out on this sir, so you also are already tracking similar facts around that score?'

When Henry rose and studied the board, he took time, then said, 'Now, we face arduous business. Need you to take great care and do not even discuss this with each other as a team at this stage.'

Glowered, then softened. 'We all face instant promotion if we uncover fraud. Or, by botching this up, career breaking material may leak into wrong hands.' Soon, back to sternest approach. 'This does not leave this office, nor does it form part of any email, computer, paper trail or telephone conversations.'

Gave them the most powerful CI raking stare ever received. 'We as a full team meet here on Tuesday morning at nine.' Stood and studied information boards again. 'Excellent work. Start by fleshing out this draft, except,' Took them into confidence, 'when discussing both reports, I,' Bestowed a fleeting smile, 'may lead you deeper into major things.'

As Mamad's confidence grew he cautiously divulged evidence Henry and Alroy searched. 'Also, worth mentioning Superintendent Gordon's name features.'

Still nervous, compunction to protect fellow officers, touched unfolding sensitive information with concern. 'But sir, admit only gently, without as yet, hard evidence.'

As Brooke took over, Henry remembered days as a sergeant, when colleagues steeped conversations in innuendo and gossip. Yet, how often that led to them hitting on valuable information, useful leads.

Brooke interrupted his musing. 'More background, factual now, declares he and Assistant Commissioner Flynn were an item in the past.'

When that raised Henry's eyebrows, Brooke's growing poise urged him to reveal more than intended without first discussing strategy with Alroy. 'Although we do not wish to race on into weak conjecture, time to investigate top brass.'

Notwithstanding how their information rang noisy bells, Henry said, 'Your research digs deep. But I agree. Until proven squeaky clean, keep them in the mix.'

Slipped seamlessly into tough mode. 'However, under no circumstances dare investigate these names without my express permission.'

As Henry marched off, strove hard to conceal raging excitement.

Sergeants bestowed spectacular high fives as Frank said, 'Wow! Big stuff. Cannot wait.'

31

PAULO'S UPDATE

An impatient Morgan nailed Saunders.

A hardened drinker for years, nerves in disarray.

Since their plan to kill Heraldon backfired when it caused Shaun's death, overindulgence threatened to slip into alcoholism.

Spent two days of their impromptu holiday with Paulo and Morgan, surrounded by luxury, forbearance, and unnecessary drinking.

Now, well into his cups, defences low, Morgan sensed an opening.

Earlier, Morgan employed a master stroke when she despatched Paulo and June; Saunders' wife. Her suggestion, sound, gave June an opportunity to inspect Paulo's yearlings, fawning her valuable opinion on young stock must confirm hopes of them fetching big sale prices.

No matter she outlined her intent to Paulo, found him unsure but Morgan convinced him that by buttering up Saunders, she could ferret out information around how her brother planned Heraldon's execution.

With them gone, she, while refilling his crystal glass with Abreu Cabernet Sauvignon, a smart Californian vintage, accepted space, and opportunity to squeeze Saunders. 'Now brother. You know I cannot cope with your messing around.' Kissed, soaked him in genuine fraternal hugs then encouraged him to sit beside her.

Saunders always loved his young sister and thrived in security of her presence, snuggled into her. She, delighted in his company, steeled to business, and opened with a lung draining sigh. 'Because we distress over a valuable horse, only you, dear brother, with your famous expertise can help.'

He relished her response, released a relaxed chuckle as she, now soft, *carpe diem*, said, 'Know you masterminded an outstanding solution to your financial difficulties.'

Now, leave him a moment. In a dreamy mood encouraged by the decent vintage and what he termed his financial mastery, Saunders relished his sister's comforting presence, basked in fraternal affection.

Until suddenly, she guessed timing ripe and dug in. 'For instance, understand you manufactured an impressive plan to destroy Heraldon.'

His painful, immediate shudder confirmed she tracked a straight road, but sympathetic, winced at palpable images which flooded his psyche, supported him. *This man never steeled himself to kill farm chickens. Of course, sense and appreciate that effort an emotional hammer slapping his brain. My poor brother. Notwithstanding pain, need his support.*

Confiscated his wine glass, placed it delicately on a coffee table, then, searched glassy eyes with demanding, diamond cutting globes, advanced her argument. 'You earned big money. Without delay, insurance payouts saved your sorry ass, kept head above water.'

No match for persistent sister, as often happens when people mastermind a clever plan, they need to talk, reveal cleverness. No point in doing something extraordinary if nobody listens, pats back at your brilliance, offers congratulations, expresses their admiration.

Moreover, her approach struck right chord. Obvious. Saunders sat back, smiled. 'In truth, before losing that fine horse, things settled onto a sticky wicket.'

That tiny admission provided Morgan's opening. 'Right! Divulge your clever plan. Need names, vets who conducted this project for you, who planned the exercise.'

Overall, with her knowledge of illegal killing accurate, those remarks invigorated Saunders who now basked in success, delighted with sister's support, and found a touch of sobriety.

Despite that inner glow permeated his mind, warmed body to levels absent since they contrived to execute Heraldon and fought to show a modicum of restraint. 'No, my dear, you are wrong. For yes, I involved two vets that night. They worked hard, helped me control pain and distress experienced by those poor horses injured during that horrid storm.'

Hugged, kissed. 'Doubtless people talk. Yet we acted out a straightforward vet relationship. How sad to lose that fine animal, although my shares... phew.'

Her chuckle drew a faint grin. 'Never change. Just as I remember, when you tried to worm your way from demanding situations, could not hide truth from our dear mother.

Unable to resist, she bared your soul as precise as any scalpel wielding brain surgeon.

From a cavernous mouth filled with strong, professionally whitened teeth he issued his best laugh in months. 'Mums Mars Bars.'

Her foible. Mum ate two Mars Bars weekly. At three pm on a Friday afternoon, her *me time,* she sat in lounge, undisturbed for one hour, with a racy novel a goblet of Pouilly Fuissé and two Mars Bars.

Morgan revelled in that memory, picked up the theme. 'Remarkable. Loaded with four ice cubes, moment of indulgence.' Smacked shoulder. 'But! The day her chocs disappeared, blamed our friend Archie, the groom's son when she acted bananas.'

A gargantuan memory never forgot his only hiding.

Virginia Hetherington, smart socialite permanently surrounded by a flock of eligible suitors, loaded their steeplechasing father respectability. Captured by dashing looks and sparkling repartee, brought Saunders wealth when they married. As part of nouveau riche, he rented, then purchased stables now gracing Saunders' business.

Overall, it was a gaggle of former suiters who, following her, loaded stables with smart classic horses that led to rapid success.

Family matriarch, a handsome size twelve, five-foot eight-inch blond used classic fullness to dominate every man to cast an eye her direction.

Passed on that description and personality to daughter, but only Saunders inherited her oddly shaped ear. June, aware of that familial defect found only their son affected. A smart plastic surgeon moulded lopsided ear as a three-year-old.

He begged for his glass.

Took a strong slurp, misty eyes watered with love as he said, 'And, as mother's spitting image, suppose you gained her detection abilities.' Grinned again when he held hands out, palms up. 'Secrets impossible.'

Despite being crooks, bolstered by similar intentions, they shared special loving bonds. Soon, after bathed him in a moment of rare, enviable tenderness and twisted both arms. When drained of facts, rewarded with an irresistible bunch of carrots. 'With our venture a major effort, Paulo guarantees you will receive an enormous payoff after your people conduct our little exercise.'

Turned to her and caressed a thigh. 'Now you talk my language. So, do you mean this impoverished brother of yours may earn commission?'

With floodgates open, Saunders, now an active co-conspirator, filled out loose gaps and offered constructive advice.

Later, after jolly horse experts returned, Morgan dragged Paulo away to give June and Saunders time for intense conversation.

On their return, platitudes over, Paulo explored. 'From my side, having discussed this at length, suggest we approach your vets as follows.'

Paulo and Morgan controlled both Saunders and June as she, still shocked at how Saunders frittered finances, tried hiding head in sand when depth of fraud with Heraldon surfaced.

Now, fully aware, regularly so of their accounts, rose to suck in Morgan's offer, keen as any trout inhaling Mayflies. Agreed something significant had to happen.

The promise of a million-dollar bonus for information without   physical activity proved a significant sweetener. As Heraldon's money had cleared debts, established finances on track, Paulo's bonus promised to set them up for years. *Future secure. Now under, my control, set for life.*

'Get both vets together. Entertain them royally, my expense. Somewhere discrete where Leon can meet them and set up the event. Agreed?

After shaking hands ironed out finer details.

32

INDULGENT WEEKEND

'Decided you chaps deserved this pampered weekend.'

Hence, lunchtime on the Saturday.

Saunders, Georgiou, and Calder already into the liquid side of things, found the venue, Black Swan at Helmsley's award-winning tearoom, perfect for their al fresco lunch.

Calder said, 'What a treat. Those girls...'

Georgiou agreed. 'La, la, la. True bombs. Best night ever.'

Saunders treated vets and himself, at Paulo's expense, to a thoroughly excellent evening, steeped in such unheard of debauchery, the hotel appended their names to their undesirable list.

Unforgettable, reinforced extent of their treat. 'Prepare for tonight. Fresh ladies, better.'

In the first place, easy to soak in lavish luxury, naïve about Paulo's plans. On balance, knew Saunders already hatched another killing to knock down at least one foal, assumed that simple exercise must net a tidy profit, one to justify this extraordinary weekend bonus, an advance sweetener.

Nevertheless, Whitby crab with Dom Perignon. Exceptional food with herb fed guinea fowl to follow. To satisfy immense appetites, feast rolled on. Amid a sense of freedom and merriment rarely experienced, boundless joy knew no bounds.

Until Leon joined their table.

Calder's mouth slackened, open wide enough to satisfy a short-sighted dentist, as disturbed by the American, when they expected voluptuous company. That Saunders introduced mincing Leon, proved a shocker.

All unwanted, after introductions, perceptions changed when he led them along a most unexpected trail.

Leon: under guise of a London based blood stock agent named Percy Blackstone; flourished his counterfeit passport, exposed customs stamps from five countries then darted into business.

If feline, sinuous movements fluttered through his body, a sharp, active mind concisely informed them of Paulo's expectations. In the meantime, never mentioned client's name, nor detailed horse or its whereabouts, Leon uncovered boss' desire for them to kill him.

In time, laid bare jist of the exercise: beginning with them entering US under expertly forged Greek and British passports supplied by him. Later, in Georgiou's smart hotel room, used the latest fifteen-hundred-dollar Samsung phone to take photographs, head shots for fraudulent passports.

Employed them to kill a stallion.

Insisted they conduct slaughter with a method that must arouse no suspicion and by using preferred undetectable methodology. Necessary to satisfy insurance and forensic investigators it fell with the *natural causes* realm.

Afterwards he would ensure they were whisked back to England on the same passports.

Paulo described payment mechanism they should expect.

Gesticulated with extravagance of an Angler fish as it waved its lure, when he beamed details of payment to follow as he lodged two million dollars for each in Swiss bank accounts.

Credit due to vets for not falling off perches at such a figure.

Leon anticipated effort must take four nights.

'This session was tasty, but insignificant with what I have planned for your last night.'

Outlined how their final evening must prove an even more extraordinary example of what young men enjoy than Saunders provided. 'You probably watched the TV series Billions... well.'

After he marked where Georgiou's' expectant facial expressions darted through various pictures conjured by a lively mind, he said, 'Those scenes of three sensuous girls fawning over each man.' Left rest to imagination.

Leon's approach hooked the lads. Afterwards Calder pleased with himself, impressed how masterfully he got the fee up to the three-million-dollar mark each after which Leon advised them to anticipate secure delivery in two days of one hundred thousand pounds cash each. A signing on fee.

Despite haggling, result pleased Leon for Paulo authorised him to agree on a four-million-dollar fee each.

'We are in. When and how?' Georgiou fretted in starting stalls, keen to go.

Their meeting was a late breakfast effort at which vets barely recovered from a feast of Bacchanalian extravaganza as Leon suggested the matter held no urgency for a conclusion.

His duty to organise passports for their holiday, a five-day process including transport from US. Revealed a delay of three or four weeks before they settled everything Stateside and they must not concern themselves over trivial details, for he intended providing ample warning.

Calder expressed a concern. 'One problem presents as a potential obstacle for our firm contracted us to work in Newmarket area for two months.'

Before Leon responded, Georgiou said, 'For this money... Let Newmarket flounder. No worries.'

Calder, busy running through his mental diary, said, 'And yet, as your timing is casual,' Stared at Leon, 'we can plan our US visit around Newmarket.'

Moreover, watched as a sensitive Leon patted dainty hands together, and made Calder realise minds followed same lines as Leon' added, 'Advocate you present different, but synchronised stories to release you from business, which leaves you space to travel.'

While they debated how to approach the visit, Leon suggested Georgiou concoct a family incident. 'Why not spend a few days in Athens on your false passport, then proceed to US from Greece?'

Calder enjoyed that simple solution. 'Certain to fit in a similar something. An RTA might afford me an excuse.'

Which puzzled Leon. 'An RTA. What have you in mind?'

'Sorry Percy, setup a ruse where after being absent overnight, I may not return for duty because of my involvement in an RTA—a road traffic accident, which leaves me immobile for days.'

The longer they spent discussing killing, easier it seemed, and Leon finished the discussion. 'As my boss is the most professional of men who thinks of everything, I declare with confidence to set up an impeccable scene and solution to this quandary. Will discuss it with him and get back to you.'

33

CALDER'S LETTER

Monday lunchtime found vets discussing sordid business.

Acted under Saunders' strict instructions.

Began when they covered their trails when a sound plan whisked them home in separate vehicles.

In the meantime, on reporting for duties in hospital, they concocted stories for staff and associates around how different weekends unfolded.

On return to business, whenever rounds of stable duties and hospital cases allowed, they discussed weekend's entertainment. 'Phew, that was a holiday. Although it leaves me exhausted.' Calder, chuckled at feigned distress, still luxuriated in glow of licentious excess, ripped open an envelope and stuck nose in a missive from Margaret and twins.

As that drew out his rarer, gentle side, he as he lolled in reminiscing mood, found it natural to sigh, and say, 'Often miss family. For twin sisters and I were great friends who shared massive fun growing up.'

That brought a peal of noisy, unrestrained laughter from partner in crime. 'To emphasise your thoughts, agree. For none enjoy family like Greeks. Sometimes they wrench heart strings, make it tough to be away from them.' Fiddled with a sideburn and used a waspish tone. 'Although they can also make it difficult to,' Laughed again, 'live with them.'

Calder shared humour. 'So true.'

That said, when Georgiou noticing him brood over his letter, embraced a touch of jealousy, proclaimed disappointment. 'Mine never write to me.'

'Nor mine. But we regularly communicate via WhatsApp and Twitter, and with pictures flooding Facebook, they rarely find it necessary to write. Mind you, never scratch a pen over paper.'

Calder smiled at a photograph, waved it at Georgiou. 'But this letter lands with important intelligence because they forward me a wedding invitation, and this special photograph of Alroy, my twin.'

Georgiou took a quick peek, and said, 'A smart chap in uniform. Bet that gives him pulling power with chicks.' Strong language relaxed. 'Your twin you say and obviously not identical, but a distinctive character. What does he do?'

Calder's voice tinged with pride when he proclaimed Alroy received a grand award from the police force. 'He is a superintendent with the Met, their youngest ever.'

As a result of that matter-of-fact mention of Alroy being a police officer, it set off alarm bells in Georgiou's brain, had him instantly on high alert, physiognomy firmed into an expression tougher than Calder ever noticed, Georgiou, after fiddling with sideburns and earrings, gripped his shoulders and said, 'The police, you say.'

Shook both of Calder's arms, forced his attention. 'You never mentioned our business to him, did you?'

Calder tucked pic back into the envelope. 'Don't be daft, man.'

Still, as conversation drifted on, surprised him to find how hard it was to placate his partner, then as he remembered a recent conversation, bit a lip. *Although, odd he asked my opinion on horse injuries months ago. Wonder. No this is rubbish, move on.*

The American story captivated.

Besides, facts around slaughter for this major job demanded thorough preparation. Overall, snatched every undisturbed period in hospital to get together and focus on strategy required to establish a fail proof approach for the killing.

On edge, Georgiou proved reluctant to arrange too many planning meetings during evenings for a fine honed criminal background advised they practice social distancing as part of their cover. 'Who knows. Too much togetherness, before and after the killing, may encourage pointy fingers.'

'That weekend in Helmsley still races through my brain. Excites me every time memories flash.' Georgiou, while readily agreeing with Calder, allowed brain to race on and now, furlong in front of him said, 'Sense Dr Alex Calder is on cusp of an exceptional, well-paid career. For instance, one ensuring we work only for best people. Mean those with ready money, wealthiest of patrons.'

Doodled a pen against a desk pad. 'Perhaps only one job every two or three years.'
Even if Calder's head bobbed, his sex-addled brain still hung in the clouds. 'Helmsley style weekends on tap, for our earnings will pay for them.'

Georgiou rattled his cage. 'Now you plan on us making our efforts at strenuous pleasure tax deductible.' Despite Calder sharing his joke, Georgiou's eyes narrowed. Fine cracks emerged around them when he studied Calder's mien.
While they sat together, guessed their upcoming kills plucked at conscience. Assumed they when added to already conducted slaughter, niggling at sense of decency, threatened to float doubts to surface as fat does in chicken soup.

So, Georgiou, as he brushed away an errant, overlong curl, leaned over, and ran a finger through hair. 'Out with it. What bothers you? For I sense a troubled mind raises disconcerting notions.'
Calder, aware when he introduced the original concept, exhibited no trace of doubt, nor suggested moral issues when laying out embryonic ideas for conducting butchery, admitted. 'It's just... well, since the messy Heraldon incident, conscience pesters, encourages me to lose sleep over killings.'
Partner got firm. 'I, needing money will do this,' Cautioned, 'but should you wish to pull out, must have your answer by tomorrow at latest.'

Fingers moved from sideburn, traced a thumb alongside a spectacular Hellenic nose. 'For I know a horseman, a hard-headed trainer, who will help me with this project.'
By the time Georgiou unwrapped his backup plan, Calder, horrified at notion he could miss out, confirmed involvement, then explained unease. 'However, find this killing. Tough.'
'Agree. Hard, but stop thinking of racehorses as real animals,' Gentled tone, 'so, come on man! They are machines, only objects for man's pleasure.'
He, thinking ahead, had contemplated the softer Calder might lose focus. So, launched into a monologue so detailed and structured, only later, Calder appreciated extent of his preparation. As he repeated. 'Stop thinking of racehorses as pets. They are not fluffy toys.'

Gave Calder a minute to reflect then hit even harder. 'Reflect on bloodstock as you do chickens, bullocks, and even... pretty, woolly lambs. Besides, with their entire existence under our control,' Diction slow and firm, 'they are not pet dogs.'

Calder grasped that point, latched onto shred of wholesomeness Georgiou threw his way. 'Understand your thinking, how our attitude towards different animals is shaped by their destination.' Growing brighter by the minute, said, 'So if they asked us to take out pets, would that affect you different?'

'Come now, man. For sure. Our industry is based on thoroughbreds and race greyhounds as mere chattels, expendables.' Flung arms apart. 'We race, then dump them, often euthanising because we cannot rehome them. Ditch them as passed their sell-by-date. Rubbish.

Circled both hands around Calder's throat and encouraged thumbs to caress as might a lover. 'But pets. Never in a million years. So, ponder over how different are pets and production animals. Miles apart.'

With Calder's demeanour improved, cajoled with suggestions sticky, persistent as treacle. 'The racing industry is based on gambling. Mull over how majority of our clients function as if they are farm animals bred for processing.' Caught Calder's elbow. 'Think of owners we know who never visit stables, many who during a racing machines lifetime, never stroke one.'

'You make a valid point. For we breed them to race and when careers end, we shoot them, so, I must remain strong, act tough, and be hard on myself.'

Calder, who spent days and nights becoming increasingly unsure with the plan, allowed charismatic Georgiou to carry the day, particularly as final offering paralleled Calder's own measured approach to livestock.

'You are a farmer. Reflect on calves and lambs you fought hard to deliver, to keep alive when ill, yet do this aware you keep them alive as economic units for later slaughter?'

Georgiou's argument carried enough weight to satisfy still nervous Calder, enough to clear heads and permit them to continue working on practicalities for the trip.

Settled on a sensible plan of flying out separately from Manchester and Athens. After arriving at the airport, Percy designated two drivers to whisk them away, deliver to different hotels within ten miles of the farm.

To begin with, considered a guise as international bloodstock agents interested in buying stock.

They could only meet during the closing moments.

34

BLOOD DIAMONDS

Henry's team, flamed with passion.

Luck, skill, meant everything they touched turned up trumps.

'As we investigate these trails, I reach an inevitable conclusion.' Brooke stressed two entries on the work board. 'These relate to investigations followed by various departments highlighting how blood diamonds from various sources, move out of Africa. Relevant, they add strings to our quota of hot research.'

'Agree Frank.' Mamad drummed fingers on tabletop and continued. 'Stagger at evidence cavorting through brain when pondering same questions.'

Brooke took over. 'More evidence declaring senior officers involved in corrupt practices. The DCI will appreciate spanking new evidence.' From Angola, the Congo to Sierra Leone, burgeoning facts rang clear.

The two sergeants, convinced of funny business attacked the subject. Brooke explored. 'Notwithstanding this solid evidence, you demonstrate connections in US, China, or Russia?'

'Well, yes. And here it coagulates with remarkable coincidence. For, as list of names, suspicious and otherwise, explodes, everybody has a finger in this bloody business.' Although, shy of unmistakable evidence, journalists finger persons of interest.'

He appended a pink note to the board. 'These include Ivanka Trump, Moshe Lax, and the Steinmetz family jump to the fore. On the contrary, while people mentioned names, nothing solid proved them involved.'

'Wonder what DCI Henry will make of this? Better get his input.'

Keen, Henry organised a team meeting for nine am the following day to investigate matter at length. First up, DI Mandy, satisfied her research collaborated their findings, said, 'Boss. Remember they established the Kimberley Process Certification Scheme in 2000 to better regulate diamond trade. Important, for that by pushing blood diamonds deeper under counter, makes it challenging to quantify extent of fraud.'

Mamad distilled that notion. 'With Africa often termed as being the Dark Continent, why wonder so much emanates from there?' As Mamad spoke, Henry nodded in respect for just how much his team uncovered.

DS Brooke said, 'Zimbabwe again. Uncle Bob set up an enormous plot with communist Chinese partners to control the market. Even if poorly coordinated, new regime, proving equally corrupt continues his work.'

Henry, in human mode, expressed disappointment the great Zimbabwe nation, hopeful of a resurrection after Mugabe, rein, mired in further, self-inflicted misery of greed.

Then, homed into current business, mind sharpened with precision of echo locating bats, congratulated team on extraordinary work. 'You chaps impress.' After thanking them, asked for a gargantuan effort.

'Now Sergeant Frank, your task, a huge one, is to probe US side. Correlate position of the super wealthy and find who they work with. The four of us can meet on Thursday morning at nine.'

Ds Brooke made the discussion flow. 'Find the Daphne Galizia case of particular interest. Assassinated shortly after reporting connections between Russian mafia, Columbian drug cartels and Ivanka and Donald Trump's hotel investments in Panama.' With Henry remaining ignorant of those events, raised eyes, and motioned with a hand for him to continue. 'Assassinated her with a car bomb. Investigators marked it a Russian mafia hit.'

Henry pulled things together. 'Now we grasp true extent of how our subject agglomerates into a mix of diamonds. Drugs. South America. China. Russia. Every link hoped for, and now...' Paused. 'Must speak to my DS for we may need a concentrated effort.'

35

FIRST SHIPMENTS

Six weeks later, US vets met three Belgian horses.

Tucked away in the back streets of a colourful French village.

A resting house on the D119, ten kilometres short of the Calais ferry terminal. An extensively used rest stop and collecting site for in-transit horses.

Owners and staff were unconcerned about three smart two-year-old warmblood horses, which occupied one of six, discrete stable blocks which included basic accommodation.

Besides being tight, minimalistic, although Yvette approved of cleanliness. 'Not much of a place, but manageable for first night of our romantic honeymoon.'

Proprietors owned four identical units.

Experienced in horse transport, they appreciated and expected horsey people's paranoia over security.

Louis and Yvette; still excited over their wedding, flew in from NY on false passports for initial leg of their honeymoon. Arrived at stables at around eight pm, to a freezing cold June evening.

Unusual, even harder than weather left behind in New York. Again, impressed over Chinese planning, a dark Mercedes, with tinted windows, swished them to the unit, two hours before their custom built, horse transport; one of the cheaper, plainer ones available arrived.

When they finished checking documents and approved them as fit for horse transport within the EEC, Louis whistled. 'Perfect, these are handsome individuals.'

Yvette nodded. 'They are a decent bunch of promising jumpers.'

He agreed. 'Should earn extra pounds when we sell. Bet the bay colt winks, tempts you to take him home with us. Sure, has stamp of a decent prospect.'

'Hmm!' Yvette patted his bum. 'Shall we get on with the job? Please.'

By eight pm, they had drenched the three horses, loaded them with sparkling stones, their full payload of diamonds, under supervision of Chao who slipped into the stables at last moment.

Vets impressed with their efficiency when managing the horses. 'The first time, I have watched you in proper action. A superb job. Lovely.' Disappeared from scene.

Horses and people rested overnight.

All five of principal players were in form the following morning at six, as they prepared to load for transport to the ferry. Yvette, as she dutifully played role of groom was most careful, secretive when she collected, sieved, and carefully examined every dropping the horses passed.

Louis seemed lethargic to the few permanent staff who moved past and since he slouched around yard acting as lookout, they considered him lazy.

Although they expected no diamonds to pass through so early, vets still respected most valuable garden fertiliser manure in the world. Yvette snapped off gloves. 'Good. Nothing to report.'

Vets used false EEC passports during the twelve-hour journey by horsebox and ferry, then on to a small yard near Whitfield.

Horses travelled well.

Over fifteen hours, all dutifully deposited precious cargo and with diligence of a cat fixated on a mouse hole, they collected and sieved every dropping.

Yvette exclaimed. 'Come to me beauty for you is the one the cobbler used to kill his wife.'

Amid a noisy cloudburst, checked for and found, every tube intact, and confirmed valuable cargo arrive in perfect condition and following a simple WhatsApp message, *weather as expected,* Louis stood by the roadside for five minutes until Chao sneaked up beside him, collected package of stones and vanished.

More good news followed when a shifty horse dealer, mind you, most are dodgy, walked up to Yvette, introduced himself as Gordon Brown, explained role as a permanent sifter out of bargains. 'On the whole, as a dealer, check if you wish to sell any of your consignment?'

Explained he met most local ferries and often picked up a bargain.

Yvette hung back, asked for more details.

'Odd, but despite effort involved, people change plans. Often sell me horses for a fair price.' Asked permission to inspect their cargo and then offered to take them off their hands.

'If not quite my cup of tea, could help you out, move them on.' His manner and professionalism, even though they haggled for forty minutes, astonished Louis over how easy they sold the horses. For both he and Yvette anticipated it difficult to contact local dealers willing to take them off their hands.

Brown scrutinised and appreciated fool-proof passports which intimated decent breeding lines from Belgium Warmblood sires.

They accepted twenty-two thousand pounds for the bay Yvette liked and eighteen for a smart chestnut. Compared to the others causing smiles, quibbled at the third horse, a chestnut with three white legs, for a swelling on near hock caused concern. 'Fear this could be a spavin.'

Louis, having checked lump earlier, knew it was a reaction to a knock, but glad to move him on, accepted twelve thousand. They earned fifty-two thousand pounds from a good, quick, and clean deal. If less than the horses true worth, it never mattered. Quick. An easy, clean deal. Brown gave them his business card. 'Should you consider further trips, can meet you anywhere.'

In the manner of a modern car dealer, as they signed over the horses, and Yvette's phone flashed to indicate he already deposited the fifty-two thousand into their US bank account via eft.

As they left, Brown organised transport and mused. *Nice that one lad. Doubtless stolen, but who cares. Paperwork in order. A decent profit.*

Only two days later Yvette suggested they made an idiotic mistake. 'Slipped up. For that deposit leaves a dangerous paper trail.'

'Although acting like novices, but provided we do not err again, am sure we may pass this off as commission story. You are, however, right. Must not happen again.'

During the five weeks of their honeymoon, they repeated the exercise four times through ports at Cherbourg and Dunkirk.

On each occasion, Brown met them and delighted in taking over the horses. Now, understanding their MO and content to realise a decent profit, paid them better prices than he did for the first load.

With the final shipment, a consignment of four superb French Warmbloods, which Brown snapped up. He, happy with how fast he moved on the others for a significant profit, upped the ante, and forked out two hundred and sixty thousand pounds.

Chao, disappointed at their earlier amateurish effort when they moved money, organised for their overall commission on horses sold and diamonds delivered; eight hundred and forty thousand dollars, to arrive in usable, safe accounts in the US.

A chunk of luck arose when Chao used the money as a deposit to purchase for their NY hospital, the latest German radiography and scanning equipment, to a value of one hundred and five million dollars.

Much less than its face value, which meant their hospital the best privately equipped in the state. Installed and running within four weeks of their return, they amazed competitors.

Eventually, because others begged to hire the equipment, they employed an additional vet and a nurse. The fact it increased turnover and never showed up on books, was a welcome bonus.

36

CHERBOURG

'Know we planned our final run via Cherbourg.'

Chao reported Gregor delighted in their success.

Apologised as he outlined how they arranged final shipments. First, gave them good news, hinted at what they hoped to forecast the end. 'For now, I confirm the KLM trip, after Cherbourg, should be our first, perhaps only flight.'

Eyes lifted; confident his statement could improve sagging demeanour.

'Regardless of our increasing urgency to complete the project, a supply problem means that will only take place after your week in Paris.'

Revealed how much he enjoyed collaborating with them, appreciated tireless efficiency and professionalism.

'A luxurious, five-star honeymoon on us.'

Nevertheless, amid excitement that caused, when buzz generated by news settled, Yvette, tiring of the process, said, 'Thank you for this, but worry as trips increase, does that expose us to risk? Sensitive to us being able to escape detection for ever?'

Chao scrutinised their faces.

When content, sat beside them, and called for a second pot of coffee, then outlined feelings. 'With us spending so much time together, family almost, I express honesty.'

Outlined how the company, his masters, delighted in their expertise, now, hoped for more, dragged out process, determined to maximise investment.

'Trust, however, after our adventure from Cherbourg, this time, common sense may prevail.' Asked them to pack, for they must move within the hour.

Later, ensconced in their decent Hotel Chantereyne room, chosen as always for it being three star and therefor a tourist destination, unlikely to draw attention, discussed immediate future, especially increasing concerns around possibility of an organisation spotting their involvement in smuggling. 'Worry if their greed in overusing the system means they suspect we leave a trail.'

Pulled his arm. 'Fear they might dump us, hang us out to dry?' Impossible to detect and without an alternative plan, laid negative thoughts aside.

Louis' grandfather lost his life in the Battle of Normandy.

Thrilled him to visit Omaha Beach where his father landed in June 1944 but lost his life soon after his feet hit the sand.

A poignant memory, a trip his own father wished to make but missed out on because of a heart attack three weeks after Louis' graduation.

Mother also passed on soon afterwards, losses that helped mould man's character along self-reliance.

Yvette, with family scant and estranged, contributed to how when they got together, she and Louis wrapped themselves in each other, only family they ever needed, apart from her burning, increasingly urgent desire to birth children.

Apart from window shopping, because travelling light they purchased little. 'Let's leave that for glorious Paris.'

Thrilled to take two sightseeing trips through Cherbourg in horse driven carriages especially in a three-in-hand covered wagon pulled by three grey, Percheron-type draught horses, then back to business.

Unexpected news of two trips from Cherbourg to south coast of London unsettled vets, but with no chance of influencing matters, settled into usual rhythm, as before. But disliked making two trips from same stable base, so close together.

Yvette worried their employers, by slipping into a laisse fair mode lapsed into carelessness.

In time, they conducted their trip, with four horses, amid usual scene, and with normal, excellent preparation all proceeded as planned.

On their return to Cherbourg, lapped up two relaxed days of sightseeing, including a coach trip with six horses.

Yvette, especially concerned over this departure from normal, complained their employers added in this unnecessary complication.

While he agreed, he said, 'My dear, as we near the end of our adventure, let us rather focus on incredible value of our trip as a financial exercise.'

In usual kind manner, evinced great care when he asked her to get her head down, stop wrapping herself in imponderables, and work.

On meeting their six horses, found a similar batch and again, appreciated quality, the news of earning excellent money, reduced concerns. Until, as she approached the fourth horse to give him a routine inspection, she surprised how he danced away from her. The smart bay colt stood out because of an ugly blaze, running from an irregular, jagged star down left side of face to the end before it reached the nostril.

No slouch when reading equine behaviour, Yvette called Louis over as he finished checking out his last charge. 'Come Louis, dislike this chap. Strikes me as a horse incubating a virus.'

'So, too much to expect our luck to hold up. At last, you spot a horse fit to pose a catch.'

Louis approached the horse and after he experienced a similar reaction to the one that raised alarm, said, 'Doubtless this fella presents a quandary. Wonder if an infection affects him, like viruses we encounter back home.'

'Agree, because dilated pupils, homed in eyes staring at everything, yet understanding nothing, he may experience an encephalitis. A West Nile virus or similar.'

Regardless, without knowledge of local infectious equine diseases, they contacted Chao, explained concerns, advised they diagnosed a health concern, one serious enough to render horse unfit to travel.

Chao agreed to take advice further up the chain, then report.

One hour later, informed them provided the horse does not deteriorate overnight, they should proceed as planned.

Disappointment and concern occupied vet's minds, although, throughout the evening horse never deteriorated. So, they instigated their pre-travel business, including tubing with diamonds, as normal.

Yvette suggested they leave bay colt for last. With him proving testing to control, and only after a low dose of the tranquiliser Domosedan, Louis inserted the stomach tube.

After Yvette poured in water and tubes containing diamonds, as Louis removed the tube, the horse exploded into action.

In a display as savage as expected of any rodeo star, he went nuts, erratic, aggressive behaviour ending only when they stood back and watched in horror as he plunged and reared. Demented, fell backwards, crashed head against the brick stable wall, then collapsed.

Dead.

Loaded with diamonds.

That most valuable carcase caused considerable excitement, and since they expected horses to move onto docks in two hours, his death changed plans.

And Chao, in departure from normal, attended and witnessed this debacle. Shocked, expressed, he for one and only time, declared disappointment with masters. 'A disaster. Explained you, as experts, had significant doubts. And now.' Flung hands in air. 'A waste. Their failure to accept constructive advice may cause disaster.'

As arms conducted a hidden orchestra, he continued. 'Shudder to imagine the consequences had this happened on board the ferry? Authorities must have demanded a forensic examination. Diamonds gone.

Everyone faced jail.

Besides his thoughts, urgency around shipment found them rubbing brains together to solve their immediate problem. Only solution meant Louis to travel with consignment to Poole while Yvette remains behind and salvage the solution by extracting and saving his diamonds.

They received unexpected help while discussing this, as Jean-Paul, owner of the yard, alerted by noise arrived.

He appreciated urgency, acted fast when he produced a thin, ultra-sharp blade.

Without delay or discussion, cut the horse's throat.

Watched him bleed out, while his passionless voice explained the next step. 'Friends shall now call my butcher cousin. At least he can salvage body for meat.'

In an extraordinary example of experienced professionalism, as he left, the three stared from horse to each other.

In time, a remarkable fifteen minutes, butcher's truck arrived, and with barely time for goodbyes or regrets, Yvette followed them to a nearby slaughterhouse.

Yvette hated her first and only experience of a horse slaughterhouse, never appreciated this worse because she faced a desperate example of a backyard effort.

Under guise of a unit for destruction of horses to enter the dog food chain, appalled at condition of horses waiting for a better word, processing.

Moreover, her attitude reflected how our vets openly displayed polarity of concern, their duplicitous reactions when money involved, around animal welfare. Ran gamut of emotion, from fine, to kill them for profit, to how can people act so cruel.

Numb, speechless, watched as her charge jumped to head of the queue and two proficient workers, dressed in dirty clothes, different from expected hygiene of food workers, de-gloved his skin.

Warned Pierre, Jean-Paul's cousin they had dosed horse with Domosedan. In halting English, he delivered an unintelligible comment which she understood to mean, *not my problem.*

Yvette excelled herself when in a remarkable display of subterfuge, under guise of conducting a postmortem, collected samples for analysis including, and unseen, stomach contents containing the precious cargo.

If the three thousand francs cash she received for the animal's carcass, *take it, or leave it,* fell short of his sale value in England, it proved handy spending money.

Four hours later, Louis contacted her by phone with coded message. 'All well this side. Enjoy visiting the flower festival.' Breathed better on receiving his final, guarded reply, twelve hours later. 'Show worth attending. Stunning, aromatic herbs.'

37

ALL THINGS END

Yvette anticipated their final air trip.

Air France / KLM / Martinair Cargo proved most efficient. Doubtless, the best outfit they dealt with.

With vets set to travel on forged passports supplied by Chao, including certification for them to transit in hold with horses as flying horse groom and veterinarian, when they would replace the companies' normal professional attendants. Horse accommodation was in two pallets with each to contain three diamond loaded horses each.

Standard airline staff serviced an additional four pallets.

Vets enjoyed their experience of travelling horses by air, from Amsterdam Airport Schiphol, and despite misgivings, felt their charges arrived in New York, in better condition than those ferried across often turbulent waters of the English Channel.

On arrival, arrangements played out as normal when they stabled horses in a local unit overnight, during which they collected precious cargo, then transported them on final leg to a holding yard barely six miles from their hospital.

With superb papers, this meant Chinese protected their investment by organising to sell magnificent animals through DHT Boutique Auction House four weeks later.

Vets laughed off their experience, declared an important overseas shipping agent convinced them to do the trip. 'A free flight home and a big payout ensured we settled balance owing for our new equipment. Flawless win-win story.'

The horses excellent breeding attracted buyers and as they sold well, they accepted their carefully laundered twenty percent commission.

'So, a splendid deal.' Louis, delighted in the exercise, and encouraged Yvette to relax and enjoy her hospital and relax at home for five days before returning to Holland. Still, agitated she complained. 'Had enough of this.'

In Kentucky, safely tucked into their recently restored refurbished and stunningly outfitted apartment, and content vet business ran smoothly during their absence, discussions rolled on... and on as Yvette begged it time to close their European adventures.

'So glad you agree, but how are we going to break news? Fear they may never accept it time to drop out?'

'A fair question.' For he too remained concerned how the Chinese must react to their wishes to end trips. How would business partners react to the breakup?

Yvette's hormones were all at sea as they reacted to the ripe egg in her left ovary which demanded to be fertilised to start her desperately wanted family while she became less convinced their partners intended to allow them to break off.

As always, he provided her with the solid support only unconditional love offers, and as he hugged again, tried to console. 'Let's hope tomorrow's meeting goes well.'

Played the oft repeated big card. 'Always anticipated the Paris trip should be a proper, romantic honeymoon.'

While she eagerly anticipated such indulgence, remained half convinced.

Over a breakfast meeting in an understated suburb, Gregor brought their fears on that subject into the open. 'Our masters declare their pleasure with your achievements, but I also present bad news.'

He, because he understood Yvette's position, took a small drink of coffee, offered a plate of stunning confectionary and when he continued, highlighted his smiling delivery. 'They decided that although we have done superbly well,' Increased tension with a powerful pause. 'Declared it time to conclude our enterprise.'

Prepared for Yvette to threaten tears, he jumped in. So, we need you to do one final trip to Europe. On the same basis as this one, in three weeks' time.'

But as he sensed Yvette closer to proper tears, sweetened the deal. 'However, I bring exceptional news.'

Then, watched as a suspicion of a smile began to chase frowns, permitted her to regain control, then said, 'After your trip...' As Yvette's gasp threatened to stop him, Gregor held up his hands, motioned her to relax. 'we plan this for two weeks from now. First, fly to Paris, enjoy your honeymoon stay in most romantic city in the world.'

Hugged Yvette with real warmth, which made her appreciate how much he enjoyed her company. 'After which, take your final trip from Paris airport to New York.' Relished Yvette's improving countenance. 'You travel with six genuinely valuable two-year-olds with impeccable breeding.'

Now as she unfolded her interest, Yvette remained silent, tight-lipped as Chao picked up her hand. 'As an additional bonus this time, for with this trip legitimate, we arrange for five to be sold off via DHT, as before.'

A flicker of a chuckle slipped when he watched Louis do the maths. *And number six?* To answer his never posed question, he said. 'Yvette, my dear. You may select one of the horses for yourself. The pick of the bunch, one to be legally yours. Our leaving present for your valuable work.'

Louis never guessed she could get so excited. 'So, Chao, this time we fly back to the US on our EEC passports, destroy them... and then go on with our normal lives.' Hardly contained herself. 'Finished, then? No business?'

Chao's grin matched hers, for he also decided it time to move onto a fresh enterprise. 'Yes! Although we will destroy all papers, let us not take risks.'

Viewed smiling faces. 'We agree on this happy ending?'

Louis shook hands. 'Despite being a fascinating, profitable exercise, yes! Time to close.'

And so, their lives returned to normal... well, not normal.

Despite insisting they increase the payload of diamonds each horse carried, the Paris holiday and final flight played out as smoothly as the first.

Yvette picked her horse.

A magnificent Chestnut devoid of white, from the impeccable Furioso sire line via a Florencio dam line.

When he displayed the colossal fluid movement and fabulous temperament required to justify his fantastic value, she declared him everything she ever dreamed off to improve her riding.

The bonus.

For investing in dodgy, disgusting business, they outfitted their hospital as the best, most handsomely equipped equine private veterinary hospital in the US.

Let's not forget Yvette's egg met its wriggling partner that night.

38

VETS FACE NEWMARKET

Calder and Georgiou pondered their move.

With Georgiou destined for Newmarket, uppermost in his mind was how to perform the Kentucky slaughter.

A troubling question, but at present, purely a mechanical discussion.

Despite ongoing doubts, Calder responded to Georgiou's leadership. Harboured no negative discussions on professional aspects related to vets killing animals, well, at least submerged them in the protective layer of greed, which commissioned them to prepare the kill.

The fact they embarked on another round of indecent, criminal slaughter for financial gain unimportant.

Lunched together for the last time at their home base, one important enough of an occasion to encourage them to risk meeting in Calder's flat.

Over a bottle of excellent wine, drawn from his dwindling store, thinned before the intended trip to Newmarket. Fact an afternoon's work lay before them never reduced their intake.

Brains followed an accepted patterns suggesting where ingrained crime along one direction softens entry into other pathways. As this included driving and working when influenced by alcohol, they skirted close to the wind, although constant, higher than acceptable blood alcohol levels might have led to serious trouble.

Georgiou survived a third scare two miles from hospital when pulled up during a routine roadblock, the policeman, breathalyser in hand recognised him. 'So, doc, out playing with racehorses today.'

Waved off his partner to visit the next car in line then wrinkled nose. 'Now lad, have you taken a drop or two?' Fingered his machine.

'That's me officer, but as I have to get off and save lives, perhaps a small contribution to Christmas festivities might soften my route.' Slipped officer Docherty his papers which concealed where he had loaded them with eight-hundred pounds in notes. Second time with this officer, while it worked again, but tight.

They formulated plan after plan.

Discarded them as unworkable, rehashed others with the likelihood of them employing a massive overdose of insulin by injection lodged atop their unsavoury list.

Interrupted when Georgiou's phone beeped again. 'Our man again.'

Saunders said, 'So, off to Newmarket this afternoon?'

'True. Hope to reach farm by eight, ready to reconnoitre stud tomorrow morning.'

Pushed the speaker button for Calder to share his conversation.

Sanders' voice firmed; held notes of concern they might wish to change plans as he said, 'Although this major excursion which must go well, absorbs much of your time, still demand special attention with one mare.'

Saunders, moved into an even dominant mode, and reminded. 'Must hope her foal by Kildares Lament, due next week does not come early, beat us to it.'

That news disappointed Georgiou into sharing Calder's concerns. For with the US project taking centre spot, had lost his compunction to perform this secondary killing.

Downbeat wrinkles embracing face made him resemble an angry Shar-pei like. 'So, you still need us to care for her? Hoped with us preparing bigger plans, we focused energies elsewhere.'

Saunders voice developed a steely edge as with authority of a children's rugby referee, he broke no argument.

'That important mare deserves your best skill. When her foaling proves a success, your extra pocket money will help.'

Careful diction ensured anyone researching phone calls, must understand that request intimated desire for a healthy foal.

Because he disliked the conversation, Calder acknowledged respect for life, when, he first frowned at Saunders' hard, forced tough laugh, and made an ugly gesture with a couple of fingers, turned away, and left.

On balance, dissatisfied with the call, Georgiou left Calder alone for two hours, to attend two lame horses on a nearby farm.

On his return, searched yard for Calder.

Found him setting up an intravenous infusion on an eight-month-old foal affected by bad diarrhoea. The youngster, although tired from dehydration, acted remarkably calm, a fact due to Calder's admirable bedside manner.

Still conscious of Calder's earlier reluctance, George worried. *Shall continue to plug away, work hard on him; ensure him prepared well for the well-paid jobs we face but remained patient.*

Five minutes later, a satisfied Calder stood, scratched foal on her wither and said, 'There you are my dear. This treatment will help you soon regain your sparkle.'

As they slipped out of the stable and left Nurse Tammy to continue supervising the infusion, Georgiou said, 'Nice job, young man.'

Calder smiled. 'Enjoy this side of the business.'

Important, Georgiou, played with his earing, sensed Calder set to enter a spineless spot, demanded he act to prevent vet sinking into a joyful state of human kindness full of job satisfaction. 'That's me, loaded up and ready to go. When are you coming down?'

Calder turned from closing the stable door, switched back to thoughts of what lay ahead and as he dived into a depressed zone, said, 'As you know, with Dan's surgery backlog of surgery, he needs my help during the next two days at least, so, Friday evening, possibly Saturday morning at earliest.'

'Good. For we make a fine team.'

Steeled himself to bring up a now tricky subject. 'But are you alright with this Saunders job?' The Greek vet, toiled hard to conceal his nervousness from partner, followed him across the yard.

For fear that Calder lose focus, functioned brain to gauge his mental state, and finally diagnosed. *Odd. Never picked up his deeply engrained bipolar disease. Under this pressure, fear it may worsen as we get closer to the big one.*

Calder shook his head, extravagant as any person does when they try to convince themselves to take on an unpleasant but essential task. Flopped down on a bale of straw and said, 'Not at all. For as we are committed to this deal, cannot avoid this visit to Kentucky.'

Neck went floppy, permitted head to hang like a tired Ragdoll, and after a cough induced glottal stop, barely raised a whisper. 'Now, as we approach our... destiny. Still... becomes harder to accept.'

Because Georgiou enjoyed his phrasing, he accepted that positive sign. 'If we botch up this insignificant Newmarket job, we bid the big one, adieu. For sure.'

Turned on his heel and offered parting cheer. 'And, big. Our last. Let how that huge payout by generating a lifetimes luxury, be your motivation.'

Left him staring at the smart chestnut that watched them over the stable door.

39

DONDERLEY STUD

Donderley Stud sits six miles from Newmarket.

On the A143 near Bury St Edmunds.

A mere Ben Stokes six from the famous Barton Stud, thoroughbreds enjoy a luxurious, equine palace, less than twenty-years-old.

To begin with, its situation and development on land converted from an existing pasture farm, found the architect given a free hand to express herself. And Helen Connelly took full opportunity when she envisaged the farmhouse and associated dwellings for not only thoroughbreds.

Her outlook proved gracious and thoughtful, which ensured she designed top class accommodation for resident staff, but also seasonal workers who called the stud home during the breeding season.

Back then, smart flats housed resident vets for four months, when the two domiciled for them, deserved a four-star rating.

That said, after an avenue of impressive Beech trees, the entrance catches the eye. Pale coloured face brick match the buildings that flank the access, houses block of flats and offices and as it presented for Georgiou that early evening, his arrival, bathed in a generous full moon, offers visitors an appealing view.

After passing appropriately marked office block, the curving tarred road swung left towards two blocks of thirty mare boxes. Overall, artfully designed in ovals allowing easy access to grassed paddocks growing in spider-like fashion.

The Beech theme continues where mature trees offer refuge from major landscaping necessary to house animals with shade and protection from rain.

Bang in the centre of the largest paddock, an impressive group of five ancient Limes declare their resistance to the Dutch Elm Disease that ravaged the country. Botanists still recorded and analysed as they endeavour to breed and propagate resistant strains.

Fenced off to prevent horses injuring themselves during collisions, their presence accords a nod into the glory of the past.

Although they managed only sixty stables, the stud employed an in, out system. A feature of the equine breeding season on most farms, designed to permit travelling mares to visit farms that house selected sires.

They remain there until, after a vet certifies them in-foal at forty-five days, after which they returned to their home farms.

As a shareholder, Saunders permanently housed six mares at the farm.

With an efficient merry-go-round of travelling mares, they expected to serve 135 during the four-month season.

Two plush stallion boxes and a covering yard stood nearby to mare accommodation, offering mares a maximum walk of thirty-five yards to visit the stallion.

From breeding accommodation, road dipped downwards, then right where, behind a smart quarter acre of traditional mixed woodland, nestled forty smaller boxes for weanlings and yearlings.

Although farm conducted minimal traditional preparation of yearlings for the sport they later embraced. Fewer than twenty individuals faced their two-year-old birthdays on the farm. Others move on to specialist training yards aged around fifteen months.

Albeit for eight months, the farm holds air of a peaceful place. Granted, resident horses and caring, expert staff still ensure atmosphere loaded with thrum of healthy activity.

Unlike four breeding months annually, when additional mares and two resident stallions created a huge increase in traffic and effort.

Busier, even hectic from March to June with breeding in full swing, an experienced leadership ensured everyone conducted their business in orderly process.

Four foaling down boxes, the maternity stables where ladies give birth, surrounded a central building. Each owned a rear, large door that accessed a main area termed *The Hub*.

Facilities included central offices, a vet clinic including a knockdown box for anaesthesia, and an operating theatre.

A staircase led to comfortable first-floor accommodation for six people and two smart guest suites where owners occasionally overnighted.

This nerve centre housed a wall dominated by plethora of monitors which displayed CCV cameras in yards, paddocks, and foaling boxes. The Hub monitored all relevant activities to ensure valuable stock received deserved attention.

With everything under this degree of scrutiny, how are we expected to kill this foal ensured Georgiou' mind travelled various routes.

In two of the upstairs flats, additional monitors allowed dozing vets and nurses to monitor progress in foaling boxes and treatment of weak foals in the ICU.

A sophisticated alarm system recorded and disseminated unusual noises from the foaling boxes. Sensitive straps around abdomens detected effort mares produced when in labour.

Wide angled cameras set high on poles above paddocks and mare blocks covered most areas. Top facilities and diligence indicated value of breeding stock, and ensured expert, sympathetic care on hand for detailed management associated with foaling.

Set on three hundred acres of gently rolling grassland and ancient coppiced woodlands, a sea of white wooden post and rail fencing embraces paddocks fit for mares, foals, and yearlings to stretch legs.

This magnificent setting justifies naming thoroughbred racing as the sport of royalty.

40

GEORGIOU PREPARES

Georgiou settled into the stud.

At eight the following morning, toured with Eleanor.

A careerist stud manager and vet nurse, she outlined buildings and accommodation while explaining schedules and expected practices. If detailed superficially to ease him into their routine, tone indicated her as queen in her castle.

While he ensured himself familiar with the stud's principles, their modern attention to detail impressed.

Noted they computerised all records, including relevant details of arriving mares, including foaling dates, the foalings, and any health problems.

Those mares ready to enter foaling boxes and others with foals under five days of age had names marked in obvious, garish format and prominently displayed on wall boards. 'At present, we update this twice weekly. But from next week as we get into the swing of things, after which it changes to at least daily.'

Decided their recording system, performed by non-clinical staff, a sensible practice to free vets and nurses from clerical effort.

That ensured an accurate approach to recording all activities for accounting and processing of arrivals and departures, beginning with a nurse scanning ID chip, checking details against passports, and confirming results with a vet.

As a modern unit bathed in technology mare owners received regular SMS reports, also phone calls advising of birthings and any associated setbacks. Their accounts department issued accounts weekly.

One hour later, complimenting them on their efficiency, declared he anticipated collaborating with them. 'Not only that but also, I pick up pointers around your refreshing attitude to recording events. Your hearty efficiency, offers tips we implement back in our hospital.'

Georgiou, aware of himself clueless as to how to conduct killing, determined to maintain a relaxed pose. That also applied to him, using his considerable charms and sexual magnetism to keep others, especially vigilant ladies on his side.

When he took in Eleanor's six feet and fourteen stone frame along with sharp intelligence, spotted danger she posed. *Ms Efficiency with a capital E. How are we going to manage anything with Saunders mare under her spotlight?* 'You run a tight ship. What stage you reached?'

'As today we celebrate St Patrick's Day, the 17th of March, business picks up. Our first four foals already dropped, and eight due during the next two weeks.'

He spotted where tiredness may offer an opening as when sighing, she said, 'Twenty, even twenty-five to follow during the subsequent two to four-week period.'

On the covering side, she indicated where they expected between eight and ten mares to visit the facility daily for ten days. Professionals they preferred pregnant mares to arrive at least four weeks before their delivery date.

Mares are less well regimented than most animals and often foal ten days before or after their due dates.

He, surprised at the sudden resignation that flooded her face, and appreciated the already tired Eleanor needed a holiday.

Her fault, she never found time to take the three-week break earned during winter. *Something there to work on. Her yummy weakness offers something for us to exploit when we plan the kill.*

'Good!' He nodded his head. 'That allows us a breather to adapt to your system before things get busy, and, as Calder arrives soon, we will soon be ready to support as required and tackle any emergencies.'

'Agree. With a full and expert staff on hand, we will be fully prepared, so let us hope for a decent season.' The early part of the term often flowed better with fewer health issues when compared to the season's end.

Next, as they visited the stallion barn, were glad to escape preliminary stages of a numbing, cold evening, promising a bitter night, enjoyed that warmer environment. As they walked through substantial double doors an articulate voice instructed a groom. 'Keep him coming, but steady, steady, and yes!'

Mountjoy's Delight; the second of the resident stallions mounted his mare as they entered. Georgiou and Eleanor watched the timeless, business of procreation develop as a man guided stallion's penis through the mare's vulva. She, an experienced mare, backed into him, encouraged penetration.

As the stallion ejaculated, then dropped off mare's hindquarters, the same voice, softer this time, congratulated the effort. 'Well done, team, lovely job.'

Only acknowledged visitors, after he controlled the situation. 'Welcome, please join us.' Alfred Denning extended hand to Georgiou. 'Come inside man, escape this chilly evening.'

'Yes, sharper than expected.' Georgiou decided it already time to start wearing climate friendly clothing.

Eleanor continued the weather theme, when she declared a few snowflakes decorated the farm the day before, then cheered vet when she informed him, they expected temperatures to rise by tomorrow into a balmy phase.

The Greek vet missed native balmy Mediterranean winters.

After that brief greeting, Albert outlined his side of the business, how rare it was for them to cover a mare in late evenings. After they watched staff wash down both horses after mating, he invited Georgiou to perform a brief external inspection of both.

Then, he reacted to his satisfied nod and watched grooms lead them off to their stables.

Georgiou, while he paid respectful care to Alfred's comments, especially his hopes for how they might work together, acted his usual rake. Always more into girls than horses, he glanced at the girl who led mare back to her stable. Bulky clothes never hid a smart frame brought his normal attitude to the fore. *Now, she is a looker. Something to warm me at night.*

Besides that, thought, when he turned away and scrutinised her, a memory clicked. *Hang on, I know her. A vet student, she worked in Saunders yard.*

Back to business, the professional absorbed studs' routines and after leaving them, headed for the kitchen, hoping to scrounge a sandwich.

Mind on the girl, a ticking, warning chime advised take care. In time, we must grab a quiet chat. flatter, touch her up, establish how she and staff coped with Heraldon's death. Of course, Shaun as well.

41

CONCERNED FAITH

Faith led away the mated mare.

The horse acted a spirited creature.

Loaded with joie de vivre induced by the stallions' welcome attention, she demonstrated her enthusiasm, bounced around, pronked like an irrational Springbok, neighed furiously in sharp bursts.

As they pierced the cold evening's air, she triggered off answering calls in nearby residents. The girl, having hands full, concentrated on calming her.

Recognised Georgiou before he spotted her and unsure how to react, kept chin down, and focused on the mare, played down the chance encounter with a man who sat atop her list of those to avoid. One who, despite being the archetypical tall, dark, handsome stranger, deserved labelling as an unknown quantity, a dangerous man.

Even if Faith could not exclude him from thoughts, the sensible girl toiled to direct dynamic mind away from engaging in ideas fanciful and otherwise to concentrate on the volatile horse.

With both hands firm on the bridle, head collar combination necessary to secure control, worked to calm the mare and used a gentle, yet firm tone, while she smothered her neck with long, reassuring fleshy strokes.

Experienced with horses, knew nothing as effective with excitable horses than drenching in a constant stream of words. Even gibberish sentences help smooth troubled, small brains.

Thus, she talked to the horse as any mother soothes an infant. 'Steady on girl, please relax and I will give you a few cubes to eat when safely home.' Continued to stroke the mare's sweat covered neck while she led her and as they reached the stable, pleased her to find how fast her charge settled.

Faith spent ten minutes rubbing her down to remove residue formed by already drying sweat, then offered two tasty carrots. As the mare gobbled them down, Faith's brain whirled, dragged her back to the vet.

Impossible to avoid in that tight circle of stud workers she needed to form a plan, a method to diffuse tension, poised to flare before inevitable meeting with him set to happen soon.

She gave the mare a final stroke, pleased with how that repetitive action reassured both. 'No, dear girl, cannot allow emotion to control my impulsive brain or beating heart by engaging in silly actions. So, Faith, speak to dad first.'

In contrast to immediate fears, she benefitted to find the following morning busier than anticipated.

Whereas she and Georgiou passed each other, exchanged only briefest of nods, and thus without firm contact, necessity of conversation that might unlock doors best kept closed, meant she suppressed tension, held her tongue.

Faith found time before lunch to contact father.

And, after usual, *hi dad, and favourite daughter* greetings, got down to business. Leaned atop a railing between office complex and a sleeping, perennial garden that promised a riot of exuberant growth with splashes of ambrosial flavours during late spring and summer.

As one foot rocked the bottom rail, faith explained concerns. 'An unexpected difficulty threatens to blow up in my face. The Greek vet, the one I considered acted odd, dodgy, during the Heraldon incident is here. With amazing coincidence, they employ him as one of our resident vets for the season.'

In time, sensed father's mind before he responded, but then, after he heard her out in standard, unflappable manner, departed from his courtroom prosecutors attack, and surprised her.

Tone lifted into a bubbly, conspiratorial mood, one she might have expected from a girly confident. 'Besides, this unexpected confrontation now offers you an interesting coincidence. Envisage you already structure this as opportunity to savour a chance to snoop around.'

When he paused, she refrained from talking, which allowed him to continue. 'Doubtless, you spot an opening to engage in smart, investigative journalism, and undercover detective work.'

She eased into that upbeat manner. 'Thanks dad. Yes, I will...'

'No!'

A single, loud word brought her to a dead stop, made her lose control over phone, and after she juggled to gain control, listened intent, as he continued. 'Guessed that must be your attitude, how your smart brain would search gamy solutions along those lines.'

As he took a deep breath, she waited until he issued instructions, treated her as he should a junior officer. 'Under no circumstances engage in conversation around the accident; and let's call it so for now, at Saunders yard.'

Father's concerns rang distinct. 'Because his presence concerns me, need you to promise to do nothing silly, amateurish.'

While Faith accepted father's common-sense approach, nevertheless, she, as hopes of criminal exploration still flamed, plugged on. 'And dad, although appreciating your experience, you must agree I face a noteworthy situation, one where appeal of uncovering hard facts provides me with an excellent opportunity to investigate.'

Stricter than ever, his hard voice as he interrupted her flow, laid down rules. 'No! For my instincts as a senior investigator warn we face complicated circumstances, even bigger, wider reaching than you imagine. In fact.'

Paused, then delivered his stern warning. Tough, direct, she appreciated his sincerity. 'Dislike absence of healthy actors to cushion you in security. In that unsanitary environment, ask you to leave the farm now!'

She gasped as he continued. 'For you face a tough, even precarious situation.'

'Oh!' Faith embraced two silent minutes before she plucked up courage to express how her concerns grew. 'Risky, dodgy business, but now your tone brings alarm. For I sense you worry I face something life-threatening? Never dreamed they caught me up in such a serious situation.'

Debate hummed. Although he understood and appreciated his daughter grew into her own personality, worried his darling angel now tread the inevitable path towards independence.

That said, although prepared to encourage growth, paternal concerns, rather than legal opinion, poured out in a conciliatory tone which bathed her in concern. 'Please, listen my love, need you to think logically. If those deaths, and here we remember the groom's loss of life is under investigation, may been part of a massive scheme to kill horses and defraud insurance companies.'

Diction hardened to perfection. 'Given these points, do you understand my concern?' He picked up her strained tone when she replied. 'Gosh dad. Can I truly face a serious crime? Some horrid business.'

'After our chat with Sophia, noted her concerns, am working in harmony with her investigation and started began researching insurance fraud involving horses. Find this commoner than anticipated and especially when I detected where individual claims often achieve large financial pay outs, they raised hairs on my neck.'

Paused to allow that information to sink in and as she offered only a series of anxious expletives he went on. 'For instance, your absence missed how our local papers detailed where Heraldon's connections collected a seven-figure sum after his death, plus smaller payouts on other animals.'

Father's fears jolted Faith's sense of self-preservation, which made her already cooling body freeze further in eight-degree temperature. So, as she pulled her old, functional rather than attractive sheepskin jacket around neck, accepted his advice to act furtive, and inspect buildings surrounding The Hub.

Nervous. Dropped voice to a whisper. 'Understand your concern. Because you fear where big money is involved, these people may not hesitate to add a nosy parker to their list. Now, I appreciate, share your nervousness.'

Faith gained more valuable insight about the world of crime; the real world, during that fifteen-minute telephone call than a whole series of lectures on jurisprudence could offer.

Still, she argued. 'Impossible for me to leave this yard now.' Girl's voice developed a grainy, firm tone when she presented logical argument. 'Gain useful work experience here that must support my future studies for stud work on this top-notch level. They must prove valuable.

Conversation flowed until Faith added another valuable, considerate point. 'But also, with them short staffed, dislike the notion that if I leave which must mean letting them down.'

'And knowing and admiring your sense of decency, understand that must prove a troublesome factor.'

After they chatted for ten minutes, Faith ed up father's defensive comments and offered one final note. 'Also worry were I to run away, my hasty departure could arouse the vet's suspicion.'

'Good thinking daughter. Also, a factor.' When father paused, she guessed mind turning over ideas which brought him to his conclusion. 'Right, we function as follows. You remain on this slippery site. But avoid any discussion on Heraldon's story, although if subject comes up, express sadness over the accident.' Added a sensible note of caution. 'Do not be woolly, although express your disappointment in strong terminology. Message me often, for I need to know you are safe.'

'Thanks dad. Promise to be incredibly careful and sensible.'

He offered a final, sensible suggestion, but for a straightlaced man who never used bad language, he suggested if after talking to the vet she got an inkling of compromise, she should slip him a coded message including the word *shit*.

And, leaving that hanging, said, 'Meantime, let me chat to Sophia.'

As he rang off, romantic notions flooded her brain, enough to force a chuckle. *Now dad, is your call to Sophia for business or pleasure?*

Which as it threw up a silky mood, lips still bubbled with noisy mirth when she bumped into Georgiou. Actions boded well for her father's advice when, despite the feverish notions that stung her brain, she maintained a generous smile as they passed.

He hell bent on nourishment, never wasted time talking, but brain sparkled. *A fortuitous meeting. With her delivering me a mushy smile, doubt she owns any worries over Heraldon's death. Brilliant, means after seducing her with a night to remember, a touch of my special magic should chase any remaining doubts.*

42

CONSCIENCE AND CRIME

Decided on a simple method to kill the horse.

But contemplate what in his distorted psyche pushed him onward.

Those who serve the public by administering justice must have a reasonable knowledge of the factors that foster crime and work to improve society in such a way they diminish the necessity for wrongdoing.

Overpopulation with its attendant poverty serves as an ancient, well understood example. Typified by the savage punishments inflicted on those who stole bread to feed starving children and received diverse chastisements from having a hand chopped off to execution for stealing a sheep.

Alongside the attendant use of the barriers of prevention does such castigation keep crime levels down?

Doubtful.

Others indulge in the most heinous of crimes, particularly those against the person and at times for those onlookers who find their actions difficult to understand the *why question* often arises.

Alongside the attendant use of the barriers of prevention. *Does the punishment fit the crime?*

See prison as a means of keeping difficult people away from the public.

In the opinion of great thinkers from the past, consider how we merely hide them away because society will not implement the necessary measures to improve basic human needs.

Why do many countries dish out aid and not encourage the employment that by reducing poverty encourages those tempted to do wrong to change their mindset and contribute as taxpayers to improving the world?

***

Accept significant crime statistics reveal people with background difficulties.

Until society solves this, yes, keep them away.

But others pose major areas for concern.

These include the greedy, those who see society as theirs to manipulate, and take the easy route to superficial plenty.

Nod at this.

Accept the Greek vet Georgiou fitted this category.

Also, the one who encourages others, in this case Calder into crime deserves further criticism. Is entitled to receive, in the words of The Lord the *millstone around his neck* captured for posterity by three of the Evangelists.

So must we evaluate Georgiou.

We have marched with, possibly dragged behind him is better as he raced past significant barriers set in place to protect society. As an intelligent man he ignored, ingrained values which ensure we receive and understand basic guidelines on acceptable behaviour.

Notwithstanding the vast variation found in people's aims and objects, their aspirations, and how they fitted to produce tolerable, interpersonal relationships, understand this included where both vets deviated far from acceptable norms.

The amateur psychologist who lurks within most normal people considers manifestation of criminal activities as inherently wrong. Humanists and religious reflect on where man's development via phenomenon of *Original Sin*, causes us to hold basic, immoderate at best, heinous at worst, flaws.

Thus, within a loose definition we understand most people, when faced with prospect of committing a crime in circumstances conducive to them doing so with success, consider crime.

Worth repeating where an educated conscience certifies them to shake that off, move on, toe-the-line for common good.

Admit squishy fear of capture, and its clammy ramifications are useful deterrents. Also, reason for the sense of common decency that holds sway and relates to most people's beliefs holding it self-evident higher powers watch, observe our actions.

Punishment is inevitable.

Besides, with most religious philosophies accepting an end game associated with judgement, strive to meet pass levels guarantee entry into eternal life.

God, being God owns the prerogative to dish out reward and punishment.

Individual crime is obvious and without condoning this, even understandable, although when that involves people grouping together, their collective action poses profound consequences.

If we dismiss gang warfare and, by extension, national conflicts that end in war, to focus on the process by which one person, Georgiou, contemplated then spread notion of crime to the genetically susceptible Calder.

Although assert each, in this basic system, possessed important flaws: basic tenets of failed decency mentioned earlier, now ripe for interactive breaching.

We may argue, Georgiou, as the senior partner in horse slaughter with a familial background of deep-seated crime which including *taking out opposition*, a movie generated euphemism for those who deserve most criticism.

Accept Georgiou's powerful personality worked on the susceptible Calder, easily persuaded his involvement because of hereditary Henderson induced tendency to bend rules, owned fertile soil in which criminal seeds planted by Georgiou germinated. They, growing well, easily passed seedling stage, and produced first fruits during Heraldon's slaughter.

However, before harvesting the main crop, Georgiou nourished his partner via promise of dollar fertiliser. That said, amid what astute Georgiou recognised as weakness, he collected problems.

First, he worked to encourage Calder.

Did so, cognisant of effort required to conceal killing Senor Angelo, which occasioned in the practical sense, meant he engaged personnel to facilitate the process. First of these was Calder.

While they doubted sensibility of employing ancillary staff, aware that escalated chances of detection, Percy, and hereafter, for simplicity, stick to his *nom-de-guerre*, in confident mood, assured them his wealthy, supportive organisation could source and bribe assistants.

Overall, while he kept Paulo's organisation secret, his personal flawed character meant it impossible to be secretive and thus hinted at depth and structure of how Monti exerted control over employees.

The vets recognised this character who they had never met as a dangerous, psychopathic killer, the merest suggestion of Monti's name guaranteed volunteers, in terms of ancient naval systems, stepped up to the plate.

Those on the periphery kept mouths closed as tight as a healthy Knysna oyster.

Percy failed to remain distant, employed his considerable brain to envisage the basic route slaughter must take. Accept too, he also fitted into the fearful state where having engineered the crime by planting seeds into that fertile soil, soon appreciated the substantial risks failure must bring.

***

Furthermore, consider the charged atmosphere.

When necessity forced them to flesh the bare bones of the exercise, Paulo, in his study after one of his window visits, waved hands and in Pontius Pilate mode, delegated mechanics of crime to Percy and Monti.

'My role is to ensure you receive sufficient funds to enable process to flow and to satisfy everyone involved, of the indecently hefty rewards success guarantees.' The offer of the biggest, carotene packed carrot kept them with him.

No matter his intense dislike of, especially profound, *weak at the knees* fear of Monti, Percy, planned his wealthy retirement, his desire to escape the organisation. The essential get-out stake which encouraged him to constantly work through the modus operandi process.

The Enforcer rose to the surface.

In as near an exuberant state as possible for his deranged psyche, Monti agreed his fearful presence and reputation in controlling staff and others invited loyalty, coerced fits better, and envisaged no difficulties.

Amid background music that simmered in foamy strains of Tchaikovsky's *Swan Lake* that, incongruously in the wrong setting promised hope, declared the plan infallible.

To confirm control in unnecessary fashion, used an over-the-top display of arrogant power when he patted his ever-present CZ-75 SP-01, fitted snug on belt.

Percy, having experienced the man's threats achieve fruition during one bloody episode where a staff member who normally functioned as a heroin packer threatened to open his mouth and disclose their business, never doubted possibility of raw violence.

Also, remember how that man's brother also mysteriously disappeared.

Memories often act to clear the brain, allow for solid reflection before allowing weak minds to embroil themselves in dangerous events. Especially true now as the increasingly concerned Percy slapped at his chest in an effort to control tumultuous palpitations which as they rocketed skyward bounced fingers.

In Paulo's criminal organisation, he via Monti appreciated the benefit of owning a bottomless, secluded lake proved undeniable.

No wonder anglers regularly trapped big, protein enriched specimens.

Without delay, as Percy struggled to gain control increased levels of anxiety and nervousness forced weak knees to make him slump into a seat as Monti left the room.

Have it now. This man will kill me to protect his plans. Expendable, it is likely irrespective of the outcome he intends to finish me.

43

MODUS OPERANDI

Unique, Monti named their planning effort *modus operandi*.

Energetic as he moved out of Paulo's shadow he grew in stature.

The enforcer assumed control, dominated the scene, assumed role of the extraordinary manipulator who coordinated twenty digits, each in different pies.

With all declared to bow the knee to Paulo, they shared his confidence and so, he sourced a third special man to assist the vets, While the team received no sign of the man's identity, nor would they ever meet him Monti, managed as close to a smile as Percy ever witnessed, labelled him *The Technician*.

Furthermore, displayed unexpected efficiency when he reduced risks.

Left nothing to chance.

Monti, embraced in the cloak of deceit manufactured by a moonless night collected him the night before. Shared an al dente spaghetti carbonara pasta; cooked to perfection by Monti, then left him secluded in a locked, ensuite staffroom.

From there, two hours before he expected the vet's visit, Monti planned to release and take the Technician to meet Senor Angelo.

Part of Monti's planning ensured no personnel be in vicinity of stallion barn and associated yards. When in control he advised all staff associated with horses to work on alternative projects.

None dared doubt judgement.

Which ensured a clear field.

The Technician's role involved a single visit to the stallion.

With Monti acting as groom, a role he hated, conduct a simple exercise designed to instigate the basic technique which must trigger of the events designed to terminate in the horse's destruction.

Duties centred on him passing a mixture of three pounds of pure corn starch, mixed in three litres of warm water via a stomach tube into the horse's stomach.

The act of tubing is a common treatment method for administering bulk drugs or electrolyte solutions to horses. It involved him pushing the moistened tip of a flexible rubber stomach tube up the horse's nostril and then direct it downwards into the animal's stomach.

A straightforward procedure, and non-professionals, including trainers perform this basic procedure.

During a three-minute pour, the tube delivered that starch mixture, an overload of concentrated energy into Senor Angel's unsuspecting stomach.

Horses cannot physiologically cope with massive grain overload thus, as digestible carbohydrates flooded Senor Angelo's system, they anticipated that must initiate powerful biochemical and digestive changes.

One expected sequel of that insult is an intestinal catastrophe which manifests itself clinically as painful, escalating colic. A loose term for abdominal discomfort in horses.

The vet killers expected Senor Angelo to develop colic signs three hours after the Technician administered the starch.

After which they intended to exacerbate that colic condition with drugs.

Even if they did nothing further, the starch should continue to work inside the animal and cause other, longer acting disease as the heavy carbohydrate overload damaged tiny blood vessels known as capillaries.

Such damage results in severe inflammation of blood vessels with associated intravascular thrombosis. In conclusion, this leads to a most distressing circulatory disease termed laminitis. Clinical signs are associated with horrid pain and permanent damage to sensitive blood vessel structures in horse's feet.

Disgusting pain.

Imagine having slivers of wood pushed under your nail. Deep into sensitive tissues. Next, set them on fire. Reader now gains an impression of extraordinary discomfort affected horse's experience. Because of the advanced nature of the disease Senor Angelo must experience, it should prove impossible to treat.

This, over days or weeks, then results in euthanasia.

44

KILLING METHOD

Monti was the expert manipulator.

Next, proceeded to control Senor Angelo's groom, Flannery.

Manipulated the grooms' schedules under guise of staff illness and leave, made Flannery function as groom. Overworked him to collect two loads of horses from distant farms.

As this was in addition to his standard duties, he worked Flannery to exhaustion during that period of exceptionally urgent business when for two days, permitted him little sleep.

This ensured him deadly tired prior to the period during which they manipulated the horse via the Technician to develop colic.

For fear that he runs afoul of Monti, Flannery never once objected.

Vets, with Percy, explained this crucial factor.

This tiredness must be severe enough to permit Georgiou with opportunity to encourage, then insist Flannery desert his horse for two hours.

That brief period of essential rest should allow vets to conduct killing.

Georgiou would admit himself an experienced horseman but conceal his profession as a vet and could then offer to nurse the horse, help supervise him under instruction of usual vet.

With the plan set in stone, ready to implement, it required both vets to act in harmony. But having concocted the plan, Georgiou faced an ongoing, escalating difficulty.

He understood his colleague's weakness, worried over his constant battle to encourage Calder. Cajoled him to control worsening emotional status.

Maintained an upbeat approach.

Which earned a reward. 'So, two days before we fly off into millions of dollars. Then, conduct our simple, severe, and effective effort.'

Slapped a fist into opposite palm and as he emphasised each word which encouraged Calder to nod approval while he unveiled escalating humanity. 'Yes. Agree this a sound plan, should do the trick, agree with the methodology.'

Despite finding involvement in proposed killing anathema, others of a matching ilk, must share sympathy with his view. For instance, *yes, kill the thing*, but endeavour to make it fast, pain free.

Entrenched in hopeful thoughts, Calder suggested. 'But this colic method has a fault. Dislike how we must cause severe pain to do the job.

Reminded Georgiou of a hungry Pug puppy that begs for food as he outlined concerns. 'So, and still timeous, my grey matter constantly searches its data base. Encourages me to spend more time on research. How to modify this or develop a less distressing solution to terminate the horse.'

Amid the start of the end game, consider how at a time when everyone needed a clear head, disaster threatened. The Greek's emotions flared as he rapidly tired of his partner's whining, got severe, practically screamed. 'You say you agree, but what does that mean?'

In danger of losing control, paced room four times, glared hard at Calder. 'Stop hallucinating, vacillating with restless, energy of a demented, qwerty keyboard.'

Stamped a foot as if he crushed a nuisance of a cockroach and while he tried to cushion his suggestion in less fleshy terms, words jumped, hard as the punch of a blunt icepick. 'If you envisage a better plan... now is the perfect time, explain how we should proceed.'

Since he agonised for days over the man's changing condition, Georgiou, as his anger neared a fierce boil, anxiety threatened to invade psyche, with inevitable, dangerous loss of irreparable control.

The only thing that slowed his degeneration into dangerous agitation was how his genetic crime background modified, supported his desire to hold back.

Announced his unwavering commitment. 'Shall kill this horse. Even if you drop out, continue, do it alone, without your assistance.' But, saying that, stormed off to the toilet. *This man threatens to become a liability. We will never again work together.*

45

MY IMMEDIATE PROBLEM

Decision made, washed his face.

Appreciated calmness generated by the effect of chilly water.

As it caressed his inflamed skin, he with control restored, rejoined Calder.

Smooth, maintained even breathing efforts to force a lukewarm smile and conjectured how best to continue.

The decent staff bathroom, clean and well fitted how one fault. A nasty cracked series of pink, white porcelain tiles ran from the washbasin to the floor. On the repair list for months, their tardy repair irritated the fastidious man. Odd, as he ran a fingernail along the crack it helped restore his mental functions.

Looked at himself in the mirror. Peered, tidied sideburns, and loosed a faint smile.

Returned to Calder's lounge and patted his shoulder. 'Must not overplay the discomfort issue.' Allowed Calder a few seconds to grasp at that angle. 'Also remember they will summon their usual stable vet to control his discomfort, and he will manage the horse's pain as you or I do when we face any uncomfortable animal.'

Although that lifted his spirits, Calder's deteriorating mental grit ensured Georgiou's mind continued to stew with uncertainty for as the younger vet, although desperately keen on earning big bucks, experienced another of his increasingly frequent attacks of decency.

Astute Georgiou escalated his control. *Leaves me no choice. Now, time to be hard on him.*

Played the money theme. Bowed to the man's greed.

Repainted scenarios where vast funds changed lives. 'With similar approaches to life, we share matching standards.' And then, in an unexpected display of genuine affection, hugged, kissed both cheeks as he did his brothers, then said, 'Accept we cannot live as we should, as we deserve, without this income.'

Calder showed a remarkable turnabout.

Responded to Georgiou's intimate, familial embrace and after he hugged hard, moved into positive territory. 'True, and although it hits tough, we do this.'

Now, fit to react in positive fashion, knuckled down enough for them to complete the plan.

Still, they needed that extra player, a fourth member.

Their as yet unknown accomplice, should never understand his part, must act to kick off action, without understanding the outcome. That meant he, when taking on that role remained unsuspecting, innocent.

Needed a professional.

Had to instigate nature of circumstances necessary to lead up to the horse's death, knowing their best chance was to involve the farm's usual vet.

To bring him on board the horse's groom, at first sign of the horse becoming ill, should summon his help in normal manner, as he did for any ill horse.

Introduced a smart part of the process. One which insisted Georgiou be on the farm when the vet arrived.

The vet must, during the initial examination, consider Senor Angelo's illness as a colic case, for this common lifestyle disease of thoroughbreds, meant he daily treated cases with similar signalment.

After the vet evaluated the horse, the would-be killers understood how he should treat him in standard manner, as per normal protocols.

Since the value of the animal would not, at the time of the examination, increase likelihood he demands specialist treatment, initial management could unfold on the farm.

A horse is a horse!

Irrespective of the dollars that crossed hands to bring the horse into the world or stable, it does not know or understand the importance of those funds.

After he assessed the horse's response to treatment, they faced an imponderable for then they need the vet to confirm Senor Angelo horse should react positively to pain control with flunixin or similar analgesic drug.

Integral to their plans, it depended on the vet, satisfied horse's condition progressed as desired, would then depart from the farm, and leave the horse's care in capable hands of groom.

At this point, Georgiou, if he played his part right, should soft-soap the vet, make him confident they could monitor the horse. Modern technology would allow them to update him by phone.

Another imponderable assumed the vet had other patients to consider.

vet made regular patrols in the area and dodged from one yard to the next.

Next step must follow when Georgiou encouraged Flannery the groom to take a couple of hours rest.

During this, when Calder arrived, the two vets could sneak into the stable.

In clandestine fashion administer the lethal injection.

Their talk stretched into a lengthy debate on which killing agent to use.

Insulin or succinyl choline.

An overdose of intravenous insulin, the same type used in management of diabetes, causes convulsions and death.

Succinyl choline is a powerful but tricky anaesthetic with an impressive knockdown effect.

When used clinically, physicians monitor the drug with care to prevent overdosing as it paralyses muscles of the chest which may result in respiratory failure. Death is possible.

This phenomenon becomes easier to understand when reflecting on its widespread role in the culling of buffalo. After darting animals with succinyl choline, usually from a helicopter, they die from suffocation.

Both drugs are difficult to detect in the system after death without immediate and intense forensic practice.

Decided on insulin.

A principal factor included the safety aspect if they pricked themselves... a problem rarely high on their agenda.

With them involved in unusual stakes which featured a high-profile target with associated nervousness, made them extra careful to avoid injuring themselves.

Leon assured them he could safely obtain and deliver insulin and syringes to one of their hotels.

Plan seemed fool proof.

So simple Calder wondered. 'Clean and simple. Wonder they do not get local people to manage the horse's death. Cheaper.'

An impressive wash of pride ran over Georgiou's face,

His confident voice boomed the answer. 'Remember why trainers use our vet practice and not the vet next door who attends riding stables.'

At last, brought a flicker of a smile to Calder's face. 'Yes. Dead right, for when real money is the target, experts always insist on the best available resources, and with our reputation for getting the job done.

'So, we are simply the best.'

Calder enjoyed his confidence. 'Nice one Georgiou.'

46

KILL THIS FOAL

Georgiou swung into Donderley's routine.

Spent thirty minutes doing fertility scans on mares.

Mares never reacted as he placed a long, thin probe inside the rectum.

Watched immediate results of the sonar readouts on a computer monitor placed beside the examination crush. In the hands of an experienced operator, interpreted the smart 3-D visualisation of their ovaries.

Good imaging permitted him to record size of ovary and follicles inside the ovary and their consistency, which allowed him to predict time of ovulation. The point where a mature follicle discharged its egg to move along the fallopian tube.

In conclusion, these changes suggested the state of the mare's cycle, its health, and when she approached optimum time for them to cover with the stallion. Important, for that meant they never wasted horse's time, energy, or semen.

With each stallion booked to breed ninety mares during that season, they desired to limit each mating to when the mare ovulated and released egg at the most opportune time for it to meet semen.

In the meantime, he, with a nurse, checked out status of four foals already in residence. As usually is the case, they found first of the crop in excellent condition. Smiled at how the treatment administered by Calder to the tummy troubled foal paid dividends.

When the onsite kitchen fed them lunch, it proved better than decent.

Granted, he continued bending over backwards to act his most pleasant self, but deceit proved unnecessary. 'Could embrace this system. If you plan to feed us this well and work us so gently... then this breeding season will be a dream.'

'Share your view. Also, a joy for us during this calm period.' Eleanor spluttered through a crust of quiche. 'But that dramatically changes when foals in abundance end this drought.'

Eleanor enjoyed her job, and being competent, farm owners shared her annual success. She said, 'After a few complex mares and a handful of weak foals, we shall find ourselves up to our ears in it.' Georgiou agreed, for having experienced the breeding season on four different studs during former seasons, he expected it to toughen.

The eyes of a prowling hunter took in everything and as conversation continued, Georgiou who never stopped searching, assessed every opportunity as he wondered how best to do the nasty on Kildares Lament's foal when born.

Two hours before, when she superficially checked the mare, Eleanor declared. 'Saunders is one of our practice's biggest clients, and as one of Donderley's shareholders, insists we take special care of this mare's foal.'

'He intimated that to me also, although must question why he excites over her.' In response to Eleanor's comment, he guessed an exaggerating Saunders in danger of bringing the mare to everyone's attention, when he should have treated her as he did every mare.

Georgiou stroked brown neck of the strong, well-rounded mare beside him. 'This lovely mare gets close to popping, although what she might produce worries me, for thus far the stallion's progeny do not shine.'

'His first crop to race disappoints, for as yet, they offer no encouragement, for sure.'

Eleanor continued. 'Also, stallion's owners own the stud farm.'

'Guessed it involved Saunders, but to what extent?'

'Earned 15% on basis he put expertise into the project and agreed to train owner's progeny. The rest, as everything is these days, is down to an Arab family dripping in oodles of oil money.' 'Nice way to go.'

47

FRANCESCA EXPLORES

Francesca snuggled up to Niall.

In dreamy mode, long after supper, they barely spoke.

Lay embalmed in the contented state that forecasts bedtime.

Until as Francesca lost control, she risked raising difficult subjects given prominence by Angela during their last meeting for the curiosity that nagged at girls' intellect demanded answers.

Despite being aware the last hour of a long day offered poorest timing, she had ago. 'Dearest, know you dislike talking about your father, although you never hint at why that should be so.'

Snuggled tighter, nervous for pressurising him and offered a bolt hole when without looking at him, as a lone finger caressed his chest, she whispered. 'Much too late now, but sometime, when you are satisfied timing good, well, yes. Love you to share your family history for it may be important for me, for us.'

As his right arm encircled her shoulders, Francesca winced at where stiffening muscles ushered in a minute of dead silence.

Until she felt him relax and run fingers of left hand up and down her bare left arm. Albeit he began with the slow, ponderous manner of a relaxed elephant as it ambles toward the next tree. *At least my questioning causes no distress.*

He never rushed to reply,

When Niall got going, she never sensed any of the anxiety or even depression she forecast. 'Comfortable talking about him. But honestly, understand little, and when I try to dig into his history with mum, she distresses.'

Followed that with a significant mood change as fingers dug deeper where his right hand rested on her thigh. Felt it tense over the loose wrapped Japanese kimono she enjoyed wearing after her soaking evening bath. 'Because mum reacts so intense which causes a sad, slow impasse.'

Obviously, the question affects mum more than Niall. Must have been an ugly marriage.

'And what about your Aunty Deirdre? How does she react?' The lack of any obvious defensive posturing permitted her to probe. Except, as she intensified her queries that triggered more reaction which she felt as muscles bunched.

Francesca decided growing tension suggested the discomposure which often precedes unease, when he said, 'With them estranged well before his death, for mum that still proves a definite no-go area.'

Released one of his familiar sights, the characteristic, lingering, slow exhalation of air associated with tension... and something else. His method for releasing pressure but stronger this time and she alarmed when he ended it with a huge gulp of breath to charge empty lungs.

Guess he may now begin to divulge potent information around family secrets.

Opinion proved correct when he said, 'Bitter enemies at worst.'

Quiet for five seconds then suddenly, he reacted, indicated how tough he found the situation and as he withdrew his arm from her, she felt his pain when he sat upright, straight, focused on a family photograph mounted opposite them.

Niall unfolded his long body from the couch and as he prepared to leave her, changed tact, returned and in absent minded fashion, permitted one finger to toy with a rope of her hair. After he twirled it in circles, for a full minute, offered a half-hearted smile, walked into kitchen and as she remained seated, a click hinted he switched on the kettle.

On his return eased a small smile through still tense lips, which she interpreted as a moment of sadness one that flirted with deep seated concerns around maternal motions. Which triggered a need to nourish and protect strong enough for her to rise and wrap arms around him in a warm embrace. 'Sorry, my love. Never intended opening old wounds or cause distress.'

For a big lump of a man, he could be gentle and that overflowed when he took her hand, led Francesca to the shining mahogany dining room table that dominated the room which served as their everything.

Despite the gravity of the moment, she managed a small amount of humour. *Goodness. Feels like he prepares me for a potent discussion on family finances.*

As he stroked two fingers over her cheek, he softened that effect as did a warmer grin. 'Will fetch coffee, and then, we can chat.'

As she blew over coffee, he sipped a hot, chocolate laced version, then seated opposite, forced himself to open, begin. 'Right, time to explore.'

Cocked head as though he asked permission to proceed and when only powerful, empathy shone from her delicious eyes, began. 'As yet, the full story remains misty, laced with various, complex situations, insights, and confusing thoughts. Innuendo collected as a boy, but never clarified, impossible to drop.'

Until now, emotions suppressed, but never dormant, he, after another lung emptying sigh followed by a noisy inrush of oxygen, plugged on. Squeezed her hands together and expressed hope in their special love. 'Admit for us to properly unite as one, you and indeed I deserve to share the complete history of my parent's dysfunctional relationship which clouds my history.

When he leaned over and squeezed her hands, she felt how he outpoured a depth of affection never experienced from another man which must have melted any heart, although he already had her in a soft centred, delicious fondant spot. 'Hope we will always share everything.'

In synch as her heart fluttered with love more intense than ever, she clutched an arm then clung. 'Yes. We always be open and honest with each other.'

Over an intense, session he remained calm, logical as a chronically distressed soul allowed as he filled her in on the background of half-truths concocted by family to create hope he once owned a loving father. 'Back then, guessed at manufactured stories meant to placate, although asides, bits, and pieces gleaned during looser family moments suggested a bleak, different picture.'

When he slowed to sip, Francesca decided it time to risk a deeper probe. 'Sorry to pry but discussed this with Angela. She offered me a, what she termed as a widespread notion of events around your father's actual death.' Watched for any reaction and with Niall slow to respond repeated what she thought he already knew. 'Some feel Aunty Deirdre played an... well, active part.'

Now, as he reacted, guessed she may have travelled a road too far but could not leave it alone. How does that fit?'

Mouth opened, stretched wide as Clyde estuary and when he stared at Francesca, she guessed, too far. *No! He is unaware of this information! They concealed this from him.*

As he dropped her hands, Niall sat upright, shrank back and afraid, dared not catch her eyes. Took sneaky glances, fascinated, as hands slithered away, to fall off edge of table into eternity.

Until, as confidence returned, eyes probed for solace in hers and oozed sufficient intense pleading to encourage her to risk making a detailed study of his face. Guessed eyes now puzzled, loaded with pain.

After two stunned minutes, he asked. 'Where did you hear that?' Alarmed, she shared confusion, and reaching out apologised. 'Sorry, my love. Never meant to spring this.' As Francesca, exercised her strong will, she never retreated but dived in, poured out information gained from conversations with Angela.

Soaked everything up, sponge-like, then said, 'So, you, after barely two minutes in my life,' Managed a weak boyish grin, 'uncover strange events unknown to me which admittedly fits with my impression of him as an unpleasant character.'

Disclosure leaves parties better or worse for revealing unpleasant facts, and as this partly answered Francesca's prayers, her pulse settled when she realised continuing expose must create a better atmosphere for both.

Confirmed that when he found a voice. 'Now that clarifies the intricate, impossible relationship between him and Aunty Deirdre. Even worse than anticipated.'

But, and unexpectedly, Francesca's confidence took a sharp, unnecessary knock and in near panic mode hideous possibilities reverberated through her brain stem. *What have I done, and will this turn him against me?*

To counter this in the meantime, he rose and looked huge, strong, and powerful when he paced to and from the window.

From being initially fearful, her demeanour changed, when reassured by a fresh, confident voice. 'For me, irrelevant as it cannot affect our relationship, our future. But my poor mum. Her life has been sheer hell. Every time the past came up, she must have cringed for fear of me learning something bad.'

The big man flopped, mellow as a sleepy kitten limp off its mother's nipple. Until an impossible to forget memory washed over him. 'Remember a hideous incident from childhood days. One that exerted a powerful effect on me.'

Required two minutes to find composure, then explained how Deirdre reacted when, after spraining his ankle, Niall, had for the only time, cried for a father's support. 'Aunty Deirdre's horrible reaction upset everyone. Powerful it affected me, still lingers as an unpleasant moment in a loving childhood.'

To sum up his distressed state, a bout of sobbing associated with him banging head into her bosom meant she gratefully held him until tranquillity eased his hard body.

When in control, he said, 'Never repeated that story.' Caressed her shoulder, 'it reflects how much you mean to me, and can at last open that scar.'

In conclusion, Francesca lost all evidence of the gritty determination that made her an analytical person, a deal broker.

Shared tears then spluttered. 'Love you Niall. Your honesty means everything to me.' Bathed each other in tears that began bitter, but she sensed they diverted pain and must flush out hidden frustration and disappointment. 'We will be stronger for this.'

When he kissed her fingertips in agreement, at last offered a great smile to break down barriers. 'And you, my love will lead me through this, become stronger as problems open.'

She returned his kiss and offered even encouragement. 'Can you imagine how your mum will grow? When she breaks free of her shell of containment, must be stronger.'

'Hi mum, we need to talk.'

'Why Niall that sounds secretive. Can I guess at a wedding?'

Unexpected, he laughed. 'On the cards, probably next year, but not yet.'

48

FAMILY OPENS UP

Nial and Francesca took the short road trip to Dumbarton.

Although chatting as always, bathed in different tones.

Fiona sensed him uneasy, guessed Niall skirted some crucial point, although at that time never knew what to expect.

As they eased along into a conversation as pleasant as walking along the pebble strewn side of the Garlock in bare feet he confirmed her suspicions.

'Mum, now I begin to understand my father's role in your life.' Speechless, almost choked over concerns he knew must flood her with that unexpected delivery, and to ease pain gripped one big hand around tiny ones.

Watched as tears dripped into a potentially bottomless well. Silent.

'But mum, now knowledge knowledge brings freedom. Leaves me happy.' Kissed her again, a lingering one with a soft hug as Francesca joined in. 'For with knowledge comes opportunity to remove unpleasant sadness from the past, allows us to clear away distasteful memories.'

Another hug, this time associated with a huge grin as he announced hopes of family gaining from truth.

Fiona's brain experienced a melange of emotion. From initial anxiety and disappointment at them unravelling her secret, disappointment grew into a positive phase where through excitement and relief accepted the fact her son, wee boy Niall, was now a man, capable of making sound decisions.

'Yes!' At first used a hesitant tone, which soon sped up and rushed into a babbling expose loaded with relief and hope. With need for deceit, too strong a word, concealment better, she said, 'Wonderful news, I suppose. Although having guessed much of the story, best I crawl from under the stone that sitting astride my shoulders, always threatened to crush me and your aunty Deirdre.'

Without delay, issued a strong peal of genuine laughter, warmer than Niall remembered hearing. 'Mind you, it lay as heavy as Dumbarton Rock itself.' With rounds of mutual laughter offering healthy interruption, ongoing satisfaction added to already building relief.

The new, improved Fiona amazed Francesca, whom she thought leathery, staid. *Got that wrong. Now, with the burden of pain drifting away, see her afresh, rejuvenated as the true woman who is Niall's mother.*

'We need tea, while I unload the uncut version and clear away what is a horrid, unpleasant tale, ripe to open and flush away all poisons.'

Niall surprised himself at how eagerly he awaited those revelations. 'In some ways mum, think on this like a forensic audit.' Now, hugging again, offered fresh example of unravelling laughter.

'Goodness me, an interesting thought.'

Amid a three-way hug, softened by happy tears, he said, 'And mum. This involves Francesca. So, please, let us get it out, cleared away... one time.'

Francesca raced to the kitchen and to a warm cry of thanks, dear one, she organised their drink.

As a result of Deirdre being elsewhere, Fiona entertained them to grimy history, until what could have been an unpleasant experience turned into a fabulous expose, an uncluttering of cupboards. Cathartic allowed Francesca to add to her opinion of the power of the woman, *the true Fiona.*

With tears and laughter, a plenty, often mixed, in the end they gained, as with barriers dropped, and now united, Niall found his real mum.

Francesca and Fiona bonded.

Niall and Francesca blended in rare oneness all couples aspire to share.

Agreed, that while none were party to the complete story they could not blame Deirdre over Henderson's death, for while suspicions abounded, insufficient to judge her executioner.

Even though Francesca, agreed to drop that subject, she nursed lingering doubts planted by Angela. Despite sharing family's joy, an unpleasant aftertaste left her unhappy to shelve further investigation.

Determined only disappointment, even dangerous sequelae could follow should she try discussing the past with Deirdre.

Dropped that theme, gone, kicked underneath the bed, family deserved their love and support.

When news reached Patrick and Holly, they rejoiced and, in softer form, outlined Henderson's history with children Sarah and Padraig.

Of course, Sarah, intuitive as her mother, took it well. 'Thanks mum. Always sensed an ugly background, and now, as families must, we should accept this, grow, move on.'

Padraig, with his father's softness, hugged parents. 'Dead information. Embrace it with love.'

Three days later, Holly, amid rush of preparing Patrick's birthday party, said, 'Well, because our friend Angela worked wonders with Francesca and contributes to family harmony, shall invite her to your birthday party.'

49

PATRICK'S BIRTHDAY

Logic declares varied reasons for indulgent family gatherings.

Pain, pleasure, or possibilities.

For instance, in the Cairn's case, their meetings revolved around them enjoying each other's company.

Blessed with solid, parental stability, excluding the part Henderson played, or rather his nonparticipation, if excluding cruelty over Fiona, they melded together with enviable, tight knit bonding of a flock of sheep.

While matriarch Holly ruled the group, she worked her tight reins with fairness and humour and understanding how wit, determination, and ability to accommodate advanced with age, so too did her inordinate capacity to spread inexhaustible glue of love.

In time, we may have downplayed Patrick's role in lives of those he touched. For sure, we earlier underlined his academic brilliance and medical flair, confirmed his innate determination to conduct himself as a healer who used standard practices. When often describing him as a big, soft lump, a feature passed onto his children and by genetic extension via shared genes, via Fiona to Niall, we missed key features.

He, as world's best proponent in dealing with personal relationships, and here touch on his extraordinary, enviable relationship with Holly, mastered technique of using essential trinity of insignificant words to ensure marital harmony.

Without being blasé, his expertly constructed use of *yes, my dear*, besides the accepted I love you, avoided unnecessary confrontation.

Since he understood how, in most matters Holly's opinions proved accurate, he bowed to her excellent, common sense, and managerial abilities. By doing so, that meant, on the rare occasions he doubted her accuracy, she bowed to opinion.

On balance, after they digested fresh, welcome information around Fiona and Niall, they listened with sympathy as Holly, glorying in these changes wrought by honest declarations, determined to research the subject. 'Now, I move to tackle Angela. For by explaining her feelings, which will help me understand how her reading of Deirdre's situation led to this expose of Henderson's miserable personality.'

As Patrick rose from his chair, he led her to the bay window which overlooked the River Clyde and prepared to offer seasoned opinion in an oft employed tenor. 'Now, my dear. Pause for a moment and reflect on how my River Clyde, my friend from boyhood, reacts to imponderable questions.'

Content, Holly snuggled into him, prepared to enjoy a rare sojourn into philosophy, and remained quiet as he continued. 'Look at that mighty body of water and appreciate how, as tide turns, it ebbs, unstoppable, marches towards the ocean.'
Tickled her fancy, when he encouraged her to follow him from the house, through the garden and onto the riverbank. Waved his right arm in ponderous fashion to allow it to sweep downstream from west to east and follow the river's course.

'Find here the unending sweeping away of nature's problems by a master of relationships.' Kissed her. 'My dear, much as you, in your splendid life, share a smidgeon of my river's expertise, accept she has exercised cleansing functions for millions of years. Well, at least since the Ice Age.'
She laughed. 'Also enjoy and respect the special place your Clyde holds in your heart, but' Aware when he allowed one of his rare introspective phases to engulf, which stretched her patience, 'move on. Explain your thinking.' Tapped palm against his chest.

He hugged with a warmth that made a passing lady who walked past smile and greet them. She, in her forties, thought them a mature couple gripped in the throes of recent romance. *My turn to find the perfect man soon*. That happy thought generated sufficient warmth to keep her comfortable for the rest of the evening.

Holly outlined thoughts on why she should, deserved to pump Angela for information.
His markedly strong reply surprised. 'Ask you to note my river's attitude, and never discuss ugly history with anyone, especially Fiona and Niall.' Voice joined arm encircling her waist in firming to the touch. 'Never.'

Holly, being Holly, instantly launched into a series of what she considered valid reasons for dissecting the question with her old friend.

Niall exercised one of his rare veto rights. 'No! Drop this.'

Satisfied, he, having exercised unusual authority, turned homewards. 'Now that you have me alive, let me act naughty. Please spoil me with a slice of apple crumble and chuck in a handful of those magnificent raspberries.'

Her turn to exercise control. 'No. Your expanding waistline demands I refuse your request. Instead, let us savour an early night and a warm snuggling session.'

She, and despite renewing their warm friendship, Holly accepted Patrick's advice and never discussed Henderson with Angela.

The following morning, as Patrick's birthday approached, he accepted Holly's unilateral announcement they deserved, as earlier agreed to celebrate the occasion with a family get together.

As their lives settled into normality, Patrick, appreciated in matters relating to family her advice solid, nodded in agreement. 'And why not, for old farts such as we may not have many parties left, so let us relish a bit of a splash.'

Holly, far ahead of him, already annotated a guest list of around forty. 'Not to worry my dear.' Moved behind and, wrapping arms around shoulders, kissed the top of his balding head. 'Can leave this to me.'

50

UNEXPECTED CONSEQUENCES

Holly chose a Sunday for Patrick's celebration.

As noon arrived, it found Patrick low.

His demeanour flat because of a combination of tummy bug and initial stages of geriatric mental deterioration. While never serious enough to bandy around diagnostic terms including Alzheimer's and related weaknesses, she, planning on specialist advice, booked him for a detailed examination by Prof Schultze at the Vale.

With guests rolling in and bringing cheer, they brought back a touch of his sparkle with hugs, wishes, and kisses more effective than copious doses; almost toxic, of B Vits already administered.

A factor incompletely explored relates to where family gatherings, centres on their healing power, how mental stimulation, when positive, improves neural transmissions. Forthwith obvious when an incredible melding of minds between Deirdre and Francesca occurred.

The girl, displayed her usual bouncy self, infected everyone with excitement, and played her part in working with Sarah and Holly to organise the function.

Fiona's early arrival threw family into concern when she explained to Holly. 'Our sister is having a dreadful day for Deirdre, amid one of her mind funks, refuses to join us.'

Which triggered off a generous, unimaginable reaction in Francesca, who as she still stewed in family revelations, jolted Holly's mind when she revealed the depth of her numinous side. 'My awakening mystical innermost being compels me to reach out to her.' As Fiona's eyes popped. 'Shall visit and encourage her to join the family, but first, need an excuse.'

Holly, dumfounded, for only third time in her life, stared, remained silent as Fiona said, 'You are a dear girl. Forgot my handbag. A cerise leather one, it sits on the hall stand.' They hugged. 'Please be a dear and fetch it for me.'

Francesca jumped into her Golf before Holly's mouth closed.

'Sorry for disturbing you, Aunty Deirdre, only me, come to fetch the busy Fiona's handbag.'

Her kind attention staggered Deirdre, who impressed at the well-liked girl calling her aunty, changed her attitude and reached out. 'Must cadge a lift with you.'

For she regrated her surly attitude when refusing to attend Patrick's celebration, and seized opportunity to redress that failing, felt a comforting, unexpected warmth for the girl. 'Before we go, let's chat over tea.'

One hour later as Deirdre encouraged the girl to embrace her Catholic Christianity, and as both shared an unexpected level of transcendent awareness, they cemented a new, firm friendship. Found in Francesca a route to express herself, albeit they avoided tight questions around difficult Cairn's history, left them forever.

Cairn's family jaws dropped as eyes opened in delight at extraordinary sight of the ladies walking into the room, arm in arm. As they commanded every eye, Holly whispered to Patrick. 'God blessed us when Niall introduced this child to our family. For only one touched with the insight of the Lord Himself has the power to work change like this in Deirdre's demeanour.'

Just as the sick patient who walks different pathways before finding a suitable remedy or medical system, so too in Francesca did she absorb extraordinary, celestial power.

Thus Deirdre, who rarely showed sparks of normality, when in Francesca's company bathed in a promising future of improving mental harmony.

Francesca also gained, just as she hoped with Angela, in Deirdre she doubled her family members when she gained the second aunt who led her to appreciate the truth and beauty of Catholicism, shared its healing balm.

With Angela also in top form, and delighted at them including her, enthusiastic thanks and praise boiled an already bubbling pot with warmth and love. 'Thrilled at you inviting me to this special occasion. Not only that, but also, rarely get opportunity to thank you for the wonderful part you special people played in my professional development.'

Hugged Holly again and said, 'Those formative early days when we three practiced together at Overtoun hospital.' Patrick and Holly, reminiscing in happy days, appreciated a brief catch-up session.

As Holly left to welcome guests, Partick outlined how he still considered them his best times. When sharing sentiments, hugged Angela with a warmth she rarely experienced.

In the meantime, a promising start improved when the much taller Francesca greeted Angela, enveloped her in a powerful hug as though intent on drowning. 'Rejoice at your presence. A joy to find you here as an important part of my family.'

Then as she stood back, she continued to hold the older lady's hands and said, 'And now, intend pushing on with my well-intended plan.'

Released one of Angela's hands to wave at Sandy and encouraged him to join them. 'For now, here comes your special man.'

At that point, Sandy, thrilled to greet Francesca for whom he already felt a special affection, breathed fast when she took him by the hand and made it join Angela's and when she held them together, said, 'You two need waste no more time.'

Hugged both. 'Beg you to greet each other as not simply old friends, but as two who need,' Wrapped arms around both, 'and deserve to form a stronger relationship.'

Her joining them together worked.

Not only did they greet but did so with extraordinary enthusiasm. Sandy, finding her presence at the party unexpected and joyous, hugged Angela and then as he intended to kiss her cheek, reacted in spectacular fashion and they, ignoring how their togetherness attracted attention, kissed properly on the lips.

Angela, heart beating faster than the swallows that dive-bombed them on the lawn, whispered. 'So, what caused the delay?'

When they hugged again, she responded as he, pulse racing in tandem, kissed her again.

Holly spotted them and opened her mouth as wide as the yawning chasm that disfigures Dumbuck.

Speechless, Francesca forced that mouth even wider when she declared. 'Nice one from me, Holly, guessed them the perfect fit.'

While she expected family to gasp with surprise at their obvious show of more than platonic affection, Niall hugged Holly and Francesca.

Francesca, without peeping at him said, 'Now Niall, told you them ripe to match. And, had your uncle Patrick been on their toes, they should have been an old married couple by now.' But postponed further discussion to involve themselves circulating among what Francesca already designated her family.

Holly, two hours later, still shocked and in danger of becoming emotional about finding the new couple inseparable, said, 'Come Sandy, put this woman down for a minute and indulge yourself in... well different sweet things.'

Winked at Angela, led them to the desert table. 'You have first dibs. Of course, baked a famous Cairn's family apple crumble especially for you.'

After leaving them, chatted to Patrick. Never did I suspect this closeness between those two.' Shook her head. 'How come we, especially me as the queen of relationships, missed this? Never in our careers, during the years we worked close, did Angela ever hint she enjoyed this man's company.'

With the party flowing, snuggled up to Patrick, asked how he missed their mutual attraction.

His reply added to the list of her astonishments. 'My wonderful lady, always guessed at their attraction, even questioned why they never acted on their feelings.'

'Tell you, Doctor Patrick Cairns. Unbelievable. Aware of this, yet you mentioned nothing.' Slapped chest hard. Twice, enough to make him breathe hard. 'Unbelievable I missed this.'

***

Angela, mind racing onwards as fast as pulse of earlier.

Wrapped both arms into one of Sandy's.

Already convinced them a couple destined for marriage, apologised. 'Missed your feelings, but also your fault. Because at no time did you ever suggested possibility, I attracted you.'

With Sandy experiencing and sharing her happiness, thoughts tumbled. 'I always had feelings for you, but hopeless at romance, never plucked up courage to release them.'

In a bashful moment, face flushed as he eased out another thought. 'Always considered you too special for me.'

Her mind flickered back to formative years. 'Often reflected on how poorly Patrick reacted to Holly's advances. And yet.' Kissed him again, then administered a sisterly slap on cheek. 'You are even shier than he.'

'My dearest friend. On balance, it takes two to tango, and so, let us share blame.'

Squeezed her arm. 'So, with time urgent, let our romance now blossom with passion absent years earlier.'

Laughed, deep enough to halt nearby conversations with a thunderous mirthful peal. 'Silly let us. Forget the past, take this further.'

Followed him to the desert table. 'Time to load your plate with delicious things, and then toddle into the park for a serious talk.' But as Angela reflected on her untidy waistline, she collected a mere tablespoon of fruit salad for herself.

Left Holly still shaking her head in disbelief at how she who always considered herself streetwise, a marriage broker of note, stared in disbelief at their disappearing backs as they retreated into the garden.

Hugged Francesca again. 'To think you spotted this within two minutes of joining the family.'

Two romantic pensioners strolled, left the garden, hand in hand, holding plates, into Levengrove Park.

In time, tarried by a bench beside the monument, sixty yards from Patrick's home.

In silence, with Clyde and Dumbarton Rock watching over them, hip caressed hip as he failed for the first time in memory to relish his crumble as before.

Unable to eat, she toyed with her fruit salad, made pretty patterns round the plate until he fed her a tiny spoonful. 'Gosh, this crumble is delicious, it matches Fiona's superb standards.'

After rescuing bowls and spoons, he placed them on the path at their feet. 'But I neglect you.' Then, picked up Angela's hand, fingered wrist and arm with same gentle, firm touch used on sensitive neck skin gracing an equine patient.

And yes, after missing so much time, they deserve a quiet moment.

51

AC FLYNN

The Met operated a Specialist Crime Unit.

Assistant Commissioner Geraldine Flynn headed the team.

At fifty-five, her six-foot-tall frame disguised femininity and because the AC's build followed structure of most male tennis players which acted against her and not all men found her attractive.

In thoughtful mood the AC found concentrating on work arduous.

Drummed fingers against a bland desk pad devoid of doodles but meticulously annotated in the three colours which indicated her complex schedule of appointments. Today, however, digits danced in time to a restless brain excited over what lay ahead. For the scheduled two-month period promised a change in lifestyle.

Various scenarios flittered with an immense intellect, took contorted paths which reflected darting movements of bats as the small furry mammals forage flies around a spotlight.

Seated at her smart mahogany desk; only quality piece of furniture in her otherwise functional, plain office, she glowered at the hefty pile of documents that swarmed over her in tray.

Surprised. For they steadily accumulated over the past five weeks when most admired Flynn, respected the ruthless approach to timeous documentation she forced on herself, and those who reported to her.

Flynn sighed with the begging desire of restless air as it escapes a tiny hole in a pneumatic tyre in a tireless effort to obtain a speedy exit.

Next, gulped a breath, rose and slapped a thigh and whispered. *Enough Geraldine.*

Sighed again, slumped back into her chair. *With plans nearing completion, must hold this together.*

Still restless and unsettled, traced circles on back of an unimportant circular. Never wasteful, recycled where possible, exceptional behaviour followed when she allowed pen freedom to doodle back and forth, as she needlessly drew wavy thick lines any zebra must approve of.

A further series of whispers outlined how she prepared to end her successful career.

In time, forced herself to finish a document and as appended her signature Flynn issued yet another plaintiff sigh. *Over. This office will become someone else's responsibility, and bad luck to them.*

Flung the document forceful at the out tray and missed. Watched, smiled at its wayward floorward descent. Left it there, and after she belled in her pa, greeted her with more enthusiasm than she felt. 'Inspector Brown, here is today's final list. Check them for me, then you may go home.'

Brown, after bending to retrieve the errant document, made to hand it over but Flynn waved it away. 'Also, one for you.'

On balance, as door clicked closed, a mere hint of satisfaction flickered across her face until fatigue chased it away.

Sat back, stretched arms and shoulders to ceiling, then rested forehead on backs of hands, closed eyes for thirty seconds until she appreciated where tiredness that fought against genuine fatigue tried to drag her into a deserved sleep.

Shivered, and without delay, beginnings of a smile creased corners of her mouth. Until, stimulated by a small thought, a happier one, which stretched full lips into a proper, attractive smile which unveiled reasonable top teeth, not the wayward lower incisors that stubbornly refused to obey expensive orthodontic treatment.

An unfair statement for those who saw the original radiographs which indicated near hopeless malalignment.

Although the sharp upper jawlines indicated strength and power, well rounded cheeks softened what might have been considered a masculine face and resulted in what a friend; in the days when she owned more than one, described as deserving of a swimwear model. A fair description as testified by her still amply filled bikinis.

Chuckled at the thought of her new costumes as they shared their inaugural but soon to be regular Mediterranean dips, then reminded herself how colleagues often got it wrong. 'Who says crime doesn't pay?'

Wallowed in conjecture and self-satisfaction as she removed a secret, personal phone and indulged herself when she studied the lady's face, her favoured wallpaper.

'Well, my love.' Touching two fingertips to lips, blew the portrait a kiss, and said, 'Patience, my love. Almost there.'

Flynn's first flirtations with corruption occurred fifteen years earlier, when, as a freshly promoted DI reporting to Superintendent Groves, her then boss, he initiated her into dodgy practices.

Soon made her appreciate how she could earn money well beyond her salary by bending rules; what he described as *gentle tweaking*, here and there.

At first, reluctant but fearful of his powerful presence, she accepted what he termed slush cash earned when his team creamed money confiscated during raids on drug lords. Of course, understanding it dirty, illegal money, they as gangsters never deserved, accepted the regular five or six hundred pounds that fell off the piles which soon amounted to thousands.

Notwithstanding, she acknowledged his instructions to use the cash wisely. Revelled how those small sums often surfaced and escalated into a few thousand. But then, over six months, when she realised bags escalated to packages of twenty thousand pounds, indicated she settled on a downward spiral without hope of recovery. Fears increased when she stumbled on him when careless, he dealt in a huge payback of protection money for a well-heeled narcotic distributor.

Gulped at money involved when he slipped her a fat, brown packet that contained forty-five thousand in untraceable notes. Only then realised events escalated beyond common sense.

When she mentioned her discomfort, he agreed, suggested it time they went clean and arranged to meet her in a smart, but out of the way hotel. Designated that as opportunity to plan their retirement from fraud and naïve, raised hopes of a clean career.

Rohypnol spiced gin, and tonic proved its efficacy as the date-rape drug.

Although he only seduced her once, that alongside two leud photographs sealed her future. For fear he intended declaring her a criminal, a life of crime not only beckoned but also, as blackmail encouraged Flynn to embrace her new lifestyle, which set her out on the road as a supremely successful, bent copper.

Flynn's criminal activities soared ten years earlier.

When DS Groves moved on, she at first considered that opportune to revert behaviour and control her actions. Until then, as a DCI, when she reported to DS Opperman, her new boss, remembered the DS's exact words when she baulked at notion of continuing to take backhanders.

He, tougher than ever imagined, dressed her down, brought up her past, recorded the list of her criminal involvement as passed down from Grimes and got brutal. 'Right! Enough of this idle chat. Do you wish to climb the ladder or is CI your limit? Because should you not work in harmony with me, shall leak these and also,' Nailed her down with his next comment. 'out your gay involvement with Sergeant Pastor.'

Seems a brief time ago and yet the force only recently learned to cope with same-sex relationships. And his remark raised alarm, for fantasy declared their relationship concealed.

One forceful Groves' comment became her constant companion, a mantra-like phrase used to control doubts when her still active conscience tried hard to strike. 'Never forget. We cannot control the substantial industry that is the drug trade.'

For the only time he ever softened, when as he caught her by both shoulders, offered a glorious chuckle. To usher in his potent conclusion. 'But we can live comfortably alongside and off the bastards.'

Used wisely, three hundred and seventy thousand pounds earned under his wing and tutelage during that three-year period was of excellent value and that exploded when he, getting too greedy, met a wayward, unmarked car.

Those knowledgeable declared it a hit job.

Early earnings proved a mere pittance when compared to how she accumulated significant safe wealth since then during tenure when promoted to DS Flynn and later as AC.

Now, fraud seemed part of her DNA.

As she, comfortably well off with the side packages that amounted to much more than her good salary only reflected on the positive side.

For she continued to exhibit her extraordinary flair for management to manipulate staff and their ability to hunt down criminals.

Hmm! Did the good justify the bad?

Also, learned from the past.

The AC never deliberately involved or awarded junior officers for toeing the line.

Even if suspicions increased, a lack of concrete evidence, and more importantly a shortage of decent senior officers willing to get involved, allowed her to expand criminal interests founded by predecessors.

The most significant factor on her side related to the numbers of senior officers who, as they were involved as well, meant she swam in a pool surrounded by even more sharks than South Africa's ANC politicians.

Often consoled herself by reflecting on how her fraudulent dealings were never associated with harmful situations involving people... or so she convinced herself.

52

FLYNN AND PASTOR

Flynn stood, palpably shook herself.

Restless, paced back and forth, dangerous as any menagerie lioness.

Doubtless, as queen in her environment, rarely content as she constantly searched for anything that might conflict with her intentions to control her environment.

Thus, she faced an endless barrage of imponderables, the *ifs and buts* that hammered at her psyche and prevented desperately needed respite.

Notwithstanding she desired the relief she normally gained when she barked orders, restraint checked her until only thick beige carpet that floored her office took brunt of captive energy.

Although its excellent condition, suggested her fidgeting unusual, since no tracks that might have been caused by the constant cycles of repetitive footsteps that damage pile surfaced.

My last deal. After this, we ease back, escape.

While seated at her desk, Flynn pulled a postcard sized mirror from top left-hand drawer and checked out makeup. Then brushed back naturally coloured chestnut hair with the merest hint of grey fibres; expertly maintained to sweep over ears, every two weeks.

Revealed standard feminine vanity when she marvelled, as she often did, at unusual, drab brown eyes and relished how they permanently sparked, owing to four obvious, yellow diamond-like stars that marked the left iris.

Two larger but less potent ones underscored its partner.

They caused remarkable glitter, scintillated as though residue left after a bling filled night on the town.

So, my beauties, are you ready to twinkle for me as I take you away from this frothy, depressing town?

Eyes emphasised a strong face with high prominent cheekbones and eyebrows, too thick, and close together for most people's taste.

Permitted herself a tight smile of satisfaction when she reached for her memo pad, then employed a smart fountain pen. The Parker *Duofold Prestige*, model chiselled in metal black, gifted to her five years before by her lady friend, her permanent, secret life partner.

A good, smart pen. If not most expensive available, when she rolled it between fingers, luxuriated in how it fitted hand and style perfectly.

Back then, within days she adapted its use when it instantly became her writing instrument of choice.

Not only had Parker crafted the instrument to be smart, but the company's determination to stick to uncomplicated engineering meant its workings never disappointed.

Crafted a simple message.

Site C. 9pm tonight.

Satisfied. Smothered face in the look of a cat when it steals creamy top of the milk as she passed her PA, fingered the ten signal, then walked through a busy corridor.

Confident in her role, barely acknowledged subservient bows and smiles of four junior officers.

With door to the Commissioner's outer office ajar as was that to his own office, which suggested him not in residence, she smiled on finding his PA bent over Her loaded desk.

Flynn's long-term lover and intended life partner, Inspector Diane Pastor focused on her computer monitor.

Their relation factual, they scarcely found time for more than four nights per Month.

Enforced separateness contributed to their establishing their relationship as a tight, faithful one. Also, the promise of what they faced, the knowledge their hidden partnership was ripe to soon blossom into normal affiliation, was further powerful incentive to cement them together.

Busy, Pastor responded instantly to slight cough offered by the AC with a thumbs up sign indicating them safe.

Flynn surreptitiously slipped Pastor the note and fled her office.

After an instant reading, Pastor killed paper when she plunged it into a secure, effective shredder. Thus ended their brief messaging system. No hello, nod, handshake. Nothing.

The C code indicated the meeting should take place in Whitehall Gardens, by the Statue of Henry Bartle Frere.

Pastor arrived bang on time.

Bundled inside a plain brown anorak two sizes larger than suited her slight figure, for that, and the ridiculously bulky hood that covered head and shoulders aided disguise.

Flynn, also camouflaged, covered by an enormous, plain, dark blue umbrella that supported cavernous, scalloped edges fit to grace a golfing brolly.

Aided concealment with the forced painful gait of an elderly man who dragged to his destination when encumbered by chronic hip arthritis.

Perhaps overkill but the heavy walking stick added to subterfuge as it fitted her acted movement perfected after hours spent in practice, then through regular use.

Initiated discussion with a business-like question. 'Any concerns over activity of the Commissioner's new team yet?' No greetings, comments, or tenderness expected of life partners. Only business.

The DI echoed her attitude. 'Still cannot fathom what business engages DS Stewart's team. Know little about them or what their brief is, although horse orientated. My only contact with them is DI Pauline Castle. Know her from way back and although I sounded her out,' Took care to emphasise, 'have not picked up any problematic vibes.'

When she hesitated, they both turned away from what they considered an untidy yob. Probably a hangover from the distant days of *Flower Power* but always aware of need for solid secrecy, took no chances, avoided unnecessary risks.

As the man drifted off Pastor continued. 'Still, until we unblock his situation experience warns to continue subtle probing.'

Flynn shared Pastor's concerns. 'He remains my most significant loose end.'

Reached a hand across to caress Pastor's cheek. 'And dearest one. Nor have I found anything interesting from that direction... and yet. Odd. What occupies his team? Why does nothing obvious surface?'

Pastor, having been around expert detectives for what felt like a million years admitted to a lingering doubt, one which threatened to fester in the depths of her criminal mind. 'Do you think, even for a single alarm flashing moment, Commissioner set the DS up with a single theme?'

That got Flynn instantly alert. 'To investigate us, or internal corruption. But you know me, how I am,' Leaned forward and gave Diane a peck on the lips, 'more suspicious than anyone.'

Fought to hold herself back when her mind raced with the notion to tear off Pastor's clothes and share passion that must break bands of tension embracing them. 'Yet I feel no threat of anything from that direction.'

Again, as a couple strolled passed, Pastor said, 'Still, must acknowledge your intuition is never wrong, which keeps me uneasy, nervous we may miss something.' AC peered around, and as time drifted on, stamped cold feet to improve circulation.

That said, when she took up Pastor's theme, worry lines around eyes intensified, more marked than normal. 'Okay. Foolish of me to ignore your alarm for respecting your detection principles, suggest leaving this to me. Will keep digging away, gently.'

Used two fingers to tease bridge of Pastor's fine nose. 'Have a trustworthy, well-paid man who will explore one or two of his team's cars. He also continues to monitor a telephone line.'

We may find damning.'

Flynn scanned the street, searched for one of the many dodgy meetings that regularly took place throughout London, and continued to express her concerns. Her final, agreeable suggestion toughened even further the worry lines which strained her face. 'Afraid we cannot meet until our much-anticipated weekend away in Brighton.'

'Yes, my love. Cannot wait for that.'

Flynn smiled properly for the time. 'Now for good news. Decided to accelerate end game by increasing pace of events.'

Risked a suggestive kiss and embrace. 'After this last deal falls into place, we can cease business. Need only one month to wrap up everything my side, and then, after handing in my resignation, with leave overdue, can empty my desk six weeks from now.'

Flynn leaned forward and kissed Pastor, properly, passionately this time as tongues caressed. 'You then wait just a month and follow me.'

Pastor skipped with uncharacteristic enthusiasm. 'Retirement. Off to the sun. Lovely.'

They somehow, kept their hands and lips off each other, and then drifted apart in different directions. Pastor's step held spring of a younger, medal winning athlete. Embraced this accelerated prospect, because of Geraldine trapping her in various money-making intrigues during the previous six years, mental exhaustion, intensified by constant need to look over her shoulder fast approached.

Also tired of their subterfuge, fearful her mental constitution might not hold up as required, should they continue much longer.

After a second, sneaky bus change she glorified in Geraldine's promise when she convinced Pastor they already salted five point four million pounds safely away. A nest egg that had to prove more than they could ever find time to spend and excluded values of decent homes crime already earned.

But Geraldine. Can she ever say enough?

53

FLYNN AND THE ATTACHE

The AC hated the thought of her meeting.

Met him in an out of the way place.

For fear someone notice, the Chinese attaché selected a select spot to treat, well hopefully soften up Flynn to a magnificent meal in a discrete China Town club.

Expressed his disdain for her, but to himself. *Patience. Relax with these ugly people.*

Only after enduring correct drawn-out preliminary etiquette, Floyd at last opened. 'So, your connections are prepared. With suitable protocols in place, your side are satisfied, they have the shipment ready?'

He, while anxious and expectant of offered support, barely hid his disdain.

for her. While he took care not to offend, skirted close to boundary when he adopted a paternal mode, and surveyed. 'The full resources of the Zhāng family are behind this. The deal is imminent.'

'Good. Although my sources express doubts, increasingly so around the newer ones, younger family members.' In this delicate cat-and-mouse interaction, each tried to declare their importance, to maintain control, as though two criminals desired recognition or vied for the gold medal in London's sleuthing championship.

That statement induced a perfunctory nod of agreement. 'With their newfound wealth, we learn the twins indulge product to dangerous excess.' Here, risked leaning forward, as though to exert authority. 'Thus, drawing interest to themselves, uproarious behaviour risks damaging our delicate, important relationship.'

Then offered faintest bow, sufficient to indicate dependence on his supply and command chain. 'Yes, and no!'

Paused, peered at Flynn, and tested her resolve with an intense stare.

Happy she survived his test he said, 'Concede newer players on the scene cause our family's only slight concern.'

Flynn tried to conceal disappointment as she said, nodded. 'Americans are big players. Although that risks FBI involvement. While superb news, they still make me nervous, for at this stage, their propensity for indiscretion must make waves.'

'My dear lady. Listen.' If not the condescending, *look lady* people subjected her to in younger days, she shivered at his ongoing attempts to dominate. *One last time. If required, shall eat off the floor to push through this deal.*

Confident he had masterfully secured the deal, the man touched palms together. 'To me, not a catch. Because my source in the FBI is an Assistant Director. Smiled as he gave the tabletop three sharp taps. 'Thus, confidence reigns we face no worries.'

She managed a small, tight smile, one he noticed as a gradual softening around corners of her eyes. 'That news impresses for moles inside the FBI are rare, useful. If they are happy, then that should keep twins safely out of our hair for the present. Good.'

Now has me wondering if his man may also be my contact. No, time to get out Geraldine, for this becomes too involved.

His concerns almost floored her, chipped away at her composure and as he continued to explain Chinese unease, disclosed how his FBI contact expressed alarm around suspicions of an unknown Met group who investigated diamonds and horses.

'At present slight, but if this holds water, insist you conduct a deeper, thorough search through colleagues' departments for a shift in emphasis, anything unusual or untoward.'

She tensed for that point triggered the same alarm bell to ring inside her head touched on by she and Pastor. *Diamonds and horses again. Is Diane right. Are the Chinese into this deeper than us? Damn. Better dig deeper into DS Stewart.*

Next, he decided it time to begin their meal and did this in elegant fashion when he offered a bowl that contained a flavourful, grey salt-water fish dish typical of the Zhejiang province.

Accepted this offered welcome distraction.

Only after following correct rituals, he said, 'Notwithstanding our concerns, your personal commitment satisfies my masters.'

She added the single necessary statement which allowed him to continue. 'It is your history of profound professionalism that allays any trepidations we may initially have faced.'

He accepted that opinion and began to outline the process. 'The good news. We have expanded our consignment to where it now contains top-quality stones amounting to over eight hundred carats.'

Surprised her with a break in tradition when he offered a dainty hand clap.

As his approach continued to soften, he continued. 'Own eyes examined several of the stones. World's best. Clear, cut by finest artisans throughout Europe. Ready for mounting. Unbelievable value.'

His looseness led to a further softening in Flynn's attitude as smiling inwardly at how the considerable volume of alcohol he consumed exerted its effects.

They worked together over five years, and she appreciated, now in his seventies, he aged, and faster than he or his masters appreciated. *Now understand where his loose tongue comes from can use this to my advantage.*

Whereas he mellowed fast and confided. 'This consignment will bring our harvest close to a market value of around one hundred and twenty million dollars.'

Then, as he enjoyed expressions of greed that swarmed across her face, tapped a single digit four times on the tabletop, leaned closer and whispered. 'A successful conclusion to this consignment must grow your already comfortable Swiss bank account by at least an additional six million dollars.'

Enjoyed how that further increased those already prominent levels of greed.

While he smiled, forgot his lack of discipline when he criticised her slip. Despite needing her, considered Flynn still a barbarian.

But continued as agreed and made the AC's face light up when he reached to the floor and opened a smart, red attaché case and withdrew a thick envelope. 'Your documents as promised.'

Opened the envelope and passed Spanish passports, ID certificates, driving licences and permanent residence documents plus collaborating papers. 'So, Ms Yvonne Baker, you, and your friend Sencha Perez, are now Spanish citizens, uncatchable. No one will ever question these. Perfect.'

'At last. Thank you for your skill in producing these.'

In addition, promised him as agreed, when settled in Spain, to contact with name of the officer primed to take over role in the corrupt practices that seemed never ending.

In conclusion, as that engineered both into the state of being nourished by the sweet flavour of greed, Flynn savoured the rest of her meal.

Even if eager to leave earlier than propriety demanded, attention to detail ensured she entertained, fawned over him as that incredible and unexpected doubling of her Swiss bank balance deserved.

At last, she got away.

Two taxi rides later, Flynn soaked in a bath in her splendid flat in the development that once housed former Met offices.

Success legitimised her to luxuriate in matching candles as they burned bright around her bath.

Until heady scent of expensive perfume and crisp champagne encouraged her to inhale deep and laugh aloud. 'Assets of twelve million pounds raked in over ten years, and no one suspects. While I should enjoy ten, further deals... too dangerous.'

Yes, my dear Sencha, here is to our retirement, togetherness.'

54

ALASTAIR GORDON

AC Flynn set off on an early morning jog.

Part of a determined plan to manage weight and fitness.

Geraldine often managed a four-mile street run near her home.

Furthermore, luxuriated during those forty minutes, as a phone free time when she never permitted calls or external agents to disturb concentration. Her *me time*, a jealously guarded hiatus when this morning person's brain collated her day.

Today proved a special effort, as thirty minutes in, on one of her irregular morning efforts, she stretched not only muscles.

Since, she contrasted this with her routine runs as during this one arranged a secure meeting to feed her prodigious brain.

Albeit this session lasted longer than normal.

With timing perfect, exemplary as always, when she turned a sharp, concealed corner between Savoy Place and Michael Faraday's Statue a fellow jogger intercepted her.

'Greetings Flynn. How are you today?'

'Good Alastair.' Moreover, both aware time and concealment dictated speed and concealment, they stepped closer to the statue and in faintest of shadows cast by a precautious, eager sun, got into business. 'Besides, happy to report all fits in with our aspirations, so on target.'

Superintendent Alastair Gordon and she shared colourful history. That said, went way back in the force to a time when heady mixed up youthful days united them as a couple.

Until she convinced herself the Welshman, whose Scot's born father donated only name and sperm before he disappeared without trace, faced no future together.

For instance, even when both were sergeants, she developed the tough, insular streak that committed her philosophy of Geraldine first.

Neat, severed relationship with precision of Patrick Cairn's scalpel when she ended the relationship. Tough, left him stranded, added insult to a man whose naïve, fatherless emotions floundered, when convinced of their long-term future, took years to recover.

Met made her DCI before him and a lingering soft spot encouraged her to influence his career from a distance, and unknown to him, encouraged his promotion. After making DI, he blossomed and enjoyed that unexpected success that often accompanies responsibility.

She found even when engaged in various parallel and conjoined projects after arriving at the Met, found provided she kept him distant, they clicked as teammates, useful allies in fraud.

But, under her influence when desirous of a safe, supportive officer to complement her spectacular success in crime, she seduced him. When a significant project loomed, she desperate, hoped to convince him to follow her path, engineered that tricky step when she took him to Majorca for a five-day break.

Bitchy, even called it a reconciliation trip.

Nevertheless, convinced herself they were compatible bed partners, that trip solidified earlier thoughts, firmed her opinion, he never suited.

Seduction has been described as conquest, and indeed it proved, for she manipulated him into joining her in extensive, corrupt practices. Soon, and despite him sharing only part of her greed, she hooked him.

And with skill of a ruthless Cabinet Minister, coddled, but aware of his never ending ongoing subtle spot for her, kept him at arm's length by ensuring weighty projects occupied her mind and time.

Inasmuch as years passed with minimum social contact, he appreciated nothing as dead as a dead love affair and thought he escaped her greedy clutch.

Within this scenario, she pulled him deeper into bigger projects, and as this, their fourth meeting generated required success her whispered demand caught receptive ears.

'The Chinese are finally ready. Committed to the big one. This shipment will find me retiring, escaping from this cauldron.'

In a soft illogical moment as she dropped her guard that fact tumbled out. Mind bubbled with hopes of her escape plans amid a whirlwind of excitement caused constant restlessness since that potent meeting with the attaché.

Had she considered the effect that news must have encouraged she would have kept her retirement concealed but erred when she revealed a touch of basic humanity.

Unable to check emotions, plans overflowed into a deeper trough. 'Time to end my involvement in these games.'

Smacked lips together when the full portent of her disclosure hit home. *Fool, Geraldine for functioning as a teenager?*

He almost choked. 'You prepare to retire from the force. Get out, leave me for good.'

Which left her with no choice other than to continue with the major fact, the one she intended to reveal only when settled in Spain. 'Yes, yes. The big one.'

Tried to cheer him by disclosing intention to hand over all contacts and unfulfilled plots already in the pipeline. 'So, good news for you. Since that information, by establishing your financial future, softens the blow.'

With his mind in topsy-turvy, he saw only disappointing points, then as a skilful negotiator she needed only two precious minutes to convince him of upcoming benefits.

In time, steered him as a farmer does with a bull's nose ring until he began to accept her reasonings, yet Flynn, aware of his distraction, assumed it due especially to personal side of things and worked to keep him on track.

'To begin with, as this accelerates, you must clear your desk, for I need a special effort. For the deal goes down week. Without delay, I will complete the details before we meet afterwards. Same time Friday.'

Granted, news left him hung in an odd place, on the fence or Ockham's razer, but never fathomed that out until later. Manipulated him as always by working him hard with unnecessary minor projects she claimed necessary to settle unfinished business, with his contribution important.

Flynn exaggerated scant information to hand. 'Our plan has a shaky element.' Relished how that emphasis swung his mind back into gear and continued. 'Have a worry that may prove unimportant.

'Stood upright, swung back into detective mood as essential discipline encouraged him to remain patient, attentive to ensure he absorbed pertinent details as she elaborated. 'This DS Stewart concerns me.'

Dug a lone, firm finger into his chest, 'As the hot kid on the block he astonished everyone, exploded through ranks into a senior position, his actions prove him elusive, perhaps a dangerous character.'

That same finger tapped twice. 'While he does nothing untoward, fear his team may hide in plain sight. For they appear to do... well, nothing.' Flynn pushed a touch of sincerity into her voice. 'Because I cannot pin him down, we worry he conducts surveillance work. Ask you to dig into him and team's background.'

Gordon embraced her trust when she delegated this to him during this crucial time and gripped bottom lip between teeth. As a hand ran through the auburn, curly hair that first attracted him to her, he said, 'That DS indeed puzzles more than us. Since, as you remark he experienced an almost meteoritic lift to the top.'

Outlined how gossip among fellow officers reached levels even she found unexpected. 'Odd, for as yet none of us have enjoined with him in any social activities we cannot even begin to understand his function.'

Hopeful this effort divert attention from her, Flynn agreed. 'He does not fit in with other superintendents. Even my inside contact in the Commissioner's office, his PA, DI Pastor, who warned me of his hush-hush visit with the boss, found nothing of interest.'

Left Gordon astonished at information around DI Pastor. 'Goodness me. Your net trawls subterranean levels fit to drag up clams from bottom of the Mariana Trench. Will she be one of mine after the transfer, after... you...desert me?'

Hangdog look plucked at heart strings, surprised her with its strength and how the pulling power of that dejection dug up fond memories. Enough to continue her effort to placate and then played another ace. 'You will also have ear of my FBI man, Leipzig, at your disposal.'

'So, you still involve him. I thought that line ran dry.'

Explained how after taking heat, he took a back seat, but now comfortable, wished her to involve him for another year. 'His strong Chinese connection makes him important.'

Remarkable information swung Gordon into positive frame. 'Wow, Geraldine, so much heady information. And yes. Important to put considerable effort into researching Stewart.

Spent ten minutes tidying up miscellaneous items.

Until, as she turned to leave, Gordon did something unexpected, reacted foolishly by acting out an unintentional fantasy, something they agreed should never happen.

Bared scars of their past when he allowed simmering, repressed affection to come alive, demonstrated how deeply he maintained his emotional connection.

Rough, pulled her to him, kissed mouth, then pulled back and pleaded. 'After this, loaded with money, we could still be a couple. Take me with you.'

Knew nothing of her plans with Pastor.

'Alastair... no!'

Pulled back, tongue-lashed him. 'You bloody fool!'

Erred again when at a time when normal deception skills should have placated him, she leaned heavier on that original surgical knife. 'Stupid. You and I are over, dead. We must maintain a purely business relationship.'

Allowed no right of reply when she jogged away, emotionally disturbed, and anxious convinced herself she began the separation process, although concerned that rough abuttal left him floundering, dangerous.

Although their planned, busy meeting lasted a mere eleven minutes but proved one of the longest of his life. Day ruined. Tortured mind meant he remained home; the tummy bug even works for those in senior positions.

Diligent, spent day torn between reminiscing and planning, although unsure in which direction to take.

55

A PRACTICAL PROBLEM

Four days and four fresh foals later.

Calder arrived at an increasingly busier scene.

Georgiou pleased to greet him. 'Welcome to Donderley, and your timing sits perfect. Glad you join me. With business exploding, need your expert help.'

With Eleanor engaged elsewhere, vets stole an hour for Georgiou to orientate Calder around the farm then pulled up at the box that housed Saunders' mare. As her kind face greeted them, she turned up her top lip, delivering a generous soft whinny of friendship.

Georgiou said, 'So, here she is. Our timing perfect, for I expect this lady to be ready for a foaling box within three days.'

Calder cast his experienced eye over the mare and while he stroked her soft muzzle, exposed the thrill of working with animals. 'Agree with Georgiou my gorgeous friend. For with your udder swelling and that vulva slackening, we can expect your imminent delivery to produce a delightful baby.'

In time, as Georgiou's' concerns over his partners' softness escalated, the facility impressed Calder. 'These cameras operate as an early warning system which enables staff to detect changes.'

By the time Georgiou pointed out extent of camera coverage, he modified his opinion. Quick to spot danger from their viewpoint, their widespread placement added to already high stress levels. 'Otherwise, amid this efficient set up how do you envisage us doing the job? For these cameras worry me, and working on a farm with efficient, dedicated staff, guess at obstacles.'

'We will find an answer.' Regardless of him exuding air of confidence, Georgiou sighed and tapped teeth. 'You keep motivated. Study the environment, camera setup and monitors yourself.'

Exhaled again with an emission of enough slow, steady air for Calder to sense concerns as Georgiou said, 'Moreover, act unobtrusive.'

Tapped same finger against his axe-like Mediterranean nose. 'Detect the two-hour period post lunch as most peaceful time on the farm. Indeed, that is when staff often grab a quick kip, so we may use that to spot a chink by investigating possibilities. Let us meet around three.'

Thereafter, Calder's mind gathered and processed information, illustrated how his unusual psyche drifted back into the uglier version when he released an opinion. 'Aside from our snooping, we should concentrate on finding a solution to target the mare in the foaling box. Need to kill this foal during the sensitive twenty-four-hour period to prevent Saunders forking over covering fee.'

Two o'clock and chicken salad behind them, they investigated the foaling boxes, drug room, laboratory, and all aspects pertinent to The Hub's workings relevant to not only business but also as vets searching solutions to their conundrum.

Altogether perplexed, sat down the following day at three o'clock and pondered findings. Even if into ever increasing, although not yet hectic business, same question inundated both minds and threatened to deluge them into a lost fee unless they found a solution. 'How are we going to get around these things?'

Georgiou's inability to find an answer stimulated Calder and after a session in the stallion barn with a successful covering, caught up with Georgiou. 'Find their surveillance system most impressive, best experienced. Does it ever give problems, or maybe even does it hide a quirky nature?'

Georgiou repeated that nose tapping thing and suggested he should discuss this with staff while Calder agreeing suggested caution. 'Do not ask Eleanor or the nurse. Let me explore it with Alfred in the covering yard.'

Paused as a nurse passed. 'Picked up he talks rarely with Eleanor for they experienced a tricky setback.' Chuckled as Georgiou eyes lit up. 'Not the usual boy girl type. Yes! We could take that route.'

Later, in as nonchalant manner as ever managed, Georgiou talked to Alfred, wondered. 'Admit to being impressed by your surveillance system. But what if someone pulls out a plug, or if you experience power outages, does it take time to reset after you restore power?'

'You surface an interesting poser. And yes, at present, problematic. Because a power loss stops the videos, a design flaw which means a blank spot where they do not record as expected.'

'Follicle at five by five, ready to go.' Georgiou withdrew probe from the mare's rectum. Cover her this afternoon.'

Alfred nodded, 'Good. That will suit the horse. Excellent.'

Business over, Georgiou pointed at the wall mounted camera. 'You mentioned snags. I believed these modern imaging systems foolproof.'

Yard manager nodded again, happy to explain his tremendous system. 'They work extraordinarily well and record high-definition videos.' In expansive mode, as he enjoyed the vet's company, explained the stud's philosophy. 'For example, these days, with security paramount, we keep a detailed record of everything.'

'With colossal money involved in this business, condone your approach.' Georgiou smiled in agreement. 'Anticipate an efficient backup process protects you against power cuts. So, the backup system works well?'

With Alfred, well into the process, he snickered as a horse does to attract attention of others as they walk past its stable door. 'Interesting you mention that as the company claimed their battery backup system ideal, but it disappoints, has a weak spot.'

Used two hands and ten fingers to indicate nearest camera. His look affectionate, Georgiou suspected he might kiss the camera could he reach it as he continued. 'In truth, our local council electricity supply is excellent, causes us few black spots. Our difficulties are because of human error.'

Georgiou chuckled. 'Afraid machines become more reliable than people.' When Alfred paused, Georgiou watched face tighten as he sank into a thoughtful moment.

When he continued, failed to laugh as most do when they admit error. 'Did something stupid day before you arrived. When changing a plug, Eleanor distracted me.' Georgiou picked up the same theme of animosity Calder earlier detected.

'With her chewing my ear she made me lose concentration and I... slipped up, caused wrong wires to touch.' Frowned, then whispered. 'Blew the system. Bang! Just like that. Entire scheme crashed.'

Georgiou permitted himself a sly smile.

Picked up on that weakness and stored it as an area worth exploring.

'We know how electrical systems demand consistency, so, easy to imagine your faux pas caused some consternation. But when you switched the mains power back on, it surely restored the feed, the supply.'

'Kicked into gear as expected. Except for the surveillance system.' In a down moment shook his head. 'Established our system has an inherent factory weakness in that department for our computer system objected to mishandling.'

Blew a shallow, mysterious breath out through nose. 'Upset a few people, including owners and particularly she who must be obeyed.' Inclined head toward the foaling area. 'For it needed almost forty minutes before it came online again.'

Got it. Georgiou' analytical and criminal mind sensed opportunity. Fought the urge to show pleasure, concerned Alfred might note keenness, and followed up on what promised to yield useful information. 'But the company, being aware of this defect, have an answer. A specialised chip, a software update?'

'Of course. They apologised profusely, advised someone else reported a similar disturbance. Their software engineers found a glitch and are confident they corrected it.' At last managed a small smile.

As Georgiou remained quiet but interested, the man opened up. 'Information so sensitive they refused to install the upgrade via the internet. Already couriered from Korea, we expect it in two days, no more. They are confident the system is smarter, easier to use.'

Georgiou's renewed laughed rang out as he slapped Alfred on the shoulder. 'In a year or two perhaps the Chinese will develop a system to make us unemployed.'

Had anyone noticed, depth of his grin and jaunty air must have raised eyebrows. *At last, this super sleuth has news to share with Calder. Sure, by tweaking the electrical system, our combined brains can fool these people. Nice one!*

56

DEATH

As they shared opinions, heads almost touched.

Closed off their discussion when Faith walked into the room.

Both noticed the girl flush at their warm greeting and assumed it because she flustered at appreciated looks from two men loaded with obvious masculinity.

Georgiou tried to charm, and as Faith pretended him successful, introduced the Heraldon incident.

Forewarned and prepared by her father, Faith conducted herself as directed and satisfied them she sniffed no problems in that direction.

Smart, she diverted them along equine matters when she asked well-rehearsed questions around horse breeding.

Thus, they found nothing in that brief conversation to cause alarm.

'So, we are positive?' Georgiou still concerned if Calder's principles threatened to resurrect over planned killings. For fear that he mounts a serious objection to them killing the foal, he quizzed. 'You know how to proceed?'

'Yes, yes and I will do this, but after our America trip am finished for good. Done and out of this.'

Timeous, ran through their foal killing plan until Nurse Jessica joined them.

At thirty-five, with a decent horse rider's body and strong brown hair that danced when she walked, similar coloured eyes flickered over the vets.

In need of a partner, her sassy stare indicated availability.

With taste in women watered down by a shortage of ready subjects, Georgiou slipped an arm around her waist and pulling to him, caressed her hand. 'Now then, stunning lady, is your bed as cold as mine?

She laughed, reached up, and kissed his forehead. 'If that is a come-on line, I say a decent effort, so watch this space.'

Brazen. Took his hand and said, 'Time for a... roll in the hay. For the boss' prize mare is on her way to box three. Groom reports she has been sliming since early morning, and now with teats leaking, on this evening's list for sure.'

Georgiou rose to follow and giving a special, explicit hug, kissed her brow, which left Calder blowing kisses as they moved off to the stable.

That means my best bet is Faith.

Calder reflected on how earlier he tried his luck with the third nurse. The attractive blond girl Bronwyn laughed him off. 'Now then, vet. None of your nonsense with me, for while I enjoy your flattery, please note I swing the best way.'

'What a pity, sad indeed.'

While Georgiou checked the mare over, he again demonstrated his fondness for horses. 'Well girly, you are making fine progress and should have a lovely foal this evening.'

As protocol demanded, they checked markings out against passport, noted the number 26 on the thick yellow collar around neck. Protocol demanded a staff member fit collar as soon as horses entered the yard. A priority completed as soon as they left the carrier.

All thoroughbreds sport subcutaneous, neck computer chips inserted for ID purposes, but garish collars ensure them easier to identify for local and immediate purposes.

Also checked computer chip with a hand-held scanner and when satisfied, formally advised Vee; senior of resident secretarial and administrative staff, he found evidence to corroborate the passport.

Vee captured that as fact when looking up at camera, used a clear voice. 'Dr Calder and I confirm this mare is Sweet Connemara.'

The four, two vets and nurses continued with various duties.

First up they supervised a delivery that proved easy: an immature chestnut filly from an experienced mare.

Even Georgiou surprised when Jessica looked at her watch and allowed lust to bubble over. 'Well, lover boy, with forty minutes to spare,' Rubbed body against his, clasped him tight as mating frogs in spring, 'so, time for a quickie?'

A mutually advantageous system, and loveless, it kept them warm during the appropriately termed breeding season after which without regret they moved on.

Eight pm on the dot. Calder engaged with Jessica and Faith in box four with a mare, while Georgiou was in the adjacent foaling box.

Soon satisfied all well with his big mare, the Saunders one, he stood outside the box and watched. She, happier for space, turned circled the box three times, presented rear end to him, then sunk down into still fragrant fresh straw.

As mares do, she, an experienced mother, galloped into a powerful labour that found her pushing out front end of her colt foal, then she lay flat on her side as her sweaty chest heaved.

Georgiou smiled at the groom. 'Thanks John. With your expert help, we coped.'

'Thanks, doc. A fine mare to deal with. Easy.' Calder kicked off the initial stage of their killing plan.

Anxiety tortured his face as he popped his head through the door and implored for help. 'If you are under control, need John and both nurses to help with this difficult mare. Please guys, join me in here.'

Acted with unbelievable callousness when unobtrusively, he stuck a large-bore needle repeatedly into skin over the mare's chest. Forthwith, his intention to irritate her, achieved remarkable success.

Her sudden and unexpected discomfort at his disgusting treatment caused her to react. Angry, anxious, and intractable, she raced around the stable and kicked out with both legs.

As she was normally a thorny character to manage, his unpleasant tactic compounded with natural irritability worked her up into a lather.

With actions fractious to control, they worried she might trample her foal.

John and Jessica picked up the foal and placed her behind a swing partition inside foaling box. Because they often experienced complex situations where mares, usually timers, struggled to bond with their new foals, they exercised that well tested system.

Which permitted Georgiou to release his nurse and groom. 'In control. Go.'

They reacted in routine manner and left the vet with the Saunders mare and foal.

Calder followed them to foaling box one.

Georgiou said, 'Will join you presently. But let me grab a quick drink of water.'

He entered the adjoining staff room, filled a glass with water then performed a planned manoeuvre.

Lay down on the floor, cried out in simulated pain, and smashed a full glass of water over the plug socket by the fridge.

There was a click.

Power tripped, and they lost power, as demonstrated by lost lights.

A most concerned Faith raced to meet and helped him struggle to feet.

When satisfied he could walk well, thanked her, but as Calder's mare screamed, Georgiou instructed her to return and help. Reassured his injuries nothing, and after removing the wet plug from socket, moved to the fuse box.

When Georgiou reset the trip switch, lights flashed back into play.

As Faith remained with him, he gripped her by putting an arm around shoulder, grunted in pain, and said, 'Thanks and sorry. Bit sore, but please get back to Calder and that difficult mare. You can get on with things. Leave me to check this pair.'

Georgiou picked up his own cue and slipped back into the foaling box to re-join the Saunders mare. Grimacing at what was to come as he considered how they lay peacefully, foal's hind legs still inside the resting mare.

Without delay, after taking in the kafuffle inside the adjacent box, pushed on with the hideous part of their effort.

Georgiou pulled a shopping sized thick bag from his pocket. After a furtive inspection, placed it over the foal's head.

Used a similar system to the one that worked well with the unfortunate Craggy Moor.

As expected, issued a mixture of smiles and grimaces when he noted it worked faster and easier with the foal.

Now for the tricky part.

As he tightened the bag, Georgiou placed his knee on the foal's chest and one hand on the plastic covered muzzle and studied his watch. *Need a perfect three minutes.*

Never intended to suffocate the hapless creature, one whose loss of potential he reminisced about with a verse from Thomas Grey.

Full many a flower born to blush unseen.

And waste its sweetness on the desert air.

Incorrigible, brutality of the situation meant little.

Counted out time, rejoiced in the three solitary minutes that passed before he partially asphyxiating the foal.

Mare rested, oblivious to her foal's slaughter as it struggled, and flashed legs that were inside the mare's uterus, which encouraged her dam to rise and separate the umbilical cord.

As the mare stretched, then turned towards her foal, Georgiou declared his timing good as he watched the foals original desperate and ineffectual struggling efforts weaken.

Called out. 'Quick, someone. Need help. Get oxygen and the emergency kit.' With the second mare suddenly relaxed because Calder stopped stabbing her chest, which freed him and a nurse to join him with Saunders' mare, leaving groom John and Faith to monitor them.

The box was soon awash with equipment and expert in the management of neonatal emergencies; they conducted a rescue attempt in exemplary fashion.

Crime went unnoticed.

Especially important, it went unrecorded, as videos needed time to come online.

Later, it collected pertinent information on how hard staff worked as they attempted to resuscitate it and how the vet student and the nurse did their best.

With skill of all experienced criminals, they conducted their work in an atmosphere of precision and, as much as we hate using the term, dedication. For so it seemed to patient, devoted staff. But to no avail.

Georgiou never intended to kill the foal outright.

Planned to deprive it of enough oxygen to assure it became a *dummy*, colloquial name for the Equine Perinatal Asphyxia Syndrome that readily develops after any incident compromises oxygenation to the brain and vital tissues.

This usually happens when early umbilical cord separation causes a disruption in blood supply from the mare to the foal's circulation.

They housed the foal and mare in the adjacent state-of-the-art ICU.

Fast, professional, they set up oxygen, drips, and drugs and used them expertly, as they did with any compromised foal.

Georgiou's timing was perfect.

Had he permitted only ninety minutes of oxygen deprivation, the foal may have recovered.

But with three minutes to conduct his foul business.

Spot on.

Damage done.

Oxygen deficiency produced a cascade of irreversible pathological changes, which included brain damage and multiple organ failure.

These ensured the foal developed regular seizures.

Died within the critical twenty hours, to vets and Saunders satisfaction, well inside time before the stallion's covering fee was due.

57

FAITH AND SOPHIA

The incident left everyone upset.

Faith was particularly disappointed.

Her first hands-on experience of losing a patient.

Also, as she sat up nursing the pathetic creature throughout a long, horrid night, loss hit hard. Failure, after a round of exemplary dedication expected of a budding vet, ended at four pm, when foal finally expired.

Calder tried to comfort with a generous, sympathetic hug. 'Now, you understand why vet schools insist on students seeing practice.'

Tone and body melded into her firmed. 'In truth, you should be grateful for opportunity to witness this case, this loss. Because it must fortify emotions, strengthen character to help you cope in future cases.'

Although he offered genuine sound advice, it was insufficient to improve the girl's demeanour, and she threw arms around him and squeezed out remaining tears from already overworked tear glands.

He held, then gave her a suggestive squeeze, associated with palms caressing her back then bum said, 'But in the meantime, take six hours sleep. Need your help with the two, three foals expected tonight.'

While hopeful of pressing his suit later, walked away.

Faith moved slow as any automated snail when she climbed staircase to the staff rooms.

Until excited chattering caused her to pause and peer through an elegantly formed one yard diameter, circular window on the landing halfway up the stairs. A custom-made stained-glass window depicted a mare as her muzzle nuzzled her sitting foal's ear and fitted the scene.

Even in her exhausted mood, happy voices, which could otherwise have drawn a smile, raised alarm. Through the unmarked glass to left of the mare's head, she watched, puzzled at where Calder and Georgiou chatted in a discreet and freezing corner of the yard.

What makes these two share big smiles and high fives when they should share and express my sadness over us losing that valuable foal. Bizarre.

Exhaustion claimed Faith.

Worn out, tired after her marathon nursing effort, sleep attacked.

Until her alarm clock dragged her away from the allotted six hours.

Showered, dressed warm for the coming night.

But vets' unusual behaviour lay trapped in her brain where it caused intense mental deliberation, again, as they left her increasingly concerned over the unusual circumstances she detected after losing the foal. *Cannot avoid this. So, let me call dad.*

First things first, ravenous, tucked into a delicious, nutritious lamb stew with a savoury rice salad but resisted digging into more than a sliver of tempting apple upside down cake and cream.

Moved back to her room and when satisfied the corridor empty, phoned her father.

He was most unimpressed with the story she reported. 'Dislike this turn of events. Must contact Sophia, although no! Best you pass this information on yourself to Inspector de Freitas.'

As he replaced the receiver, her face changed. Twice.

First, thought of Sophia which brought out a soft smile.

Then, barely two seconds later, lips tensed. *Faith, what are you mixed up in? Please stay safe.*

'An excellent idea. Promise to take care.'

Faith never got time to begin as Sophia, after she ended a conversation with Alroy, moved on. 'How nice to hear from you. Hope this means you and your father accept my invitation to visit, for I look forward to entertaining you, showing you chaps around town.'

'Now Sophia. Suspect you mean dad should visit by himself as your burgeoning friendship means you hide things from me.'

After a mere five minutes, while they only began exploring the start of something special, Faith launched into her description of recent events.

Sophia, now again a smart police officer, shared delight to receive that information and barely gave Faith time to pour out her unexpurgated version of the dead foal and how death thrilled the vets before she demanded. 'Odd. Now Faith, need you to repeat the story in depth.

Satisfied she soaked up all facts, she said, 'Agree with your father, not pukka behaviour, but tell me. Can you find any connection between the vets and the foals background? For instance, the owner.'

'No!' Faith spluttered. 'No. Cannot believe I discounted what may be valuable information. Saunders owns the mare. Same trainer who killed Heraldon... and poor Shaun.'

'Yes, indeed! Solid information.' Sophia's increasing fondness for Faith, and her father, reacted. 'Promise to take immediate action. For your excellent information pushes this to the top of my in-tray.'

Thought for a moment. 'Must pass on your phone number to a local police station. For fear that you dig into something major, dangerous, we need someone, a big brother watching over you.'

Faith paused; gasped at thought Sophia should consider it necessary to take that step. 'Shall now phone your father.'

'Hi Jermaine, trust you are well.'

Twenty minutes later, after she closed the call, Sophia pressed her back against a wall in her lounge and encouraged a soft breath to slip from moist, open lips.

While she caressed them with a finger spoke to the wall mirror. 'While I worry over Faith, that man attracts me as none in years. Hmm! Let us hope this case, and my increasing involvement with Flowers family proves a success.'

58

YORKSHIRE DETECTIVES

Sophia rushed to update Henry.

Sensed a crucial element to Faith's information.

Despite years targeting serious crime with Interpol, since working with Alroy's team, their dedication and superb investigative skills added a different dimension to her efforts.

While unexpected, she grew with them, as they did her, and under Alroy's influence, how he bathed them with a sense of family, not only a workforce, but they also reinvigorated her career when she never appreciated it necessary.

Yet, as a career officer, and content in single life, sensed inexplicable possibilities in relationships with the Flower's family.

Unsearched for affiliations uncovered needs hidden for years.

As a hibernating hedgehog awakens after a hard winter, with an urgent, pressing need for growth to replace condition lost during its long sleep, so too Sophia appreciated inner emptiness hidden in her bedroom cupboard.

No, silly woman. You do not wish for nor desire a family.

Repeated and reinforced opinion of no time for effort, dependents, or similar human distractions.

With power of any determined and focused individual who appreciated and acted on vocational nature of her profession, she slapped down those notions.

Go girl. Forget that worthless notion. Concentrate on snaring naughty people.

Given these points, she, rooted in normal solid life, joined Henry, then they enlisted Alroy's opinion.

Their brief discussion about two vets and the dead foal, left him concerned the increased amount of information they faced threatened to overload their force. For this, although he still considered that part of the investigation a lesser important case than their hunt for corrupt officers, remained significant.

Accepted their keenness and planned to collaborate with them.

Altogether, with that intense discussion, freshly fuelled by an almost girlish approach from Sophia's sparkling eyes, opened doors more significant than Alroy imagined he summarised.

'Sense Faith presents us with smart information. Her desire to help us is a significant help, although,' Issued Sophia with a silent, empathetic instruction, then vocalised his concern. 'we must protect her.'

How time unfolds secrets hidden in fatty lump that is the human brain. Tucked inside its hard bony shell, with humanity far from using its capacity. For instance, the growth of the computer industry barely touches on power possibilities of an organ loaded with problem solving possibilities.

The moon landing depended on massive scientific and mathematical calculations. Their total computing capability far less than those contained in an inexpensive model mobile telephone.

So, ask the question. When scientists enable us to unlock hidden, dormant brain power, how much can we learn?

Only then may we unravel, explain, and act on the plethora of subconscious instructions that synaptic transmissions hammer us with.

May we, as evolving sentient humans, by acting on the Divine instruction, seize opportunity to be the ultimate neighbour loving designed by our creator?

Within their environment, Alroy, as one with a natural efficiency to tap into brain resources, often sensed facts and easily discarded hunches, appreciated and acted on Sophia's outstanding detective work and opinions.

Without delay, originated two steps. First, increasingly aware of Sophia's concerns for the girl's safety, affirmed her opinion around the need for special security. 'Time to involve others.'

Instructed Sophia to instigate a discrete surveillance plan with local force to monitor Faith, be aware that should she suspect herself in danger, they, while understanding bare facts could react with speed.

Her forthright, logical approach when she informed that sensitive area was under control brought nods of encouragement.

Alroy, content Sophia covered that problem, broadened their approach by suggesting while they had enough on the two vets to bring them in for questioning, wished for additional evidence. 'Much as I should prefer to send you up to York again, time constraints mean you are valuable here as we spread the net.'

Logic dictated while they wished to continue running their operation quiet and clean, they needed field support. 'Consider it safe for us to get local officers in York itself to sniff around.'

Despite how notion of further visits to York appealed, Sophia exhaled a slow, tender sigh of relief. 'Phew! Glad to hear your thinking aligns with mine. For we own too many lines of urgent investigation with our bigger fish at present.'

First, Henry contacted both teams, and despite the growing temptation to combine forces, continued as two separate units. When sounding them out, hoped to find one with Yorkshire contacts.

With his own team, via DI Mandy, got a hit; in the words of Hamlet, a very palpable hit, when she offered an item from her background that promised effective support. 'Sure thing, Sir. Know Chief Inspector George Rodin. A sound chap. Since he and I enjoyed early years working together and based in Ripon, can recommend him. Should prove the top man for the job.'

Spent time detailing how best Mandy could approach the office.

After she spent five minutes catching up with George, Mandy, she outlined their labour constraints, asked for his help.

Filled him in on their concerns over two vets, primarily potential involvement in the dodgy business associated with horses.

'While in its infancy, we suspect them worthy of closer investigation.'

With that under his belt, asked him to check into official electrical compliance report authorities issued for the Saunders training yard. Mandy caught him at an opportune time. Since their normally hectic life normalised with them closing a car theft ring and associated chop shops.

'Besides, with the number of arrests we made, my DS thinks sun shines out of my units ear holes.' That said, described himself as an animal lover, admitted to still experiencing uneasy sensations around how easily insurance companies laid down and died over the Heraldon incident.

'Disappoints me the local force investigated horse deaths.' Imagined him flapping arms. 'Why, Mandy, they virtually ignored the groom's death. If anything, untoward went down, at least manslaughter charges are possible.'

Impressed with his sense of outrage and dedication which convinced her she found the right man for the job.

Realised that triggered a tender spot and listened as he dropped the bit and stampeded for the finishing line. 'Sorry to repeat myself, but with that boy's death, they ought to have instructed a task force, a specialised unit to uncover missing evidence.'

Heard him tap pen against desk, during a five second pause. 'Gut,' The massive, untapped computing power of his brain, prompted him onward, 'tells me we must clean up that unsavoury case.'

Likewise, declared keenness to help Mandy. 'Always wished we could work together.'

Set to detail two top officers. 'Discrete, experienced, wholeheartedly my men. They can probe your suspects.'

On balance, impressed Mandy, when three days later, reported back with corroborating evidence required to guarantee their unit ready to charge the two vets. 'Money flowed.'

While he thanked her for offering them an interesting job. DI Rodin detailed investigation into the vet's financial background.

'At first, concentrated on the Greek chap.'

Added vegetables into the stewing mix when he advised her the vet, Houdalakis never completed his course of veterinary studies in Athens and had never applied to the RCVS to have his name enrolled for practicing in Britain. 'A fraud Mandy. Could pick him up on that alone.'

She, while enthusiastic asked him to hold back. 'Have not yet exhausted our enquiries there, so although I thank you for uncovering that useful snippet, expect those vets to lead us into something, as yet not quantifiable, but on a larger scale.'

Without delay, as DI Rodin warmed to the case, continued. 'Found nothing interesting or unusual in his bank records. Except he receives significant funding, legally presented, and declared to Inland Revenue from his father. He, as I am sure you are aware, operates as a significant gang lord in Athens.'

After he underscored the bogus vet lived well, much better than a professional salary could provide, Mandy's investigative juices flowed, as Rodin reiterated his regular monthly income from his Greek family.

Shared his dislike for the family, while elaborating on them as active, unveiled crooks, mixed up in diverse nasty criminal activities. 'Cannot understand how, after a few basic enquiries, my DI easily uncovered traces of downright corruption, fraud, and intimidation.'

The Houdalakis family intimidated his sense of decency and caused him to issue an uncharacteristic expletive. 'Sorry, Mandy. But this smack of sloppy, well, even dodgy police corruption. Why does Interpol not swamp these people?'

Now with that off his chest, whispered. 'A hushed word with a Vice Squad DCI from times past informed me they suspected them, and while I hate the suggestion, human trafficking is also possible. Nasty people.'

After he added minor bits and pieces to Georgiou's family, she said, 'Nice one, George.' DI Mandy, most pleased declared her hunch right. 'Knew you were the man to ferret this information. They closed off on Georgiou's form.

Nonetheless, hoping for more, she pressed on. 'Ask if you established anything useful with the second vet?'

'His name is Calder Stewart, and yes, uncovered a valuable morsel. Had a significant, recent financial windfall of at least forty thousand pounds. That enabled him to settle significant debts.'

Mandy thought nothing when he named vet as Calder Stewart. For yet, the Stewart name remained unknown to her, so nothing clicked.

'If he received commission on his involvement in killing Heraldon, could he have been so stupid as to use the cash in such an easily traceable manner?'

'Well... You know the expression. If criminals were brain surgeons.'

Mandy shared his chortles and presumed rolls of fat over chubby cheeks danced in time. 'Dead right and reflecting on our careers. How often have we nicked idiots with brilliant schemes for doing something stupid?'

Added an import pointer to clarify where Calder may have earned his money. 'DS Bothwell tracked the insurance payouts, and bingo. Stewart banked his cash a mere three days after insurance company released the funds.'

He, as officers often do, concluded his report by saying, 'In conclusion, am now more dissatisfied than ever with our handling of this case. Thanks to your prompting me, appreciate they failed to conclude the case as one expects.'

Added how, when they issued detailed electrical compliance certification, before the accident, and investigation afterward, on Saunders' yard, they correctly outlined the house and the two main stable blocks.'

Then explained they ignored the lesser yard at the rear of the premises. 'Daft. Because the accident occurred there.'

'Brilliant work. My boss will relish this evidence.'

The lines vibrated with a sense of their empathy and mutual satisfaction over a job well done.

As Mandy prepared to release Rodin to his normal duties, she took one last dig. 'Now. And will pester you no more after this. final opinion. Could that omission be fraudulent or simply negligent?'

'Possible they pressurised an aging, overworked engineer who simply could not get around to it.'

Closed off by promising to send her the detailed reports.

59

GOOD POLICE WORK

Pauline and Bernard were not yet privy to Mandy' information.

Worked in an office steeped in promising events.

Animated by events that appeared to launch towards a successful conclusion, they jabbered, shared their bubbling enthusiasm.

Albeit recent research meant both teams engaged in office work, arranged a meeting for Alroy's team.

First, travelled old ground.

Necessary to bring their wolf pack up to speed on events that unfolded fast as any Highland river in full spate after a sudden spring thaw melts snow.

Prepared the soil, ensured when they uncovered staggering evidence, they collated it formally, to ensure their team understood significant points, involved them as one.

With Bernard up, he explained how, and when taking great care, followed their last meeting, as instructed, tapped Diane Pastor's phone. They appreciated his enormous technical experience and followed his drift when he explained measures. 'Careful, it took time to breakthrough their efficient security measures. Tricky.'

Relished how, with mouths hanging open, they absorbed every word. 'So, discretely monitored her movements.' Yet, never sought plaudits, merely outlined sensitive nature of skilled probing.

Pauline's obvious excitement spilled over. Unable to contain herself, nodded at Bernard. 'In this game, sometimes we need or deserve a touch of luck. Clapped her hands, enthusiastic as a teenager receiving her first mobile phone. 'And boy, did we get lucky?'

Bernard detailed how he scored with a single, short phone call from Pastor's second, rarely used cell phone. If not a burner, hoped it secure. Recounted how she delivered an interesting fact. 'The DI called her cousin, a Susan Boyd, to enquire after her daughter.'

Outlined where the girl sustained serious injuries during a motor vehicle accident.'

After he allotted seconds for that to sink in, exhibited flamboyance and dexterity of a card shark, continued. 'Furthermore, as Pastor slipped deeper into a difficult, emotional patch, she informed Suzan how she and her friend had an escape plan.'

Paused, noticed how Pauline studied expressions on the team's faces, delighted none sniffed where Bernard's investigation led, glad to spin out intrigue longer. 'Then the big one. Hinted how with them preparing to surface big, meant success should soon find her and Geraldine together, permanently so.'

Officers paused, drank in how puzzled team members searched each other's perplexed faces for clues. For instance, shared curiosity of a dog blubbering over three-day-old lamb chop bones buried in a bin.

'Will play the entire recording for you later.'

When Pauline invited Bernard to finish, he described how Pastor, aware she said too much, ended that call. Abrupt, manner indicated obvious embarrassment at recklessly dropping hectic information.

Pauline came in again. 'Next, our super sleuth got even busier.'

Boundless energy, excitement, and appreciation for his remarkable skill... and something else overflowed when she gave Bernard a most unprofessional hug, which raised eyebrows and kicked off a creeping trail of innuendo.

'Bernard, after more searching around, produced distinct possibility Geraldine mentioned was none other than...' Milked this by asking a question. 'But first, has anyone guessed, identified this, Geraldine?'

Enjoyed them wracking brains. until Bernard exclaimed. 'Come on, Pauline. Get this out or I will expose her.'

After a wicked smile he delivered the coup de grace. 'We believe the Geraldine is... none other than, Assistant Commissioner Geraldine Flynn.'

Alroy and Henry glanced at each other.

Speechless, amazed at this staggering evidence.

In time, Alroy re-oxygenating spent lungs, asked. 'Could she be the one the boss tracks? Wow.'

With energy of flooding water as it races downstream when liberated by the opening of the barrage on the River Leven, Pauline, and Bernard, effervescent as any ever, spoke at the same time, until Bernard gave way to her.

Pauline explained how, rather than raise a red herring with premature conjecture, they took this further. 'So, and here accepts as senior officer, my decision, we organised a detailed investigation.'

For fear that she stretched authority, apologised to Alroy. 'Sorry for not keeping you in the loop, sir, but understanding your busy schedule, we pushed on.'

Bernard then described their findings. 'So, we spent three days tailing the AC.'

Alroy advised team he appreciated initiative, but cast doubt on their inadvisable, unsolicited actions, warned they should always act within comfortable lines. 'In investigations of this importance, especially when investigating senior officers, bounce all difficult or controversial subjects off Henry.

Bernard, satisfied with that slight reprimand, gave Pauline an extravagant high-five. 'Our story improves.' Advised how they picked up a US connection. 'They also discussed an FBI agent called Leipzig. Named him as valuable support.'

Bernard scarce gave them time to absorb that fact, before he recounted, they spotted the AC in conversation with DI Pastor. Again, milked the situation, went on. 'And then, a clandestine meeting followed when she teamed up with Superintendent Alastair Gordon.

Raised eyebrows when he revealed intimate things transpired between them. Although he heard none of their discussion, subject revolved around unprofessional activity. 'Now for the TV soapy bits. The kissy-kissy bits between her and Pastor blew me away.'

When noise settled, outlined how Gordon also tried to get romantic with her, but cross, she kept him at arm's length.

Henry's comments added to scene's intrigue. 'Is she having a relationship, affairs with both?' Even an experienced officer took time to adjust to crisp, powerful evidence.

Pauline indicated the depth of their exploration when she said, 'Worth noting past events. Since she and Gordon had an affair years ago.'

Alroy said, 'Can add to this. For I planned introducing comments divulged by DS Mamad in Henry's team. He reported whisperings around Gordon's name in the force as someone who raised interest as one to watch.'

Reminded them Henry's team remained unaware of who they hunted, then added. 'So, Henry, earlier than planned, time to merge both teams.'

The group snuffled along the trail and when they picked up the foetid scent of corruption, landed in pack mode. Soon, prepared for the hunt, reacted even before Bernard added fresh evidence when he filled them in on more details he and Pauline collected. 'Lip reading is good. Excellent, so can with confidence claim she arranged two separate meetings with each for Friday.'

'Sorry guys.' All, including Alroy, trembled with excitement as they entered attack mode. Take coffee while Henry and I chat.'

Alroy asked Henry's opinion. 'Am still processing implications around this juicy evidence, how it piles up around us.'

Even the vastly experienced Henry shuffled reports on his desk, nervously pushed them around. 'Big brass indeed. A DS and an AC. Mindboggling.'

Alroy unlocked his dormant, brilliant brain and allowed eyes to glimmer when they processed information, besides, he planned a logical format for the next series of steps to take them forward and reflected on inherent dangers.

'Take care. As evidence unfolds, so too does opportunity for experienced officers to pick up on our lines of enquiry. 'Have concerns, Henry, if we frighten one player away, this investigation could collapse.

With thought processes aligned along similar lines and sequences few could follow he laid groundwork. 'Now Henry, prepare to move fast. For this involves a single, huge, sophisticated group.'

Here, aware of Henry's useful and incisive opinions, Alroy elongated his pause to reflect before propounding ideas. 'Agree with you for our officers do fantastic work. Now, we face a fascinating situation where investigations come to a head.'

Tapped fingers against a palm. 'With one decisive thrust, we may wrap up several syndicates in harmony.'

In synch, Alroy said, 'I should now contact Wolf, involve him.'

'Indeed. Glad you consider that a smart move. For too much happens now, far too much.' Reflected. 'While you take on that responsibility, please allow me to unite the teams, bring them together. Need two days to introduce end game. When they merge, then we can collate updated evidence and processes, for you to fill in the blanks. Take us forward.'

60

WOLF

Alroy caught Wolf on his private, still virgin line.

First time during the team's nine months existence.

In command, Alroy decided their operations fit for purpose. *Time, to update the Commissioner.*

Used three words. 'We must meet.'

'Right.'

Commissioner closed off the phone.

Two hours later, DS Anderson almost broke her severe protocol when she smiled in the same family orientated manner as the rest of her team, Alroy encouraged and she now assimilated, said, 'So, how sharp is your golf?'

Thought little of what might have been an odd question on any other day, but now already anticipated a coded message from his boss. So, he chuckled, acknowledged, while it needs practice, considered it decent.

To which she replied. 'Admirable, for I received an instruction from the Commissioner's office. From our DI Pauline's friend, DI *Pastor.*' Nice emphasis there.

Attitude revealed further softening encouraged by excellent interaction with her splendid team, as she continued. 'The Top Man expressed a wish for his senior officers to join him for a series of golf afternoons. Furthermore, as he names you on the list, here are the details.'

She, as all were, aware of him contacting Wolf, tittered again when she handed him a piece of paper.

Memo indicated how the Commissioner considered he neglected his top brass.

On balance, to remedy this, invited fourteen of them to golf.

With his first round planned in two days and weekly thereafter, during subsequent weeks, he relished entertaining them, to listen to any gripes. Dates booked on a first come basis.

Anderson, aware of his intentions, dropped normal formality and responded to the high-five he offered.

Then, shook herself, stood to attention, reported she already booked Alroy on the first session.

Henry and team enjoyed Commissioner's skill in arranging a secret meeting during an overt function.

Further rejoiced that Flynn, herself a fair player, was booked for the following week.

61

GOLF, OR GOLF?

The exclusive Walton Heath course.

One of the world's best, highly rated by Jack Nicklaus.

Tricky to book, unless, as Commissioner of Police, you access best connections.

Four officers met on the terrace at the clubhouse for coffee.

In time, Commissioner kicked off the fun. 'Straightaway, as the most junior member, our rookie Superintendent.' Others enjoyed him nodding at Alroy. 'To begin with, sanction you to witness my humiliation during holes eight through eleven in my company.'

Turned to Superintendent Groves. 'Need to chat with you, Jack. Get your opinion on something, so please support me through seven holes. Conrad can then carry me through the rest. How does that sound?'

In grand form, expressed his pleasure. 'Must do this often, get out of the office with my team. Always savour lunch here. Although,' Rubbed his tummy, 'that seems a long way away. So, let us get on.'

Changed partners at hole seven.

Talk, because of widely dispersed shots, centred on nothing of importance.

With diligent, expert caddies, managed only idle chit chat around insubstantial material, until halfway down eleventh fairway, Alroy deliberately hooked his four iron to arrange their balls side by side.

Wolf motioned for the caddies to stand back from them. 'Report. Brief.'

As Alroy filled him in, he apologised. 'Sorry sir. Unwelcome news. We confidently implicate three officers, including your PA. Now, evidence takes a terrible twist.'

When Alroy hesitated, Wolf barked. 'Out with it, man.' Lined up his Ping seven iron and actions, if observed by those nearest, suggested him disinterested in having the younger man's company.

'The leader is AC Floyd.'

Without delay, as Wolf hit his shot it snapped a clean crack marking as loud as his cry of, 'Flynn. The whore. Are you sure?'

'Yes.' Amazed Alroy to watch the Commissioner's ball, despite distraction, land in centre of the green.

Wolf swore again. 'A ***** mess.'

Alroy continued. 'We also implicate Superintendent Alastair Gordon.'

If Commissioner's outward appearance never changed, a faint quiver ran through his voice as he attempted to control emotions. 'Gordon always worried me because of his bloody yellow handed masonic handshake. Something I cannot yet eradicate from the force. But Flynn. Never guessed her involvement.'

Then, added cream on the pie.

Alroy declared they also implicated an FBI agent named Leipzig.'

'Also, fabulous news. Picked up his name two years ago, but trail went soft. If active, that gives me a chance to get one over the Yanks. Much as I love them. Brilliant.'

After Alroy finished his report, Wolf, as he prepared to move off the green, said, 'If you need anything get it. Drugs, diamonds, bent cops. Together. Jings lad and my hunch in handing you the job proves sound. Nail the bastards; all three. Together.' Thus ended their meeting.

Alroy filled Henry in after lunch the following day.

'Right, then.' Henry rose, raring to go. Briefed both teams. Now, after our intensive, and worthwhile two-day seminar, we can work together, understand each other.'

Content they were prepared he said, 'Come boss, lead us into the end game of this remarkable hunt.'

'After lunch, time for us to appreciate their skills. Let them guide us along a sound path.'

62

HENRY'S TEAM AGAIN

On an obvious high, Sophia captured Alroy.

Anxious to catch up with him.

Determined to grab the initiative, she beat him to it. 'Morning, Sir. Can we please chat before the full meeting?'

Prepared to make everyone aware of how his updated, freshly engineered system must fall into place, he enjoyed serendipity of the moment but put her off. 'Make it after lunch, for then I can give you twenty minutes before we must sound out the others. Set this up through DS Anderson. Then, with both teams integrated, may astonish you at recent developments. So much to discuss.'

Regardless of his best intentions, he only finished with Sophia around two thirty.

When they entered the ops room, thrilled him to find officers chattered in an atmosphere as supercharged as any remembered. Reminded him of a weasel family, noisily integrating while munching a half-grown rabbit.

Alroy inhaled a lingering, noiseless breath to focus thinking. *Sense their expectancy, can feed from their enthusiasm. Here we go.*

Began by reiterating intentions from the beginning. Who formed the team and why. With everyone introduced, of preeminent importance, spotted early signs of the harmony necessary to take them forward.

Part of his talk matched and duplicated Henry's report, but that never mattered.

For fear they miss anything, outlined why they set each team off on different tracks. With their different investigative roles separate, admired how Henry's team, aided by Mandy's intuitive skills, presented valuable information.

His job demanded he collate their effort into a single, cohesive unit.

Given that, paused for three seconds then turned to the original team and issued instructions. Attitude, professional as ever, established him their true leader. One not only competent but also determined to, and capable of leading them along a road destined to transport them to achieve extraordinary success.

Stern, advised on rule changes, introduced updated operational factors to encourage discipline, leadership and maintain order. 'From now, as we enter what may be your most significant takedown ever, the situation changes. Demand you accept the normal chain of command with deserved formality.'

Surveyed the room and clapped hands. 'So, officers. Do I explain my instructions clearly?'

In synch, the *yes sirs* rang out from all, including Henry.

Content with that harmonious event Alroy continued. 'Restrict boiling stuff for later, fearful of causing so much excitement, we risk downplaying additional information.'

Invited Henry to take the floor. 'CI Higgins. Because your chaps uncovered salient information on the diamond story. Share that now.'

Team absorbed that trail of information, although most fidgeted, impatient as they wondered what route they must navigate along that avenue.

'Thanks Sir.' DI Mandy McDonald and DS Mamad Aswat moved to the front.

McDonald led them through trails they established for routes that supported blood diamonds from Africa via China and Russia.

Sharp and succinct, ended. 'It will take time to define how these lanes operate, blend together but the China-Russia connection clears.' Those new to her enjoyed listening to a smart, skilful presentation. Her odd posing, the Jamaican Rumba, caught Pauline's eye.

Next came Aswat. 'The Chinese are not as sharp in their dealings as expected of most high-powered criminals. Loose tongued, they make careless errors when dealing with clients and business partners.'

In danger of departing from standard business talk, a great smile split his face. 'From the Zhāng family, particularly twins Chun and Daquan, we detect potent evidence.'

Hesitant, for he remained concerned this must disrupt the force: excused himself for reiterating doubts which undermined authority, as he criticised how top brass failed to react in a positive manner. 'Amid increasing whispers around weak leadership at best, or downright fraud, we do not move forward as expected.'

DS Frank Brookee, proud of investigative work he and DS Abisade Kasir conducted on the China and Russian question using normal detective principles, shocked to find their techniques basic when they listened to DS Bernard Collins.

Bernard helped him out when he explained his plan to improve efficiency by demonstrating updated equipment and support structures the following morning. 'Since some techniques include groundbreaking procedures, a practical demonstration may help define our aims, outline surveillance stages of the project.'

Alroy and Henry met again. 'So, we agree on the way forward?' Alroy interrupted himself when he coughed hard for thirty seconds. Until, after he cleared his throat, said, 'Sorry. Looks like I come down with something. At an inconvenient time.'

Henry nodded but never commented on Alroy's illness. 'If only we can keep this under wraps. A matter of time. So, yes.'

When they joined the others, Alroy, protected his voice, encouraged Henry to outline shocking news of their investigations into bent cops. They already reeling from preliminary information released by Henry during their seminar, barely reacted. Soon gobsmacked as Henry when he left nothing out, filled them in on the entire situation.

An immense trail of corruption and fraud which none dreamed possible inside the force.

As he watched, the Henry glare missed nothing, absorbed how seasoned officers reeled at shocking news of how they prepared to nail three officers. Senior ones. 'Have changed our surveillance plans related to a need for an increased labour force. Because, by linking both teams our next moves will benefit from increased cover.'

Alroy instructed Bernard and Frank to team up, to prepare a foolproof tracking system to listen in on meetings between Flynn and Gordon, Flynn, and Pastor. 'Our big hope is they meet at or close to last time. You chaps can get your best, and I mean absolute top range surveillance equipment in place after this meeting. When set up for tomorrow, the whole team can attend the demonstration.'

63

TECH STUFF

Alroy never needed their approval.

Displayed the spirit of all top leaders.

Sat back, attentive, listened, enjoyed their constructive comments.

Encouraged Henry to correct misapprehensions and to answer most questions and admired his easy, off-the-cuff approach. Straightforward, his approach and knowledge of the subject established how well he assimilated, then studied their accumulating evidence. *This man understands his business. Accept Wolf's decision for insisting to involve him.*

Sat back, prepared to enjoy Bernard's dissertation on security measures and what he termed *hot snooping stuff.*

As always trembled with excitement at opportunity to introduce salient facts. 'We begin by tweaking all existing CCV telecommunication in that general area where we suspect they intend meeting.'

As he lifted his head, DS Brooke asked around dangers of discussing requirements with City of London's information technologists.

Bernard, never anticipated what he deemed an irrelevant question, appreciated how others played eager to him answer. 'Of course, my fault. Best I describe my own sophisticated computer programs, how they allow me to divorce actions from standard operating systems.'

Thanked DS Alroy for providing funds, and then DI Pauline who in her normal but extraordinary fashion sourced equipment. 'Thanks to them we own the most significant computerised system in any police force.'

Second nature to him, never understood how others reacted to his expertise.

'Thus, I can infiltrate their CCV systems and tweak them with necessary improvements. Wise operators may spot the changes but will never tie them down to being manipulated from an external source.'

With room dead silent, explained how they reinforced visual part of the process with additional local and distance devices. 'Only the US Airforce employs the detailed investigative audio systems necessary to provide our required cover.'

Overall, reluctant to reveal all, only Alroy knew Bernard tapped into their systems, piggy-backed on freshest upgrades.

Colleagues glowed at Bernard's skill.

Until he interrupted. 'Yes, we can do this.'

Alroy, dismayed at his deteriorating health, surmised he shivered because of a virus. After an ugly, barking cough, he went on. 'Repeat this will unfold as a top-notch investigation. DI Collins will source everything required.'

A splash of a smile played round his lips. 'Fast.'

She said, 'Yes sir. At once.'

This evidence and detailed technical support were new to DS Brooke, himself one of the Met's top ten computer junkies... sorry, technicians. In time, he excited not just at their targets but also rejoiced knowing where he must learn from DS Collins, whom he already designated, *The Maestro*.

Alroy forced himself to ignore a woolly throat and almost skipped for joy. 'Good.' Turned to DI McDonald, 'You, with DI Pauline and DS Mamad form the surveillance ground team will monitor their movements. You cannot be directly involved in observing their meetings.'

Nodded in Bernard's direction. 'Our boffins will no doubt employ bits and pieces to help your distance observations.' Explained their role must find them incarcerated for hours inside a specialised surveillance unit.

Looked at Bernard who accepted his cue and explained he arranged for local electricity board team to place a large unit over an access hole. 'Anyone who checks the job sheet will find this marked as an underground cable fault. They will not understand it created by my naughty manipulation.'

As he ended, Alroy experienced a severe coughing fit, one bad enough to alarm DI Castle. 'Gosh, Alroy... sorry Superintendent Stewart. Are you okay? Not nice.' Waved her off. 'Thanks for your concern. Fine. Too much work, anyway.'

Henry took over. 'The weakest area in our work is failure to identify what was after all our original remit. As yet, we fail to trace vets here and, in the US, involved in insurance scams that involve killing horses.' Managed a weak smile. 'Now, thanks to DI McDonald, and proficient Yorkshire police we establish promising information which points directly at two local vets. But need more.'

Directed his next remark to Sophia. 'That remains your primary focus, although supported by me and DS Kamir. Who are they? Where are they?' Shared her puzzlement. 'Since the story unfolds exciting disclosures, important we miss nothing.' Paused for comment.

With nothing forthcoming, developed his theme. 'Short on time, we have not yet dug into the US side of things. If you remember, we hoped to focus attention on insurance scams.' Almost pleaded. 'Need a breakthrough to offer direction. Anything.'

After coughed again, harder, excused himself then struggled on. 'We follow two active vets in England, and although not yet linked to the US, they may be key players. But if I am wrong, hopefully so, it helps us establish something along those lines. Yes!'

Laid out various possibilities that must prove valuable in that direction, then broke for refreshments.

Sophia was next up.

Her role took them into the insurance investigation. 'In all honesty, while we study big insurance claims, find it time consuming. Can I focus on them for now? Will search connections to these vets' names and copy files for DS Kamir.'

'Agree with you and indeed am embarrassed we may have backgrounded useful material.'

DS Anderson joined in. 'May I assist, for my desk is now quieter after merging both groups.'

Sophia liked that. 'Sound. Could knock our heads together.' Pursed lips. 'Wonder DS   Stewart if it now timeous to investigate Faith Flowers story in greater detail?'

Her secondary intention proved impossible to control, thus a smile traced early lines around eyes. Thought of the Flower's family brought warmth of spicy butternut soup on a freezing day. 'From DI Mandy's observations, am positive something crooked involves at least one of them. The vet Houdalakis. Hope further digging will nail them down.'

Alroy, after he initially nodded agreement, asked her to hold back. 'Yes and no.' Walked around the room as though exercise settled thoughts. A sudden, piercing bolt of sun broke through dense, low clouds and as it unexpectedly bathed him in warmth, caused Mandy's mind to wander. *Now that is a fine-looking man.*

Alroy returned to the subject. 'Because we own sufficient information to bring them in, the temptation to act is obvious and logical. We can nail them, yet I caution patience.'

With Mandy interested in exploring that trail, she interrupted. 'Sorry Sir. Do you consider these vets are either eager beavers starting their criminal career, or estimate they may lead us into the something bigger we hope lies in the offing?'

'Suggest with time on our sides, we continue to allow patience to rule. For, when we swoop and at the risk of repeating myself, hopefully yes. Moreover, am convinced they will lead into something bigger, over the pond.'

As he prepared to move on, he said, 'But DI McDonald, you impressed me with excellent work in Yorkshire. When time permits, please remind me to phone DI Rodin personally and commend his action formally to his superintendent. But for now, continue.'

64

LONDON

Sophia and DS Anderson got stuck in.

Six hours later, DS Anderson reported.

'Twice picked up the same names. Anything valuable from your side?'

Sophia agreed. 'Spot an interesting pair. Names of interest are Yvette Ghent and Louis Hennessey.'

'Bingo. Identified them as well. Bingo and bingo again.'

Anderson turned to her external keyboard and banged away. Forceful typing meant her unable to employ internal keyboards for she destroyed them with alarming regularity, which meant she maintained a backup collection of external, Bluetooth units.

After one minute she looked up. 'Now, Inspector, will you run information through the data base program Bernard set up for us in the early days of our investigations? Which will permit me to concentrate on this side, by researching American thoroughbred stud books and vet registers.'

Sophia searched Bernard's sophisticated system and soon, spat out a profound gosh, impressed at his efficiency, better than anything ever experienced. 'Bang, bang, bang, seven hits.'

Added Yvette into the mix and spewed out a further six hits. Turned to Anderson. 'Find useful information this side. How are you doing?'

'There, and yes! Got them. The American vet association confirm they share the same practice details. Nice one. Hold that thought.' Ten seconds later, confirmed them recently married.

Overall, smart, they established both vets had originally practiced from the same Florida hospital until, after a flurry of insurance claims, relocated two and a half years earlier to New York State.

With Sophia, now convinced them a couple, found, after two hours research, she could tie them down with solid evidence. 'Noted Louis' signature on three death certificates.' 'Almost there...'

She lost time with an irrelevant phone call.

Voice shared a flicker of disapproval over time wasted as she said, 'Now, uncover her signature on two insurance certificates. Confident more will follow.'

Sophia's tone solidified. 'Got them. This cannot be a coincidence. Time for Henry to hop on a plane and dig around from that side.'

Ds Anderson disagreed. We should first discuss this with Superintendent Alroy, but not DCI Henry, for Sophia, with your horse background this is right up your street.'

Pauline at once contacted Alroy with the news, and as he concurred Sophia booked a flight to New York for early the following morning.'

In the city, there was an important development when Sophia could not follow up with her proposed meeting with Faith Flowers. Had to change her itinerary because of that urgent visit to New York which prevented her from following up that lead.

Passed this on to Pauline who rang Faith and apologised. 'However, while it pleases me to understand you are well, if I deliver photographs, can you find time to examine them?'

Faith, pleased with how well she settled into her role as Sophia's willing confident, however, got nervous after Pauline explained the vet owned a high profile. For, as Calder's name surfaced, they traced his association with Georgiou.

Horror followed.

Tragic news.

Pauline needed less than ten minutes to identify Calder as Alroy's brother.

Faith, increasingly aware of Sophia and her father's warnings, concerned over possible danger associated with dishonest vets and a plethora of ugly repercussions. With trust in Sophia holding fast, she reluctantly agreed to work with Pauline after she received a call from Sophia who apologised, explained it impossible to miss out on an unexpected and important international trip. 'Sorry, precious one. This cannot wait until I complete my trip. So, Faith, my friend, please work with DI Pauline.'

Pauline laid out a safe plan for Faith. 'Arranged our trustworthy courier to make a secure delivery to Newmarket, your local Police Station. Could you be there at lunchtime, say around twelve thirty?'

On balance, she assuaged the girl's anxiety and with Faith eager to help, grew in confidence as Pauline explained. 'DI Lotter will assist you. Trust him implicitly, but only declare your code name as Helen Dangerfield, not where you work or with whom you interact. Study the photograph, then act duplicitous. Shake your head, make them believe your obvious disappointment at failing to recognise the man depicted on the photographs. Please say nothing. Nor will he expect any comment.'

To emphasise, Pauline, determined they keep the project top secret, added. 'Ask you to take possession of the photograph. Secret it somewhere or if nervous burn it. Forbid anyone else opportunity to view this sensitive information.'

Faith, amid an unexpected two day drop in the number of expected foalings, enjoyed the serendipity of the moment which meant she found it easier than expected to visit the station during her lunch break.

She found DI Lotter efficient, discrete, and most helpful.

He hardly acknowledged her comments, accepted her errand as *just another small job* and was easily convinced she never recognised the man.

Faith left the station, took two deep breaths inside her car, and drove the ten minutes back towards the Stud Farm.

Then found a safe spot, settled herself and phoned Pauline with her positive result. 'Without doubt. He is the second vet. Dead sure.'

Pauline thanked Faith effusively, then rang off.

Got upset. *Awful. How will Alroy, particularly ill, manage this news? Awful.*

65

NEW YORK

Alroy contacted the FBI.

Took Bernard's advice on how best to manage the situation.

Before taking that step, one that because of tender years in senior management caused initial apprehension, he especially used his safest phone line, then Alroy acted after he set up the office coffee machine.

Alone in the office, no one noticed the extravagant twirl of the still wet brown overcoat that had protected him from an unseen, overflowing gutter when he exited the underground garage to grab two newspapers.

Thirty minutes later he chatted to FBI Special Agent Dennis Waterman.

The man surprised, when sounding remarkably English, delighted to take his call, eased him into an extraordinary project that satisfied both.

Otherwise, when Alroy began filling him in on their findings, Waterman displayed obvious and unexpected enthusiasm then asked for a delay. 'Apologise, DS Stewart, for I must stop you. Please hold.'

Alroy remained patient and strained to catch gist of a conversation between Waterman and a second agent in his office and realised that soon involved an extended telephone conference call with another agent. *Expected this. Guess he moves my project up the chain of command.*

Only snippets of their chat came his way.

DS Anderson joined him in the office.

She remained quiet and pointed at the coffee percolator.

Since his ears gained nothing of value, he thanked Anderson and got halfway through his first, honey laced cup, err Waterman, eight minutes later picked up the call again. 'Sorry for keeping you waiting. First, the good news.'

From his earlier contact of basic curiosity, Alroy enjoyed the thrilling business-like note in the agent's voice which indicated for Alroy, his offline internal chat had changed nature of their discussion.

Eager to explore what he now termed a significant matter, Waterman explained how, after a brief chat with senior agents, his office considered Alroy's information important.

Then, even from his opening words, he indicated he was authorised to reveal where the FBI's own team's investigation ran parallel to Alroy's with one of their own lines of enquiry. 'Your valuable information adds a creative dimension to our current work; indeed, your research may help us track down something big.'

Sharp, suggested they should not discuss the matter telephonically and invited Alroy's team to visit them.

Thrilled at Waterman's news, Alroy dropped bulleted notes on his desk and as he sensed urgency and logic in the Special Agent's voice, escalated everything on hearing this splendid news.

Waterman admitted. 'Your timing is spot on. Moreover, as we have an FBI plane scheduled to leave London in three hours, and despite risk of sounding condescending, could you chaps come over?'

With Sophia's scheduled flight cancelled, and in a breathless rush she and Alroy caught the FBI jet. Found their flight more comfortable than any offered by British Airlines. With only two other passengers who maintained their distance the relaxed atmosphere allowed them peace to strategize.

***

Waterman met them at the airport.

Lunged straight into business.

Acted with proficiency of a TV character who shepherds celebrities when he hustled them into a black sedan. Although unfamiliar with the vehicle, Alroy guessed it a Chevrolet suburban.

Two agents introduced themselves, and after briefest of welcoming chats, got down to business.

At forty-three, Waterman was a lifelong FBI man.

Owned the sporty, lean frame of a greyhound in top racing condition.

Dark hair, already well salt n-peppered, hung longish, although it never concealed a tight, hard pockmarked face Sophia decided must demand hours of an expert makeup artist's time and skill before he could be fit to take TV interviews.

His easy going, bright personality more than balanced initial, off-putting appearance. An attractive, confident tone permeated his voice, a feature that oozed enthusiasm when he contemplated then commented on Alroy's in-depth findings.

'To develop the togetherness, we need for this project to garner success, begin by admitting, while we noticed a similar theme, your research places you three weeks in advance of our investigations.

Thereafter suggested logical ground rules, fleshed out his partner's involvement when he explained where she and Sophia shared a common, useful background. 'Horses are a particular interest of Agent Jane Blanchard. It was such specialist detailed knowledge which helped her gain appointment to the team.

Agent Jane was younger, around the mid-thirty mark by Alroy's reckoning.

At first, considered her modest, reserved, an opinion reinforced by a severe hair style. Mid length, fair hair, tied in a short, tight ponytail, stuck hard against her head. So tight, Sophia decided it glued down, disliked how it dragged skin of her pale face back. Close-fitting, as though fresh from a cosmetic enhancement process.

Her strong mid-west accent embraced a common, even lowish class tone that disguised professionalism and skill. Alroy enjoyed her, for as their involvement in discussion grew, sensed her whirring, powerful analytical brain dissected facts in the background.

She often pulled at her collar as if she found her jacket uncomfortable; an irritating habit, a compulsive tick that caused Sophia's focus to slip.

When they left the vehicle Sophia detected, from the way she held herself, her slim stomach owned an athletic, even masculine-like six-pack tucked under a plain blue vest. Took him only seconds to mark how both plain clothes officers carried handguns.

The solid, man mountain of a driver, clearly more than a mechanic, whisked them to the FBI's Newark Field Office.

Since flight attendant had loaded them with coffee and pastries, they declined his offer of refreshments and so Waterman invited Alroy to begin.

He moved to the wall mounted cork and magnetic boards.

Unlocked the combination on his briefcase and removed a thick file of multi-coloured coded documents.

Alroy began his presentation.

Notwithstanding his well-prepared and in-depth knowledge of the subject, took time to define their findings while he mounted copies of the relevant notes that outlined their interests.

While Sophia sat back, demurred to him, held nothing back.

Whereas, when he began talking about how confidently they prepared to arrest senior Met officers, Flynn, and Gordon, Waterman, in an even more excited mode asked him to hold. 'If this involves such senior officers, fear this discussion sits above my pay grade. Please excuse me for a moment.'

At this stage, Alroy never mentioned he prepared to implicate an FBI agent.

Five minutes later, Waterman returned.

He followed a tall, gangly man who swung floppy arms by his sides like an agitated orangutan searching for fruit.

An obvious feature, it forced Sophia to check if his odd action caused grazed knuckles. The sensitive, weak voice that drifted from a feline thin mouth during introductions, never impressed.

But the powerful presence generated by an insightful, experienced manner when he talked, changed Sophia's mind. *A powerful figure, he catches my imagination, could be the top man we need.*

In his early forties, at least two steps up the ladder from Waterman, who, as he conducted the introductions named him as Lawrence Davidson: a Deputy Director of their Special Crimes Unit.

Intent on absorbing everything, listened with resolute, learned focus of a heron stalking a frog, the Brits barely breathed. Meanwhile, after he asked detailed incisive questions, Davidson demanded. 'Got the jist of this. Get your boss on the phone?'

Alroy waved off that notion. Patient and confident, explained it impossible. 'No! Owing to seniority of implicated officers, without yet uncovering the corrupt chain of command, cannot reveal my sources.'

Despite temptation, never disturbed Wolf's burner phone in his briefcase. 'Instructions are clear. This sensitive information demands complete silence until we set our evidence in concrete.

Alroy grew in stature, 'No, and that is final, cannot allow you to contact the Met.'

Although not himself, despite his struggle with a now galloping throat infection, displayed the confident attitude he worked hard to hold together. 'Deputy Director, assure you I have commissioner's confidence and trust, and am instructed to act on his behalf.'

To reinforce the weight of his evidence, Alroy, unsure who else might listen, and determined to lift seriousness of their discussion, slipped into furtive mode.

Without delay, Davidson, unused to people undermining his authority or who failed to respond to obvious instructions, leaned both palms on the table.

Alroy, sensitive to a possible, significant impasse, took a positive step.

Disguised his memo from others, wrote out the name LEIPZIG in bold capitals.

Slid it over the desk to land between Davidson's palms.

When the FBI agent skimmed the paper, he grabbed it but demonstrated no further evidence of disappointment or interest.

To withhold information from others, folded the paper, tucked it inside a pocket.

Overall, Alroy imagined with his mind in top gear, the others displayed a touch of embarrassment but to play down interest, so he allowed eyes to wander, stared at his notes, calendars, feet, and floor.

Davidson, reacted.

Alroy noted he disliked whatever implications the name Leipzig raised, as he sat upright. Rude, the man stared at Alroy for a full forty seconds. Used a penetrating Henry-like attitude that might have equalled his CI's delivery.

Alroy ably returned and matched his stare.

Did so quietly, without fidgeting.

In conclusion, with that proving a watershed, Davidson gave Alroy faintest softening of hard eyes, turned to Waterman, and said, 'Hate these chairs. Let us move along to a more comfortable room.'

Without delay, the three set off.

Travelled up two flights in an elevator, then Davidson conducted them inside a plush conference room, sizeable enough for eight people.

Davidson's manner changed as fast as a flock of roosting starlings heading for their roosting trees.

Invited them to sit.

Next, turned on a wall mounted recorder, stared into it, and said, 'I formally give Special Agent Waterman complete authority to investigate this case with DS Alroy Stewart from London's Met. His team may access our level three files.'

Strict phrasing indicated they recorded their conversation.

Forthwith, that formality over, he removed Alroy's scribbled note and displayed it for his agents. 'While you may source others of this name in our data base, after considering DSU's Stewart's interest and careful manner, I suggest the Leipzig referred to here is one of our Deputy Directors.'

Agent Waterman exhaled, slow and deep and offered pertinent information. 'And sir, as he is in the building at present, his name adds a different dimension to our investigations.'

Davidson advised Alroy how Leipzig, while he aroused earlier suspicions, none tied him down to any actual wrongdoings. 'In fact, carried through first-rate research and, when he put away a top Mafia unit, which restored the agency's confidence in him. Almost!'

Even though he never formally thanked Alroy for his update on Leipzig his body tone said as much. 'But now. Seems you are ready to disclose important evidence which may implicate him in major crime, both here and in Europe.'

As they continued Davison expressed hopes that after Waterman unlocked Leipzig's FBI files, they with the Mets facts should help them work together.

Authority matched tone and Wolf's no-nonsense approach as he said, 'Take him down.'

Stood, thanked Alroy warmly for his help, and waddled away from them.

66

FBI HQ

'Superintendent Stewart, you make my career.'

A smiling Waterman leaned over the table.

As though he recently perfected grinning as an art form, his boyish smiles created rare instant empathy. When he shook Alroy's hand, a firm, warm clasp confirmed them in synch, which encouraged him to bounce on. 'You heard the boss. So, here we go.'

At once Waterman brought his agent up to date when he exposed Blanchard to crisp, additional information. Admitted these developments related to problem areas within the FBI which normally were only discussed in senior positions.

Treated her as a close colleague, never a subordinate, when he instructed her to conduct Sophia to a secure operations room, where under her guidance they must set up a special task force.

'Because of the Leipzig name.' When he mouthed the name to her this highlighted significant security factors. 'Do this on level three. Need it tight with a fresh, innovative team.'

Numbered off names on fingers. 'After closing off that fraud business, you should find Agents Fraser, Scrivens, O'Malley, and Jones available.'

Blanchard gave her head a series of rapid head jigs, a three-card shuffle, which Sophia accepted as her odd, personal method of acknowledging commands.

The agent suggested. 'Because I collaborated with Agent Stieg. Can I also involve her? For her exemplary computer skills suggest she, although new to the office, should make an outstanding addition.'

Altogether, as a crime busting team, they displayed their togetherness.

In contrast to the frenetic activity Alroy initially generated, his efforts, even if unseen flew direct to the top floor where they caused intense discussion.

In the meantime, the new squads casual approach made it appear them chums taking a catch-up coffee, during the thirty minutes the others claimed to set up. Waterman could not stop talking. 'Received additional instructions, through discrete channels to move our operation's centre.'

As he explored the corridor, tapped his partly hidden ear insert. 'We reserve this floor for white-collar crimes, but it guarantees we remain clear of Leipzig and any potentially dodgy agents connected with him.'

Alroy supported that logic. 'Of course. Agree for we understand corruption is unlikely to hinge on just one dodgy, crooked officer and it may lead us to at least one other who collaborates with him. Even if not at director level, at least a special agent.'

They relaxed into a pleasant discussion around related matters which included Waterman's hopes this meeting heralded a future where they could expand and improve weak relationships between the Met and FBI. 'Understand how, by clearing out senior corrupt officers on both sides that must soften our often tougher than is necessary interaction.'

Alroy, owing to his fast track through the Met, had not yet enjoyed intimate contact with FBI senior officers, and knew little of their inner workings. Silently thanked Bernard for his rushed introductory seminar especially where he illustrated similarities in their operations.

While he enjoyed prospect of extending skills and experience, accepted the lucidity of Waterman's open approach. 'Obvious. We, both organisations that is, may sit on information when, with an honest, open exchange, a combined approach may have already garnered success in our Big Game hunt.'

Waterman giggled at his terminology, as a teenage girl might, but then Blanchard, contacted his mobile, advised they prepared the ops room and were ready to receive them.

67

OPS ROOM

The nine-person team convened in a tight strategy suite.

A mere twenty foot long by fifteen.

If far from the massive units depicted for entertainment in various TV shows, this relaxed unit, never hinted at how fast they threw it together, declared proficiency and promised success.

Alroy embraced its clean lines.

Despite being stuffed full of sophisticated equipment, by hiding the anatomy of the beast's organs, except desk monitors and wall mounted screens, Alroy enjoyed how it appeared organised and uncluttered. *Fit for purpose, this arrangement could suit us.*

Insisted on patience while he encouraged the team to introduce themselves.

Blanchard returned the compliment.

Agents included in James and Scriven, two additional field operatives, two technical behind-the-scenes researchers, Fraser, and O'Malley, and a boffin.

Sophia impressed over how, in Agent Stieg, they found a Bernard clone. Albeit her curvaceous, feminine frame sat quite different to his soft, lumbering appearance.

Alroy brought everyone up to date with the part of their investigation which focused on British Police officers.

Sophia introduced their thoughts on Calder, Georgiou, and the two American vets their fraud research already marked as persons of interest.

Instruments leapt into life.

Fingers barely left keyboards as investigators caressed technical wizardry and worked furiously, even during Alroy's presentation. While this was a process he discouraged at home, he soon admitted that as it worked here, considered it time to soften his attitude.

In familiar territory comfortably allowed Sonia to take centre stage.

She described how they traced two American vets. 'They are a couple, formally from Florida and now practice in Newark, here in New York.'

Distributed copies of salient facts. 'We find them noteworthy because they slipped under the radar during four of the last five months and we let them slip, stopped tracing their movement.'

Scrunched her nose. 'Although in fairness to our team, with information so new, time proved a limiting factor.' Voice hardened. 'So, where did they go, what did they do, and what are they doing? Those are the key points.'

Agent Fraser interrupted. Heavy, sable-rimmed glasses disguised half of a kind, but plain face as she flicked a curl from her forehead, contemplated the wall, and presented fruits of her research. 'Sir. Screens one and two. Vet details.'

After a brief study of quality photographs, Sophia regarded Blanchard's cool mien and added facts. 'We established their Veterinary Practice is purely equine, so that suits our scenario.'

Held a finger up to gain valuable seconds, then added a salient point. 'When making a gentle enquiry, pleasant, helpful staff informed they were recently married.'

Alroy appreciated where this confirmed Bernard's research on them certifying their legal union and said, 'So, they took a sabbatical honeymoon.'

Surprised at the length of their absence from practice he continued. 'But during that surprisingly protracted break, when they may have been better employed establishing their business at home, how could they; when immersed in such significant change, survive financially?'

As Sophia accepted that valid point she developed the theme. 'Sense their holiday as greater than R & R time. Thus, can we trace any evidence of them being engaged in business, legitimate of fraudulent.'

Allowed that to hit home, then team accepted them now back at work. 'So, it seems they are back in the saddle, engaged in normal vet work with horses.'

When Alroy repeated a session of coughing and wheezing, Waterman noted his discomfort, recognised where he fought to regain his breath.

Albeit Alroy tried to regularise his respiration without drawing attention to himself, then suggested. 'We must develop a workable approach. Sophia, as an accomplished horsewoman, is our specialist at contacting horsey people. Suggest she visit them. Do this as a preliminary gentle, but stimulating probe, establish basic facts.'

While Waterman never commented on Alroy's deteriorating health, he concerned the DS might be unfit for purpose.

Left that aside and readily agreed his suggestion offered a positive way forward. 'Will go along with your approach. Straightaway, as a foreigner, and smart. Sure, Inspector Sophia can fabricate a story, something catchy, to get them off guard.'

After another funny giggle, he said, 'Encourage them to relax. Open to even a snippet of positive evidence which may point us forward.'

Sophia shared his humour. 'Funny you suggest that approach. For we have already embraced a similar theme, developed a scheme to attract.' Issued one of her delicious, upper crust, cream-licking looks.

68

ALROY'S BROTHER

FBI efficiency impressed the Met officers.

Waterman instructed Fraser to find information on Leipzig.

Their FBI officer, having survived an earlier cloud of suspicion, jumped to the head of the list.

Fraser whose her dark skin, and fine, attractive features suggested some Asian descent, had used their quiet time to dig into coffee and pastries.

Now activated, she sat up, smart and to control waist length black hair, tied it behind her head with a plain band. As fingers bounced keys, Waterman narrowed her search. 'No, sorry, search the two Met officers first.'

At once got hits with DS Gordon, found him noted as having brief contact with one of their own people. 'We recently flagged Assistant Director Wayne Rhode's name, marked him a person of interest.'

Blanchard said, 'Nice one. For when we add that to your fresh information on Agent Leipzig, which thickens our unsavoury plot.'

Sophia considered their system big and flashy when compared to Bernard's. Smiled inwardly at how faster he processed information, convinced his solitary, dedicated approach could move the investigation on smoothly if available to access their fabulous computers.

Alroy coughed. Rough and hard, enough to interrupt them and make Blanchard air her concern. 'Dislike this cough DS, for your infection deteriorates at an alarming rate. Can you cope?'

As she said that, when she stripped two heavy elastic bands from her hair, a rich, thick chestnut bunch, bounced, glad for freedom, framed her tight face with in an altogether softer look.

Unable to hide his illness, Alroy coughed out disappointment over deteriorating health. 'This throat infection of two days earlier seems to work its way downwards.' Because everyone now shared that diagnosis the thought it might attack lungs alarmed everyone in the room.

Field Officers Scrivens and James, snug in back seats, remained understated, but frowned in harmony.

When he coughed harder, and clutched at his chest, he sat down and after an obviously painful session apologised. 'Sorry team. Nuisance. Hoped a head cold but now feel quite ill. Should consult a doctor.'

Waterman sympathised. 'Yes, and we can help.'

Raised a hand, acknowledged the stricken officer, and brought conversation to a precipitous halt.

As Alroy rose, and prepared to leave the warm, stifling room, Waterman commanded the others attention. 'Sorry everyone, important.' Invited them to concentrate on three screens.

Agent Scriven, a burly, late forties researcher, displayed information on British vets, including excellent head shots and biographical facts.

Sophia barely blocked a gasp, flabbergasted they quickly found more details than owned by their team.

Waterman, who missed nothing, noted Sophia's surprise at how she impressed over FBI efficiency for producing clear body shots that illustrated detailed features and managed her with an exhibition of proficiency.

'Now switch to facial recognition. Your initial area of interest is JFK airport.'

Alroy again spluttered through another coughing fit, apologised and left the room.

Sophia studied her phone in silent mode and gasped. While she placed a hand on a chair back stared at the name Calder Stewart but remained quiet. *No! Alroy's brother is a vet called Calder. No. This cannot be.*

Besides, Agent O'Malley, who worked in parallel but with different search parameters added her contribution when she handed Waterman, a note.

All watched him scan, then listened as he reacted, detailed more instructions. 'Search following dates as a priority.'

Turned to Sophia, face covered in genuine concern. 'As this will take time, the interval offers opportune space for us to consider how best to visit the equine hospital.'

As he switched from business, his humane side popped up as he shared his concern over Alroy. 'But first. Shall organise for DS Stewart to visit our physician.'

Sophia hung back to take a brief call from DI Henry.

Two sentences confirmed the brief note.

The gist came when he named Calder as Alroy's brother.

She replied. 'Not here. Also busy this side so, so best deal through me.'

69

BARONESS FELICITY

Sophia developed her idea.

'Our well researched plan follows a neat, logical approach.'

First, presented agents with copies of her smart business cards. 'Note, on these I am the Baroness Felicity Fortescue.' Natural, never emphasised her normal posh voice.

To begin with, she rose, moved to Waterman, and with grace of her early training in classical dance, bowed. In a scene from a bygone era, extended her hand towards him, and continued. 'Of course, you may kiss my hand.'

In coquettish, flirting fashion, cocked her head to the side. 'Perhaps a delicate bow is also in order?'

Everyone enjoyed her attitude, a unique presentation, and when Waterman executed the regal greeting expected of a mere mortal in the presence of royalty, it went down well.

Meanwhile, because they lost minutes, during which the team clicked together, Sophia hung back until Waterman indicated she could continue. 'Contact details, phone, email are dedicated numbers. Our team will process all enquiries correctly, with standard efficiency.'

While Sophia proved her expertise in manipulating people with that impression of a flouncy socialite, when required, she conducted herself as a business-like officer.

Waterman thrilled at her presentation. 'Perfect.' While Blanchard, amid another example of her three-card shuffle, issued wholehearted approval.

As Waterman grew in confidence with her approach, he said, 'That card, your accent,' Impossible not to, looked her up and down. 'and, well, the whole package provides you with the perfect disguise.' Nodded, agree with himself.

Sophia continued. 'We present me as a new player in the local horse industry, someone from Europe who fronts an important player. A fabulously wealthy man investing in a new enterprise.'

Here, began to outline how she hoped to attract interest in crime. 'He, disturbed by some recent, American-based and expensive fraud, desires to poke a finger in the eye of US equestrianism.'

As Waterman contemplated her performance he suggested. 'A useful, unique opening gambit. Next, how we help you develop that theme?'

'Will be subtle. Begin by suggesting my company needs a US vet team to go to Europe. Need their help to select the best horses for this,' Long, elegant arms waved. 'our local market.' We need their regional knowledge to vet horses.'

When satisfied, them still with her, she elaborated. 'Desire someone in accord with the local situation. Because their intimate knowledge of the industry means them better placed to understand what buyers find attractive.'

Waterman held up a finger, then turned away to consider a note handed to him by Agent Fraser then whistled. 'Interesting snippet. One that confirms our suspicions, for one of our vets, Louis Hennessey, deposited thirty-five thousand pounds sterling into their personal bank account when on sabbatical in Europe.'

Tapped his nose. 'Senses suggest this may not have been from a genuine source of income by treating continental horses. This may prove a useful slip up.'

'Nice one. Earning decent money during a trip disguised as a holiday. We all wish to emulate that practice.' Sophia hit the nail head hard. Everyone decided Sophia constructed an excellent opening gambit.

In harmony, Waterman, then Blanchard questioned Sophia. 'But where are you going with this?'

Agent James had been content to remain on the sideline but now probed. 'While I like your approach, find it quite fragrant, it needs detail. What angle will you used to hook them?'

Sophia gave him a sparkling smile; content she could add flesh to the skeleton of that concept, said, 'Presume you will wire me, load with decent surveillance equipment.' After that her cocked head brought a swift thumbs up from Jones, then she said, 'I proceed softly, then delicate, introduce how we hope to bring ten, superbly bred two-year-old warmblood horses into the country. Will indicate they, the vets that should place them in fashionable yards to start off their initial training.'

Will intimate this required expert advice of the chosen vets, 'Our team members will supervise this process at a distance. The object is to offer them for sale one year later.'

A couple of frowns indicated she must continue to clarify her thoughts. 'Later, with them already into training, even if preliminary, that will still be sufficient to expose potential talent, make them a sound investment.'

In the meantime, Blanchard, familiar with sport horses, accepted where she headed, while Waterman exposed deficiencies in matters equine. 'This I understand but need help. How will the promise of decent performance horses encourage them to open up to us?'

Sophia played with the crimson collar that picked out her smart, expensive verdure suit, then eased it away from her cream, frilly necked blouse to expose a tanned throat and raised hopes with sparkling eyes.

As keen as any hound hard on scent, she led them deeper into her explanation. Offered a small clap of hands as she said, 'Need to get clever with them.' Aware of where researchers tapped keyboards hard, without delivering fresh facts, took her time and, knowing how it melted hearts, dazzled them with her sweet smile.

Artful, she caressed strong cheekbones, dropped twenty years in age, and captivated everyone. 'Will then arrange for a longer meeting. Early in the day, if possible, and then over a decent lunch or dinner.'

Furthermore, having established control, explained she then hoped to talk money.

Jones issued a small peal of laughter. 'At last. Thank you. For the money angle always works, fraud responds to the impeccable carrot.'

'Must explain where and how we source the horses. And then.' For the time, aware he sat in the background, directed her remark to Agent Scriven. 'Only then, again gently, shall I explore their attitude to dishonesty.'

During a tight pause for effect, watched as Scriven, and James exchanged impatient glances. Then as she understood her delivery slower than suited the Americans homed in on the crucial part of her approach. 'From their history and admittedly this still conjecture, when they rise to the bait, declare horses are part of our European fraud ring.'

That unexpected twist brought them back to her, on their toes, raring to go.

70

DOUGHNUTS

Waterman called a halt.

Offered Sophia a bow.

'Now officer, you take me into a never experienced scenario,' Repeated the bow. 'I, as am sure you do, need a break, so let us find sustenance. Afterwards, if you could take us through this again, from the top.'

That said, he led them away, suggested they adjourn next door for coffee.

Sophia was happy to accede and said, 'Done deal for me. Ready for your famous doughnuts.'

As Sophia looked around, she appreciated from the agents propitious pause, they sensed her ready for a tease.

Blanchard laughed, introduced a light-hearted moment. 'Now, CI Sophia, surely you cannot believe those stories about us American lawmakers craving sugary doughnuts. Surely, not.'

Doubtless, her humour helped.

Until, on opening the door, Sophia clapped her hands on spotting a generous boxful. 'Yes, Knew it, Doughnuts for Africa.'

'Delicious. Chocolate and raspberry jam. Whoever developed this twist to classic confectionary, achieved their aim.'

Sophia, although blessed with the figure of a dancer, shared metabolism of a racehorse, and ate like the fastest.

After she delivered two doughnuts into history, wiped her lips, sighed with content, and said, 'Outstanding and enchanting. And now, ready for the finer points?'

Agent James, after agreeing on the quality of doughnuts, said, 'While your delivery fascinates, ask you to elaborate. For I cannot understand how you intend sweetening the deal. Moreover, help me understand how you can convince them enough money is available. How do you flash the tangy dollar signs needed to hook them?'

'Here we go then.'

Sophia, after a longing glance at the still loaded box of doughnuts, turned up her nose and dived into the subject. 'The story depends on inexpensive horses, because of moderate breeding, arriving Stateside.'

Offered a small handclap. 'Will emphasise how our excellent certification establishes them as being from good, yet modest bloodlines.'

Explored the group's faces. 'Only when I sense them thirsting for additional information shall I introduce the fraud we constructed, by informing them registered mares produced these horses, while certified as covered by ordinary stallions,' Another gentle handclap followed. 'when they were in fact mated through AI and ovum transplantation to the *best stallions* in Europe.'

The emphasis got them sitting to attention.

'Ah!' Blanchard, further on the others, followed where she headed with this twist in her plan, as Sophia moved on. 'Explain how my team, at significant expense, organised this in clandestine fashion via a process which involved masterful substitution by highly paid stud workers under our supervision.'

'Yes, I grasp this.' On balance, with Blanchard admiring how this must cause excitement, grasped Sophia's masterclass in deception. 'Instead of bringing in batches of young horse's worth one-hundred and fifty to two-hundred thousand dollars each, you bring in individuals with, on paper, a lower value.'

She stopped, licked her lips as Sophia did when she nibbled doughnuts. 'And then, as their training develops, obvious class, if not paperwork,' Applauded. 'must show and when that proves outstanding. Their dollar worth rockets skywards.'

Which pleased Sophia. 'Well done agent. Then again, as we horsemen understand, while buying on pedigrees is important. Nothing, however, has the pulling power of horses when potential purchasers watch them work.'

Introduced the second part of her system, the one that led to her explaining how the vets earned easy, safe, and regular money.

'Now, I must involve them. Encourage the vets to consider how best to develop the system for me. Besides, as professionals, they must relish the idea of importing quality stock, then exhibit them as potential champions.'

Agent Scriven, the quietest member of the team, had his say. 'Parents are Wyoming cattle farmers. They raised me on horseback, although I never enjoyed the creatures.' When no one interrupted, he continued. 'Remember when corralling young horses for breaking, we took bets, based on their conformation, when deciding which were likely to work out best.'

Shook his head. 'That said, difficult, but after only two months' work, we found it easier to assess them. So, I am with you. A superb idea.'

Sophia thrilled to find them on board, how her presentation excelled as she lifted them to her level of excitement.

'Then I act fair. Notwithstanding, my company conducts the shipment trial with a reduced expectation, we hope annually, to earn three to five hundred thousand dollars.' Progressed by explaining they earn reasonable money from professional fees and commission. 'Hammer home this as a risk-free venture.'

Until now, hushed, Agent James enthused over Sophia's skilful trap. His melodic, Southern voice suffused the room when adding his congratulations.

Gracious, while she took pleasure from his confidence, Sophia continued. 'Of course, repeat, my aenigma reflects on convincing the vets to appreciate how easily they earn regular commission. Shall constantly reinforce it as a safe, fool proof system.'

Raised her arms. 'When managing them with kid gloves, as opportunity grows... they must find this irresistible. Nevertheless, in conclusion, easy money from their protected,' Flashed arms, 'practically legal involvement.'

Waterman complimented Sophia. 'Whereas my minor knowledge of the horse breeding industry makes understanding finer details of your concept, difficult, but when dollars are involved, anything possible.'

Sophia agreed and repeated that well-known truism. 'Greed pays our salaries.'

As Waterman's interest grew so too did his pizzicato pitch, and already attracted to Sophia, said, 'They should be gone forty minutes, so, time to check what information our veracious computer flags.'

71

A DIAGNOSIS

The doctor's opinion perplexed Alroy.

'HIV? How? Impossible!'

To begin with, he towered over Alroy, who remained seated on the crisp, bleached sheet of a standard exam table, as the doctor squared massive shoulders.

Doc Freddy flooded the room like a line-backer, rather than the archetypical middle-aged in-house GP Alroy expected.

He said, 'Let me take you through what we know.'

Tucked his stethoscope around the neck of his lovat green, tailored clinical jacket. For fear of alarming his patient, he stretched a generous smile to encourage calm. Must lead you through this.' Without delay, he suggested Alroy dress, then join him in his adjacent office.

Two minutes later as he encouraged him to sit, Doc Freddy showed his human side when he took time to ensure him comfortable. Next, after he had relaxed his patient, said, 'Bear with me DS for as a result of my scientific mind, I work better when making lists.'

Without delay, having often faced doubts and frank disbelief before, he, expecting Alroy's concerned reaction, got straight into it. 'You are normally a fit, well exercised man. Although you find your usual fitness regime tougher than normal.

You drink little. Tobacco absents itself from the equation. You lose weight; agree on six pounds in two months. Not sleeping as well as before. Gay, even if faithful to your partner.'

Nonetheless, after exploring his bulleted list in detail, he approached his diagnosis, explained how Alroy's respiratory infection may be a secondary problem.

Doc eyeballed him. 'Dislike this chest.' Jabbed a fat thumb on his desk and flicked through notes.

On balance, as mind firmed on how to approach the case, he asked permission to proceed. 'If you agree, shall run the full range of tests for haematology and biochemistry, and also request bacteriology on your throat swab.'

Thumb jagged again. 'Experience points to importance of early diagnosis when faced with this virus, the one I suspect, or at least must rule out, as we begin treatment.'

In a formal tone, reminded Alroy he taped this part of the consultation, asked for written permission to proceed. 'Also,' While pork sausage fingers, collected needles, syringes, and swabs, requested additional permission to run an HIV test. 'and routine, in cases such as yours, it means neglecting duty by not offering that option.'

In time, as Alroy worsened by the minute, he agreed to a second more detailed examination, as well as routine blood samples. Remarkable dexterity for a bulky man followed when he adroitly manipulated collection materials, as fingers flirted with dainty movements more appropriate for a concert pianist. Collected four vials of blood.'

In the meantime, Alroy phone Waterman and surrendered. Asked him to inform the others doc collected bloods and samples, then said, 'Sorry guys. Cannot cope, must get off to bed.'

Followed that up with a similar call to Sophia. 'Have informed Waterman you have my full confidence and the investigation must proceed.'

Thirty minutes later, in his hotel room, Alroy; still unaware of Calder's involvement phoned Trevor.

After briefest of catch ups, said, 'Had to get off to bed. Inasmuch as this virus leaves me in a mess, get this.' Paused as his worst coughing episode racking through weak chest brought on a light-headed spell. 'Doc worries my condition is AIDS based.' 'Feels I may have AIDS. How? Why?'

Alroy's coughing truncated the conversation and, agreeing to call again, collapsed into bed.

Sophia visited him three hours later.

Not only was she concerned for his health but also eager to bring him up to date. Forthwith, he shared her excitement over the excellent progress made by the task force which suggested their investigations on both sides of the Atlantic reached remarkable levels of intensity.

Her eyes shone when she brought him up to speed with everything discussed after his departure then finished. 'Waterman says with regular jets flights to London, they wish to deliver you home.'

Sat on a chair beside his bed. 'Agree. For, should this vicarious infection worsen, best our own doctors treat you at home.'

'Good. Also, on my mind. Contact Henry. Place him on standby for a swap tomorrow.' Coughed hard and long. 'Cancel that. Instruct him to swap, take my place.' Head flopped onto pillow. 'Even if we hope these drifts off overnight, doc is convinced it may worsen.'

When Alroy's condition worsened overnight, an FBI driver conveyed him to the doc.

Doc Freddy hardly took the time to greet him before getting straight to the point, razor sharp as military training demanded. 'HIV tests positive. You have AIDS. No doubts.'

Staff swap went like clockwork.

An FBI car delivered Alroy to the airport and in London, a police car took him to a hospital.

As Henry integrated seamlessly with the FBI, it relieved Waterman who recognised him as a true professional.

72

ALROY HOSPITALISED

Sophia stressed Alroy's serious condition.

On hearing this, Henry made calls.

Even as he packed to catch his New York flight, organised for a police car to conduct Alroy direct from the airport to the nearest hospital.

'Remain faithful to you.' Trevor and Alroy tried to discuss his condition, especially how he may have contracted the virus. With that difficult, Trevor, released Alroy's hand, rose and walked to the window and back again.

Alroy, even if connected to drips and oxygen, and sick as the proverbial dog tried to understand his partner's odd reactions, so, he motioned him over.

As Alroy gripped Trevor's hand, he scrutinised his face, searched for clues to explain his hesitant attitude.

'Sense a *but* coming, for it seems you keep something from me.'

Trevor, shilly-shallied under a cloud of deceit and concern and although desperately concerned for Alroy, came to the party. 'You will remember my trip to South Africa... Well.'

When Alroy coughed fit to burst, Sister Prendergast interrupted. 'In this ward, you take orders from me.' While she fiddled to remove the transparent, tacky, ashy mucous from his mouth, she waved Trevor away. 'Go. For your partner is unfit to talk with me never mind visitors.'

To negate all chances of conversation, fitted a see-through mask over his face and increased the volume of oxygen that flowed through his nose. Checked the oximeter, the instrument attached to his finger, and waved questions away.

She said, 'Your oxygen level sits at only eighty-four percent. No talking.'

Alroy caught Trevor's arm, but Sister ushered him away when she used her most bossy voice. 'Need you, young man to wait in the waiting room, while I ask Doctor Dingwall to visit. So, get out.'

Amid the desperate scene, only when Angus Stewart arrived Trevor explained how his son Alroy presented with AIDS.

Nevertheless, said words best left unsaid, might have been stored for later.

Overflowing grief stole his normal eloquence which caused him to blurt out how his careless actions resulted in Alroy's illness.

Aside from Angus' concern over his son's condition, and during a challenging time when he attempted to calm his distressed mother, he stared, listened as Trevor poured out his heart as he explained how his irresponsible actions threatened to kill his partner.

Despite his profound, sincere apologies, only the doctor's intervention stopped Angus punching him.

As it must, the story came out.

Hillbrow in Johannesburg is one of the naughtiest, most dangerous places in South Africa. A fact that holds true during the day, but the dying sun exposes its seedy side as the city's sin capital.

The Sandton Terriers who hosted Trevor's rugby team, the Camden Warriors entertained them in true, unparalleled South African fashion.

Meanwhile, after the final game, they visited one of the so-called men's clubs, a Lollipop Lounge. Red-hot boys, warmed by a superb tour, mirrored their crimson, iridescent rugby shirts.

Even drew the gay Trevor into the hectic party, and despite the beautiful Zulu girl's prompting, for some inexplicable reason he refused to wear a condom, and!

In the hospital, he tried a one-sided confession with Alroy.

'Our conversation prompted me to visit the doctor and explained your, well, our situation. He confirmed the infection I experienced last year, six weeks after my return from South Africa, was due to contact with AIDS.'

Even if Alroy could hardly talk, his wide-eyed stare, when added to his already distressed breathing, suggested he tailed the jist of Trevor's story as he continued. 'He took a blood test. Expect the result to come through tomorrow morning.'

Trevor attested to be one of the lucky ones.

Despite contracting HIV, his immune system responded in exemplary fashion and protected him from developing overt illness.

Alroy failed to reply.

Trevor turned, fled the scene.

Wracked with what he termed unforgiveable grief; Trevor ended their relationship.

Regardless of how well he coped, and while he showed no sign of developing a fulminating infection, he remained capable of passing on the virus. Notwithstanding a decent level of immunity, his system contained enough active virus to mean unprotected sex with anyone, placed them at risk.

Virus hammered Alroy.

The guiltless one.

As his condition rapidly deteriorated, within one week he was hospitalised at the Kings College Hospital.

***

Her favourite child was desperately ill.

Margaret entered panic mode on hearing her special child was not just ill, but in critical condition.

Doctor Dingwall, appreciated his case needed intensive therapy, so, organised for transfer to specialist care at the Royal Free Hospital in London, whose reputation for the management of HIV in children and juveniles jumped them into first choice.

They accepted Alroy as a patient.

Margaret and Angus booked themselves into the nearby Church Street Hotel, although Margaret spent three nights at the hospital. 'Shall sleep on the floor, for I cannot leave him to die without his mother holding his hand.'

Mr Sing: consultant in charge examined him in detail and following extensive testing including further chest Xray's and CT scan, confided in parents. 'His condition remains critical, for Alroy's pneumonia settles into one of the most serious variants and threatens death. Moreover, as a purely viral induced condition with insignificant bacterial involvement, we treat him symptomatically.'

They acknowledged his humanity at a time when many others haphazardly criticise doctors for being uncaring.

Overall, exhibited great dedication which included how he updated the family twice daily. Gentle with them yet never hid his concern.

Margaret was a mess.

While Angus did everything possible to support her, she sensed her in danger of slipping away.

Only on the third day of their vigil was Angus able to make her shower, dress well and take a bite of lunch with him.

Altogether at sea, as she picked at a citrusy, prime Dover sole, dismembered and strewed it around her plate without much of it reaching her mouth, they revisited the same ground. 'And, having explored every possibility, my dear, I am at a loss for consultants agree he is in best hands. So, what can we do now?'

The always perceptive Margaret caught a hint of a positive note on Angus' face, as the kernel of an idea made fertile by a recent memory brought a sudden thought. 'Wonder.'

'What? Do you suggest a novel approach?' Flung arms around, begged him to offer hope.

He took her back to Patrick Cairns' last visit with them. 'Given how he enthused over his nephew, you may remember he outlined his career, glowed over success in medical research at Glasgow University.'

Impulsive, Margaret's grabbed and hugged in an abstract fashion which meant she distracted him for two minutes.

Only, as she calmed, he reflected on Niall's work with homoeopathy against HIV.

She cried, loud enough to alert a passing orderly. 'got it now. Said his nephew Niall's latest experiments meant him close to a breakthrough.' Excited, decided her compassionate God rewarded her for praying to Him.

'Call him now, for his number must be in your contact list.'

'Hi Patrick, it's Angus Stewart here.'

'Goodness me. How nice to hear from you! How are you all?'

73

NIALL'S CELEBRATION

Irrelevant niceties slipped past.

Angus dropped his manners.

Quicker than ever in recorded history his wife's escalating anxiety forced him to bypass normal courtesy and beg for Patrick's help.

Inasmuch as Margaret's background plaintive sobbing rushed everything, their approach raised alarms Patrick had seldom faced since he retired from medicine. 'Your sad news also stabs my heart. With us firm friends and our history of surviving through illness, how do we face this? Need to please explore every contact in the hope you can help find us a solution.'

The kind, generous man rose to the plate. 'You bring us terrible news. Share your pain and commiserate with Margaret.'

Angus got to the point, declared as Alroy had HIV, they hoped Niall may point them towards a solution and offer at least a glimmer of hope.

When she took the phone Margaret emphasised their despair, poured out her heart. Dived in, reckless as any kamikaze pilot. 'You recently enthused over Niall's wonderful work against this frightening disease. Can he or you help?'

Patrick added balm to her troubled mind when he said, 'Not only that but also, we are lucky for Niall is here with us. With your call propitious because we enjoy a family celebration in honour of their latest trial results. Will fetch him to chat with you. But warn he has also been down for a couple of days with a horrid virus.'

Because he heard his name mentioned several times, Niall had already joined his uncle who handed his cell phone to Niall. Without delay, memories of Deirdre swapping children flooding back made him whisper as he moved into the bubbling lounge to call him.

There it goes again. Another bout of the sympathy pains these children share. Gosh, but this could be awkward.

Niall, despite his own bronchitis, coughed through an involved conversation with Angus and Margaret.

Francesca, soon aware of an extraordinary event, joined him and listened in to their chat. After spending those informative, desperate minutes chatting to Angus, the news of another's distress lightened his burden.

When he put the phone down, his own condition improved, as in an odd, inexplicable way, their news, made him respond to this unexpected shift in their research subject.

Unknown to him, miracle of twin relationships meant he embraced an unknown factor that with increasing health, meant he had no choice. Had to consider could his team's research offer a solution.

As a result of Francesca hitting the sweet spot serendipitously with Margaret's aspirations she said, 'Niall, what if?'

In synch, both walked the same track.

For something else about Niall's chat with Angus Stewart heightened both sets of senses.

'Francesca, we should help. Feel this man reaches out to us through the ether, for he, especially Margaret, touches me in a most special, intimate, inexplicable way.'

As always, Francesca publicised her oneness with Niall when she demanding he act. 'Know by now that when you have these profound intuitive thoughts, they often prove right.'

She hugged him. 'And bingo! From research to treatment. A wonderful opportunity to treat a dying man jumps into our psyche at the perfect moment.'

A mother's love carried the day.

Even Francesca, increasingly hoping to follow that path, responded to innate factors that drove them onwards. 'My brief chat with Aunty Deirdre opened my eyes to God's power. Believe He prompts us, pushes us on to intervene.'

Niall, agreed, accepted his responsibility to act.

Now obligated and empowered to help, brought the family up to date on Alroy's illness, then excused himself.

***

At once, he phoned Evan.

'Agree with you.'

Niall listened to Evan's logical comments, then interrupted. 'You are right for sure. The Prof will say that when we talk to him. And yet!' Punched an edge on palm against the wall. 'If we phrase this well, can motivate him to at least try to influence the board.'

Together, as always, Evan broke in. 'For sure, we stand up as a special case. Because, if the man is dying, we can do no harm. And!' 'Imagine if we save his life. How a single successful case could do more to justify our research better than another year and dozens of experiments.'

'Good, leave this with me for now shall bring in Uncle Sandy, use him as a sounding board.'

Evan reiterated that positive thought. 'Also, consider how this case could throw our research forward by eighteen months.' Evan and he often finished each other's sentences and understanding his friend better than any lover, he accepted Niall not only animated but accepted his determined frame of mind made him age ten years into a newfound maturity.

Thus, as Evan closed off, he appreciated where his friend's sudden growth took their discussion to the next level. 'With timing critical, shall contact the Prof now and explain our position, ask him to reflect, prior to us meeting him early tomorrow morning.'

His concern over Niall's wracking cough made him say, 'But with your voice so rough. Will you be up for this?'

'If I cannot get there, bring him here to my mum's house, or I shall get Francesca to drag me there.'

When he returned to the lounge, Niall prised Sandy away from his beloved Angela, and led him into Patrick's study.

In time, Sandy enthused over possibilities, even more so than Evan.

'Dead right. As sure as God gave us the healing gift of homoeopathy, we can save this man's life.'

In conclusion, as Sandy returned to the festival atmosphere, Niall's growing confidence made him agree with Dire Straits magical guitar work that oozed from Sarah's collection. 'Yes, we are indeed Brothers in Arms.'

74

PERMISSION TO TREAT

'Agree, this is an unusual request.'

As Niall's health improved, he matched Evan's opinion.

Began by stressing the unreasonableness of Niall's presentation to the Prof.

Then, interrupted. 'You are right for sure. And were it not for these extraordinary circumstances, could never risk your wrath by even hinting at what is *an impossible request.*'

That unexpected emphasis made the Prof stare at him over his desk.

With only a simple, thin in-tray, and a burgeoning one for exiting documents, on an otherwise empty desktop, Niall guessed at his efficiency.

For the Prof, having digested various scenarios, continued to dislike how each played out and used Evan's negative words to explain why they, with hands tied down by protocol, had no case to make. 'Under no circumstances can I present your extraordinary, admittedly well-intentioned request to Ethics Committee. Which means risking credibility that has taken years to accumulate.'

Evan, more perceptive of the two, imagined the Prof's mind churn as he continued. 'With barely three years before my retirement, cannot sully my reputation.'

However, and now the manipulative side of Evan's personality struck a light chord when in a masterstroke he empathised with the Prof's powerlessness. Watched as the older man's face hardened.

For he, despite himself, disliked Evan's implication that as a departmental head he was powerless. Besides, it is one thing to accept your weaknesses, to roll over for the tummy tickling session that marks surrender, but when another puts you down.

So, my loyal workers believe me impotent!

Niall understood Evan's approach.

Hung back when he saw the first glimmer of fight. *Because Evan has this, I can stand back, leave him to dig.*

True to form, Evan landed a sucker punch, a right cross that punched home. 'Sorry sir, for disturbing you and I accept you are powerless, and although disappointed, wholeheartedly accept you blameless.'

Niall popped in a sigh and a simple statement. 'Advised Evan not to even suggest this route. Unfair and unreasonable. We knew you could not get involved in university politics.' Hung his head and whispered. 'And yet. When I reflect on that young, dying man. In his hopeless condition, only his family's despair suggested we bother you, sir.'

Continued their Laurel and Hardy image when Evan said, 'Cannot remove this image from my mind where our research produces fruit by saving his life.'

'Hold that thought.' The Prof opened his contacts list. 'In danger of becoming stymie, fuddy-duddy in this august centre of learning, well, hell's bells, have nothing to lose.'

After three calls, he tracked down the responsible person and invited, but his strong tone suggested a demand.

She indicated her intention to at once visit him.

Niall thought best to excuse himself, bowed to Evan's skill.

At first, the Prof shared sympathy for her difficult, now rigid position as she, after taking barely three seconds to weigh his argument, emphatically denied they could proceed. 'While I understand your position, my role as deputy ethics coordinator is unequivocal.'

Rigidity in Helen Lambert's diminutive, five foot two, seven stone body marked her tone, how she never shared the Prof's enthusiasm.

That firmness fully matched the severe lawyer's garb of blue suit and white blouse, her constant companions when she stalked the famous academic halls of the university in the garb of a restless prowler. Denoted her mistress of the university's correct moral veins.

He frowned, disappointed at cold, unambiguous facts of how necessary controls governing medical trials made his position impossible.

Be fair, public deserves protection from cavalier, unfounded experimentation.

After a ponderous moment passed the Prof enquired. 'Agree and sympathise with your noble view. Still, the urgency of this case,' A fist slapped into a palm. 'the chance to save the life of a man destined to die, this sanctions us to use this as a fulcrum to do something special?'

Even if a cliché, his argument *fell on deaf ears.*

Her pale, stringy face certified a negative stance.

Devoid of makeup, when she was one of the few women who could benefit from decoration, went hard, tense and used flavourless, insipid words to express discontent. 'Impossible. Even if time proved propitious, with required paperwork correct, in order, University Senate will never allow this. Unfeasible.'

Evan, whose experience with the Prof garnered how he reacted poorly to her tone and body language, was unimpressed. *Difficult lady this. She may stamp a foot any moment.*

Prof plugged on. Gentle, keen to avoid unnecessary, potentially damaging confrontation. 'Agree with, respect your opinion.' Opened both palms, placed back of hands-on desk, and leaning over, pleaded as Evan had never witnessed him do.

'Besides, by taking this historic step, our research must gain invaluable lessons.'

A palm in front of her nose prevented intervention. 'Ms Lambert. Offer you the unique chance to play God. We may save a man's life.'

Evan winced as she positively bristled, then from a wide open, tiny mouth she issued a coherent stream of negative thoughts decided to dominate the Prof, instead she brought out the Prof's rarely seen toughness.

This set rigid as she said, 'First, in a centre of excellence such as this, a source of human driven, scientific advancement, we should ignore the nebulous God thing.'

Prof's face dropped when faced the sheer audacity of her making a declaration against a man proud of his efforts as an Elder in the local Presbyterian Church

She now made Evan cringed as she, unable to hold back missed obvious warning signs and said, 'No, no, and no! This will not happen on my watch. Never.'

Evan had touched sides with the lady three times before and tried to send her a message through the ether. *Girl beware. You go too far, and I fear my Prof prepares to eat you. Do you know the power this man wields? His standing in our community?*

Somehow the Prof held it together. Remained patient. 'Suggest a break for coffee or tea.'

As impervious to granite her attitude hardened 'Only when we settle this discussion.'

Niall who had crept further away from the coal face slunk deeper into the background. *We get nowhere with this lady. Gosh! She is the personification of Iron maiden's* Call to Madness.

Not the Prof.

He held up a hand to stop her adding to the discussion. Voice was low, hard, and cold. 'Ms Lambert. Confirm to whom do you report?'

'The Head of the department. Your best route to follow if you need official confirmation.' Leaned forward, again tried to intimidate. 'But a warning. She has never undermined me. Never.'

Prof got stern. 'My simple question indicated a need for me to know the name of your ultimate superior?'

'Dr Morag Livingstone and she will support me.' With her name dropping, for the time they discovered a chink, a crack into which the Prof leaped. 'Of course. Morag. Time for a coffee break. You must wait here.'

Disappeared, left them confused and concerned.

Niall surrendered, slipped out of the office.

Even survived an uneasy fifteen minutes.

***

A telephone call which he dragged out, saved him from embarrassing silence. Even Evan: the lady's man, failed to charm her into a reasonable conversation, relieved to find the Prof return in fifteen minutes.

At his most authoritative. 'OK. We proceed.'

Outlined how the university offered Alroy's family the chance to have their son admitted to the Queen Elizabeth Hospital in Glasgow. Drew a noisy, grave breath and when glancing at her, Evan spotted empathy flit across his face.

Almost apologetic, continued. 'And provided we gain everyone's consent, with normal waivers in place, their physicians, under guidance of Dr Cairn's team will treat him in this novel fashion.'

'Impossible.' Ms Lombard took a flying leap onto her high horse, a ceiling grazing Hanoverian one. 'A trial of this nature is impossible. Cannot...'

Prof interrupted. 'No! Stop right there. I now explain the process in a manner even you will understand.' Without delay, patience exhausted, at the bottom of the syringe, spoke to Evan. 'Make no mention of this being a clinical trial. Nor will we record any ensuing information for public discussion... by my team... or any of us.'

Ms Lombard attempted to continue. 'Must renew my protest at this heinous break in protocol.'

But the Prof, knowing he won the day acted magnanimous, demonstrated personnel skills needed to conduct his job. 'Not to worry my dear. For this conversation never took place.'

Assumed a benevolent, almost paternal approach. At one point, his attitude concerned Evan, nervous he prepared to pat the lady's head. 'We face a unique situation.'

To her credit, unwilling to accept defeat, she tried again. 'No, sir. This cannot happen.'

With time wasting, the Prof showed his complete commitment when he silenced her. 'Notwithstanding we draw a veil over this exercise, our secrecy pact also applies to you.'

Delivered a glower brutal enough to crack open the large Clyde's mussels known as clabbydoos, ended the discussion in a deliberate manner. 'Anyway, time to move on and as of now, for your own protection, you are out of the loop, safe.'

She slammed her hand on the tabletop, collected her papers, and entered history.

75

DUMBARTON AGAIN

Holly was on a high.

In dreamy mode, rejoiced in Fiona's news.

For instance, with Fiona now able to relax when the Henderson subject arose, which lifted her as it did everyone else.

Overall, Niall's intended hit high notes when she captivated Holly, and now Deirdre, as indeed she had the whole family. Also, they warmly welcomed her interest in Caroline.

'Suggest some bonding time, a quiet afternoon as a chance for your new aunty and one stealing her favourite nephew to spend time together.' Impulsive, hugged Francesca, fiddled with a stray lock of the girl's hair as a mother does while expressing a hidden, urgent desire they left simmering for ages.

'Together we should open a fragrant pot of glue, something useful to add to the wonderful part you already play in unifying our dysfunctional family.'

The girl stood back, and as she held Holly's eye, declared. 'Now, Aunty Holly. Can a mere scoop of cement make me like you?' When it came to a spot of indulgent banter, Francesca never shied from standing up to anyone.

Holly hugged her and suggested. 'Never forget Niall is like one of my own children. So, yes, treat me with deserved respect.' Performed the telling hands-on-hips thing her daughter loved. Then got serious. 'The next time you have a couple of hours free we can visit Caroline and then do a spot of lunch. How does that sound?'

Two weeks later they studied the same spot by Loch Lomond.

Savoured a fair day. High cumulus clouds in a powder blue sky, warm enough to ensure Caroline's comfort and hopefully keep her at ease. As a result of the gentle, ever-present breeze caused by the uppermost leaves of the beech trees as they whispered sweet nothings in the language of the ancient ones to each other they added to the relaxed tone of the place, as shared confidences often do.

The padding on the benches down by the Lochside worked well enough to keep Caroline content. Snug in a tartan blanket over shoulders and knees, she demonstrated a contrasting character to the one Francesca first met.

In remarkably fine form, she put Francesca at ease. 'A treat. And to think you prepare to become Niall's wife. *Cairns*. Lovely.'

They hardly settled into their chat when matron joined them and as she fiddled with Caroline's blanket said, 'So, can you spot the difference between our friend today and last week?'

Demonstrated the magical distinction between vocational healers and financially motivated technicians, when after giving Caroline a spontaneous, tender kiss, she said, 'The specialist advised it now time to grow her wellbeing by arranging a series of appointments with a psychologist, Betty Snaith. A remarkable improvement, Catherine is quite our star patient.'

Holly only half listened, contemplated why the puzzling emphasis Catherine normally employed when she mentioned the Cairns name was still absent. She said, 'We have reached her on a decent day.'

They chatted on about this and that, until Holly recognised Caroline tiring, suggested. 'Right, dear one. Time, we got you home safe.'

As the ladies reached the home's front door, Caroline paused, motioned Francesca towards her, then grabbed the girl's arm, pulled, made her bend towards her. Took care to look around, then whispered. 'The birthmark. Does Niall have one?'

Francesca used fingers of her right hand to ease one of the old lady's nails out of the trench it created in her wrist, while she tried to prevent Caroline from detecting her painful wince and worked her voice to remain calm. 'Yes. Niall has a lovely mark. A titchy, well-formed splodge.'

'Know. Pink, almost heart-shaped birthmark high on inside of his thigh. Yes!'

Caroline paused, dropped her head, and yawned.

Eased out the next words soft and slow and dropped a potential bombshell. 'His twin has the same mark.'

Frustrated Francesca when she squeezed out the next sentences, the ones that must have contained potent facts but delivered them in a garbled hotchpotch of scrambled words, then finished. 'Then the news. The psychologist and horrid Deirdre from the past. That bad, bad Cairn's woman and the twins.' Closed her mouth and eased into a troubled rest.

Thirty minutes later found them comfortably seated in the Cruin restaurant, another important Lochside feature, near the nursing home.

With salmon salads yet to arrive, they clinked wine glasses and Holly said, 'Funny she remembers such a slight detail as Niall having a birthmark from years earlier.'

'Coped well today, and yes. To remember something so insignificant after dealing with hundreds of babies.'

After she swirled wine, Francesca talked into the glass. 'Despite that, find her insisting Niall had a twin disturbing.' Contemplative sipped again. 'Because Angela made a pointed referenced to twin births in the hospital at the same time as Niall's birth.'

Holly reacted to that remark when she set off a discussion on memory, brain injuries and other factors that affect mental health. 'Odd she still focuses on twins after decades.'

In midwife mode, shared facts. 'Yes indeed. Back then, only twenty births per thousand involved twins. Although with modern fertility management, that figure creeps up to higher levels.'

'Sure enough. I recently read where fertility drug treatments may cause twins in twenty percent of births. A significant increase.'

Holly, with memories of the old days sharpening, dug deeper and continued Francesca's theme. 'Hear where you go with this, but other factors made Stewart twins unforgettable.

Back then, my role as a midwife included special training in the ICU.'

A short gap allowed her to pick out memorable incidents associated with the next part. 'Both a Stewart twin and Niall were under my charge. Of course, with Fiona being Niall's mum.'

Cocked her head to the side. 'Are you getting the picture now?'

That said, as food arrived, Francesca laughed as her sense of humour meant she blurted. 'Now that makes sense.' Stroked Holly's arm. 'Aunty, you ran eyes over my naked intended before me.'

Holly, enjoying that one needed time to stop laughing before she could go on. 'Both children gave us a challenging time. Two days of hell.'

Sniffed at her salmon and smiled. 'Mind you. Through them, your man, I got that big lump, Patrick, to appreciate me.' Clapped hands. 'A wonderful, romantic time. Did you hear the story of his proposal?'

'While keen to listen to your story, the unexpurgated version still wonder why she confuses Niall as a twin.'

'Do not forget the seriousness of her injury. For she almost died and remains confused.' Threw hands around. 'Never mind for I love recounting my story.'

That fascinating oft repeated tale placed birthmarks safely in the background, for the moment.

Francesca realised Holly was unaware of Deirdre's comment.

Confused and concerned, left it for another day.

76

KENTUCKY

With the kill decided, vets moved.

On expertly forged passports,

Sailed through customs.

From Manchester and Athens, they luxuriated in first class.

When home, Georgiou, as one who always sought parental approval and recognition, never resisted filling father in on his plans.

Theo, in a departure from normal, collected him from the airport. Listened as intent as a Robin stalks a fly, then made him pull the car over to the side of the road.

Pride oozed as he congratulated him with familial hugs and kisses, expounded on his plan to kill the horse. 'A sure, safe, well-planned job. In and out. You are now the man I always thought you could be.'

Heaped more praise on son's shoulders in fifteen minutes, than in a lifetime of rewards.

As always, he, nervous of upsetting Georgiou's mother, finished with the big warning. 'Not a word to mother. Keep this between us for the present.'

Despite his earlier enthusiasm, Georgiou spotted a trace of doubt swim across dark eyes as serious, and after kissing him, father said. 'Her heart weakens. Doctor says it makes funny noises and is leaky. So, until specialists are happy. No stress.'

Disturbed by that news, although following their effusive reunion, mother's normal attitude never raised concern.

He, forgoing normal invitations to party, held himself in check to prepare for the main event. A clever move, it allocated space to spend more quality family time with her than normal during his calm, four-day holiday.

***

Then off to the US.

Georgiou settled into his swish hotel room in the Griffin Gate Marriott.

Even smarter than Calder's room in the Best Western Richmond, where they met to put last touches to the kill.

Georgiou stood in front of his seated partner.

Fought against raging, restless emotion as he tried to restrain himself from exposing the depth of his anger.

At one point, exercised maximum control to not escalate his loud voice to a shout.

Early days, during a lawless upbringing, taught him losing one's temper was counterproductive. The inestimable value of discipline held when he summoned self-control and pleaded. 'Come now, Calder. We do this. Promise, after this we will never take on another job. Honest.'

Despite his constant reassurance, Calder wavered.

As time approached for the kill, growing reluctance culminated with him being physically ill enough to vomit his dinner, when he only reached the toilet bowl in time to avoid a frightful mess.

After he washed his face, weak from retching, staggered back into the room, then flopped down onto the bed. Amid this his most severe bout of doubt, dug head into the duvet and whispered. 'Never reckoned my interest in animals could bring me to this.'

Uncertain how to cope with him, Georgiou poured coffee.

Watched, soulless, felt only disgust for the man with whom he shared so much. For now, on the edge of something huge, when he needed only support, the wreck he studied left an unsavoury bile taste.

'If I kill again, what next?'

Calder, in danger of degenerating into formless pit of a bag of wilted cabbage leaves, moaned. Pale face stood out against dark purple duvet.

In horror, Georgiou watched him snuggle into softness of the bed, a cat as it prepares to sleep.

Enough of this. 'Come, lad.' Georgiou's powerful arms picked him up, pulled to his feet, and grabbed shoulders, shook him hard enough to make teeth chatter. For fear that he loses support, exerted his authority as leading player in their unfolding melodrama.

'No choice. To begin with, if we try to pull out now, we face severe repercussions.'

Shook him, hard. 'In a nutshell, we face dangerous people.' No fool, the vet faced a decision. *Yes or no!*

Stuck at a famous junction, powerful as Robert Johnson's, Cross Road Blues, they ran dangerously short on decision-making time.

With the dedication his birth father Henderson earlier expressed in his pursuit, then domination of Fiona, those matching genes exerted their effect.

Change suited Georgiou, who breathed slower when he watched colour flush over Calder's face as he, fearful of losing face, aware of and embarrassed over what he recognised as his pathetic reactions, reached for hidden logic and strength to summon a forceful recovery.

Georgiou added to that resurgence. 'Fear we deal with powerful, criminal people.'

Stared into Calder's eyes. 'Friend, I worry your indecision, and weakness may impair negatively on our safety.'

When he divulged doubts, Georgiou never played out actions of the director who manipulates an actor to cajole her into a masterful performance.

Instead, acted from genuine visceral fear.

As realisation only properly dawned, appreciated pain as intense as the pre-perforation pangs of a duodenal ulcer and slapped both hands onto his abdomen in a hopeless attempt to gain relief.

Amid what now developed as heart stopping visceral terror of impending death, when a tense throat permitted speech, Georgia released words that vibrated with slow threnody of swarming bees. 'Afraid for our safety. Yes. They may do something unspeakable. For to them, we are as expendable as the horse.'

Without delay, Calder, an intelligent, imaginative man, accepted the Greek's warning and at last appreciated then shared his partners state and fears.

But before he could respond, a ringing telephone demanded attention.

Georgiou picked it up and after a ten second conversation, said, 'Yes. We are prepared.'

Turned to Calder. 'Now, please we must smarten ourselves up. Get tidy. Need us fit and in synch with a confident air to impress him. For without prevarication, he should recognise our air of command.'

Outlined Percy arrived with their drugs to help complete final details.'

Calder's mind whirred.

Not just with unsavoury prospect of horse slaughter for Georgiou's fears of what could happen if plan goes awry motivated him. Headed for the bathroom. 'Must wash my face.'

After briefest of greetings, Percy reinforced Georgiou's comments around failure. 'This is where we find ourselves. At a momentous phase. Your plan must work, for too much is at stake, and with our detailed planning laid out, act out the role of men prepared to climb the hill toward success.'

Left off his monologue to hang head. 'Failure is not an option.'

Percy: his attitude far from usual pathetic, mincing character could not have acted any more different from that he normally portrayed when he confirmed Georgiou's earlier thoughts. Again, warned them how deeply involved with difficult people they found themselves.

That said, intimated how a failed plan endangered their lives, rambled on in nervous fashion, and outlined his boss' intentions in greater detail than ever dared. Until now, conducted his boss' orders, whims, and desires without discussion or hesitation, to the letter, the original, highly remunerated, yes man.

But now, after he had noted Monti's deteriorating demeanour, Percy feared a failed plan must also cause his extinction. Besides expressing fears for their safety, scarce believed how he permitted personal fears to cascade in tumultuous form. 'Yes! We face big trouble.'

Threat held sway, as his shaken mien created greater menace than Georgiou's concerns, and as Calder appreciated depth of the trouble they faced, he investigated Georgiou face, appalled to recognise for the first time, his own fears mirrored on the Greek vet's face.

Percy's normal, mincing manner disappeared forever.

All semblance of order drained away as he half stuttered. 'You cannot understand who we deal with.'

Visage cleared, hinted at hope, and promise of reward. 'Besides, consider the other side. Generous. Forget your promised fee. Compared to what must follow with success, well, this man, my boss shall flood you with honesty and support. Most generous.'

A soft, flimsy hand flapped a delicate, pink handkerchief up to smother a sweating brow as he flopped down hard in a firm sable leather armchair.

Percy examined silk as though it held a wealth of inspiration. 'However, remain serious by reminding you this exercise cannot fail.'

Had already convinced vets of the seriousness of their situation yet now slipped into a phase of repeating and reinforcing a likely scenario of destruction.

'If we do not kill this horse as planned, because of our inadequate response?' Aim was to reinforce to himself personal danger.

To summarise, when unnecessary, searched for words. 'Any carelessness or inefficiency places us at risk.' No actor ever conducted himself as he did. Besides an outpouring of profound sincerity, drenched them in his genuine anxiety when he advised how an out-of-control Monti must react if they fail.

'He will kill you, us.'

Words and actions hit hard as any pile-driver, or in their case as the ancient poleaxes used to stun animals for slaughter.

Dead, an appropriate word.

Silence bathed the room for a full five minutes.

Shocked common sense into all three with Calder, first to break the spell when he urged them onwards. 'Now, the final rehearsal.' Rose, grew in stature, fetched the bag Percy placed on a table, brought it over to the bed, and emptied contents.

By the time he and Georgiou finished studying materials, the Greek ran a hand through his hair and relaxed enough to express approval. 'Good. As we requested.' Delivered Percy a double thumbs-up. 'Thanks. All in order.'

They discussed the situation twice more. When all satisfied, Leon turned to leave. But then he paused, pleaded with them as a Beagle puppy in urgent need of a tree. 'Please guys I am serious. One of my boss' men will be on hand. The unbelievably dangerous, psychopathic Monti and we dare do nothing to distress him.'

Like a slap on the face with a cold wet fish, Calder now fully recovered from the state of permanent anxiety that held him during the previous week, understood seriousness of Percy's state.

Shivered as Percy continued, repeated earlier warning. Did so as he plucked at Georgiou's sleeve, 'For he will not hesitate to shoot all of us if things go badly.'

Percy slipped into a disembodied moment when he reiterated the likelihood they could face Monti as a killer. Strengthened that view when he hinted how bodies disappeared in the past. 'The profound depth of the farm lake never yields secrets.'

As intense as the lake's hidden depths. Weighty silence embraced them in the deepest of dank, flavourless dungeons.

From that oubliette, Calder, commented, displayed inner strength which allowed him to make a complete turnaround. Amid threat of imminent danger as his future opened it offered two choices, pathways to either hope or disaster.

First, could breakdown completely under pressure, or, and here he surprised not only Georgiou but also himself. Calder continued to grow, exhibited unknown untapped callousness when he unveiled the usually suppressed hideous personality of Henderson, the father he lost as an infant.

Logic forced him to take the best option.

Where Georgiou now swithered, Calder assumed newfound role of coordinator, found fear summoned power to dredge up missing assuredness. Illustrated how partnerships work because people feed of each other.

Just as Patrick and Deirdre Cairns worked together, when one was down, provided the other was stable, they worked through difficulties.

Lucky for these potential killers, so too as Georgiou now dropped, Calder surfaced and dragged them on.

Calder's dark eyes reflected his father's dangerous ugly side.

He picked up Percy's theme, hinted at his own defensive mechanism where he prepared to unfold menace which matched the now dangerous, diabolic tone that permeated his voice. 'Now, we have it. Aware of imminent danger, even the prospect of death,' Grabbed his partner's shoulders. 'we must prepare.'

Turned to Percy. 'As we reach the business end of things, let me again assure you this hose will die. But to make certain need a pistol.'

Tapped Percy's cheek twice, firm enough to make the man step back. 'Let you not doubt, we appreciate the immensity of this undertaking, and excluding financial considerations for the moment, for personal safety, this venture must go well.'

Faced both. 'So, yes! I must have a gun.'

A positive step that shocked Georgiou and strengthened his courage as Calder continued. 'For if I sense danger, shall kill this Monti.'

With such words immersed in a powerful delivery he continued to surprise the earing pulling Georgiou when he stood tall and exuded air of professionalism everyone needed.

Percy had already anticipated need to defend himself and gently extracted a Velo 6.35mm Mini Pocket Revolver from the inside of his coat pocket.

Never having fired one, extended it at arm's length to Calder and displayed inexperience and nervousness. 'Planned to use this to protect myself if we get to that desperate state.'

Calder, experienced with firearms, accepted, then scrutinised the gun, dismantled it to check its working order. 'Super. Even if it holds stopping power of a hungry female mosquito, this, our protector, may at close range, buy time.'

His remarkable, emotionless, coolness buoyed them onwards. 'Although we shall not need it. For we, in a display of efficiency your boss never witnessed, shall slaughter this damned horse.'

Georgiou, whose own emotional state had steadily flagged, picked up on Calder's attitude. 'Good man. Thanks for being strong and enough distraction. We proceed.'

Rose and said, 'Let us get out of here for now.'

Others relished this suggestion. 'First, Percy, take us for a drive around the area. For a change of scene as we reconnoitre will dispel doubt, improve focus.'

The hour they spent drifting around gentle, leafy, farm and parklands convinced them it was unlikely anyone likely to interrupt the killing.

When Leon dropped them off at their hotels, Calder asked. 'Percy, you forget something.'

Without delay, Percy almost choked. 'Sorry. Shells.' Dug into a pocket and produced six bullets wrapped in tissue. Hoped they heralded fears that slipped away to a permanent, contented rest.

77

SOPHIA'S MEETING

The head nurse conducted the tour.

Earlier, Louis warned Tessa of Sophia's importance.

Business card she left earlier when booking the appointment raised eyebrows. On time, vets hung back, secreted themselves in the office as they awaited Louis planned Sophia's hospital tour to allow her to understand she dealt with a modern, efficient outfit.

With due diligence, Louis had checked up on Sophia when he disguised his voice as he rang the number. 'Morning mam. May I please speak with the Baroness?' 'Whom shall I say calls, sir?' DS Anderson affected a powerful upper crust English accent, acted smart as ever.

'Name Godfrey Frieze. Interested in talking to her about importing bloodstock.' 'Thank you sir. The Baroness may well find your theme attractive for import and export of quality stock forms the backbone of our business. Although a project to attract the Baroness' interest, sadly, may I caution you to patience? Can this wait until she returns from the United States? For business keeps her there until this coming Friday.' 'In that case, thank you for your courtesy. As my project is not urgent, shall contact her when she returns.' Gently replaced the receiver.

Bernard at once traced the call then Pauline contacted Henry. 'They reached out as planned, so bait heads down someone's throat.'

That hit, a useful sounding board, impressed Waterman. 'Well done, Sophia. First strike to us.'

'A better standard of excellence than expected.'

During her visit, Sophia swanned around the hospital, acted Queen of the Castle. 'On a par with what I expect in Europe.' Offered them one of her delicious mini bows. 'So, you may indeed be the right people to consider as partners in my venture.'

Eyes wandered. 'Yes. This place leaves me with a pleasant taste. A fuzzy feeling.' Shimmied shoulders and winked.

They stood outside the operating theatre.

Through a large, fortified glass window, watched a vet, and two nurses castrate a cryptorchid horse. Because one testicle lay trapped in the abdomen, they anaesthetised him. Now, in dorsal recumbency, on his back, vet worked between his back legs.

Despite immersing everything in a sea of green drapes and anaesthetic equipment, the scene proved impressive. Their technique enamoured even Sophia, who in younger days, worked as a student in vet hospitals. 'Most professional, human standards.' They structured the meeting to perfection.

As the vets planning deserved, they hoped to impress Sophia, keen to hear of the prospect of regular involvement in importing quality bloodstock from top European lines.

Anticipation of regular, easy money encouraged Louis to suggest a second meeting. 'Time presses today. Can we meet again? What about dinner tomorrow evening? We should love to entertain you with our US hospitality. How does that sound?'

'A splendid idea. Because, with a second hospital visit today,' Enjoyed how a flicker of dismay traced concern over Yvette's demeanour, 'also run out of time.' Extemporised when she added threat of opposition into the mix.

Sophia gave them her temporary cell phone number. 'This number is purely for my business trip, personal to me. Anticipate our meeting, soon.'

78

WITH CAROLINE

Holly and Francesca regularly visited Catherine.

Niall's lady spent an increasing amount of time with her.

So, Niall pretended jealousy. 'You never find time to for me now, as you spend more hours in Dumbarton with Aunty Holly than me.'

Slapped him. 'Love Holly already. Firm friends.' Hugged. 'Also, she gives me the low down on naughty things you did as a child, more than your doting; *he never did anything wrong*, mother does.' Clasped palms together as though in prayer to indicate Fiona considered Niall her gift from God.

Hugged her back and brushed lips. 'Love how you guys' team up. Superb. Can always beg a decent meal when your busy life shuts me out.'

Deserved the fat smack.

A Wednesday in late August found Catherine in fine form, able to take a decent fifteen-minute walk. Because brain damage left impaired nerves, that meant she still faced a conduction defect illustrated by how although she knew where legs wished to go but got frustrated when they never responded as fast as she wished.

To accommodate, learned to take care. Picking up each leg and only when she slapped that down and steadied herself did, she start with the next. Holly remarked she walked with the goose-stepping motion of a Russian soldier.

As they arrived at the home, delighted them to meet Elaine as she exited the front door. After a warm greeting, explained away their initial alarm when they spotted a cumbersome surgical boot on her left foot. Sustained a simple lateral ligament strain on her ankle after tripping over one of her Jack Russells. Even if slight, it irritated the permanently restless Elaine. 'With the hospital placed busier than ever, here am I,' Glared at the boot, 'invalided for two weeks.'

Sympathised with her, but, since Elaine's lameness and Catherine's demeanour offered them time, took tea in the house. A move which allowed her and Francesca to catch up on more of Overtoun's history.

Elaine's life followed a steady path with her successful marriage to a doctor. Fulfilling, they found it easy to enjoy each other and resist children.

Inasmuch as the usual chit-chat played out, Catherine changed the subject. 'Now, my diary, Elaine. Have you finished reading it?' Peered with the incisiveness of insect hunting meerkats.

Although Elaine smiled, Francesca frowned at the ensuing bluntness when she said, 'Sorry Aunt Catherine, despite attempting to get into it, your book it is difficult to read.' Adopted the façade of an archetypical elderly spinster librarian. 'Your depressing tone paints only the bleak, sombre side of a difficult life.'

Furthermore, when she stretched out a hand to touch Catherine's arm, Elaine settled into ruthless manner of a disgruntled literary agent. 'Suggest we defer your weighty tome for now, leave it hidden in an attic cupboard until you are fit to lead me through the work. So, still unfinished.'

As that caused Catherine to slip into a phase of the hidden, shadowy deliberations often embraced her, while encouraged by time, the ladies began excusing themselves.

Two minutes later, as Elaine prepared to hit the road, Caroline grasped her arm. 'Bring it to me.' Spluttered dank saliva while saying she wished to reread the concluding chapter again. 'For, hidden inside are my notes, loaded with potent, important information.'

With one of the remarkable bouts of clarity, her improving condition encouraged, indicated her desire to reflect on the work. 'For those birthmarks hold the key to my family's success. With my memory returning, I need to study that chapter.'

A plea which although it began with great intensity, fell away, and by the time those words slipped out, sleep claimed that still frail body.

Forthwith, as Elaine tucked a blanket over her shoulder, Catherine continued to mumble and despite being a loose collection of incoherent babble, Elaine, working hard, sifted jumbled words. Deirdre. Dragon. Twins. Psychologist.

After Elaine took care to arrange her booted foot around pedals of her automatic VW Tiguan, she stretched hands over and around the steering wheel. 'Damn! Hate this boot. Too confining.'

Restless, rushed as always, only when settled, ready for the off, thought. *Damn. This blooming diary. How to react? When my aunt displays that sense of urgency, her wild-eyed expression suggests trouble. Nevertheless, should dig into the thing. Besides, may stumble across dangerous secrets, instructive tales of grim times.*

Laughed aloud. A most uncharacteristic expression gave her fine mouth prominence and outlined hidden attractiveness. When she chuckled into the rearview mirror, criticised concerns. 'Silly girl. Only rubbish.'

79

ELAINE AND THE DIARY

Elaine sipped Earl Grey tea.

At home, rested foot on a stool.

Failed to embrace her unexpected period of slackness and coupled with almost total home confinement, that lack of mobility, linked to unused energy, was more galling for Elaine than expected.

In time, discarded yet another magazine. Straightaway, after sliding that into a magazine rack packed full of everything from home decoration to gardening, never fashion, considered what should follow.

An impossible time. So bored, whatever should I do next... The diary.

That image brightened her face, made her decide she struck a suitable time to tackle the books. *They cannot depress me further.*

Homed into her project with diligence of the perfect student.

Until Elaine, as she resolutely struggled through volume one, gradually fell into Caroline's haphazard writing pattern, but struggled with her train of thought as her rambling, aberrant style caused problems.

Thus, she failed to fathom machinations of a disturbed lady's brain, soon tired of the effort, set it aside. Too many pages related to the family's forced move.

Desperate, unhappy descriptions of Caroline's own mental state, when coupled with sadness surrounding her mother's admission to hospital, brought only distress. Pages focused on her mother's depression although impressed at supreme efforts her aunt made when she worked hard to support parents mentally and physically. Those drew sympathetic tears.

As she closed the volume, a scrunched nose indicated sympathy. *My poor aunt. Always suspected a challenging time, although at no time dreamed it this bad. Shame indeed.*

Nonetheless, one hour later, showed application of a tortoise as it reaches for a flavourful, yet distant, unreachable calendula flower, tried again to struggle through the first volume.

After Caroline's thoughts on what Elaine considered inexplicable Cairn's incidents, she appreciated how that led to a more relaxed, less stressful period.

Months jumped, passed without entries because as her situation calmed, additions became shorter, logical, less tart, and even snuggled in an aroma of content. Even managed happier entries, including joyful, scrumptious events that surrounded her nursing career.

Still, Elaine constantly surprised at complete lack of familiarity. *Never realised her such a lonely woman. Friendless. Immersed in a tough world.*

The inaugural volume catalogued failing health, how both parents entered the fabric of nature.

The following sections allowed Elaine to soften, unwind into pages of entries which began five months later, when Caroline's easier attitude suggested life treated her kind, embraced her in a hearty, comfortable state. Made her appreciate how sad the opening pages of volume four differed.

Two days later, when Elaine reconnected with the saga, the potent words, CAIRNS AGAIN, pricked ears as firm as an inexperienced horse approaching an upright. Date indicated this diary period six months after Caroline joined Overtoun.

Elaine's tight lips stretched, beamed at how at last in Sister Holly, aunt found someone with whom she could enjoy a citrusy chat.

Downhill from there. Because page after page of stagnant diatribe, indicated how her aunt recognised the Cairns family who ran Overtoun as the progeny of a particular Cairns.

Detected the relationship between Overtoun's Cairns family and the hated accountant who mismanaged Catherine's parents' removal from their beloved family croft. A nauseating period that set off her mother's illness into an ever-increasing downward spiral of misery.

Elaine staggered at the change, recognised how within space of five pages and three months, aunt's mental health deteriorated. Also, it was around that time when she became irrational, lost weight, forgot her manners. *Gosh! Now I remember, and these notes help me unravel poignant events around the time.*

Elaine brightened when moving forward she found a hiatus in her decline. Found where Elaine joined Overtoun Hospital and how she initiated that improvement, knowledge which lifted spirits.

Doubtless, during a period when she described Elaine first months at Overtoun, how familial contact bolstered reserves, brought significant, albeit brief improvement.

But only as she explored the meat of the story did Elaine uncover a mesmerising tale, one fit for a Netflix series. While absorbing, it also depressed, for it heralded the end game.

As Elaine unfolded Caroline's distorted, vicious rantings, the matching script forced concentration. Especially when she recognised aunt's unripe ravings pinnacle into one enthralling point.

After reading that paragraph, its potency demanded she reread, aloud this time. *Have it now. The key to my family achieving deserved revenge centres on three babies. Margaret Stewart's twins and Fiona's boy. Shall expose where something fishy, dishonest, even downright criminal took place. But what? Shall snoop, intensify my research efforts to find the key that can unlock the dragon matron's musty secrets.*

Elaine's husband cut short her musing when he arrived home, announced shift changes offered them a rare, three-day, free weekend.

Monday at around eleven am.

With two days left before she returned to duty, Elaine picked up the diary. Reread that same passage five times, which caused her to rotate her head in ever enlarging patterns.

Facts raced back. *Remember talk of the twins. The Stewarts. Yes, because of how Rod Stewart and Baby Jane flooded the radio at the time.*

Remembered how her aunt often mumbled, rambled on with comments around the twins, of bizarre goings on including birthmarks.

Nonetheless, with Caroline's poor writing, and her personalised shorthand habit of truncating and repeating thoughts and conjecture, her disordered style confused and frustrated Elaine. *Why, if my aunt confirmed irregular, illegal practices, did she fail in committing it in succinct fashion to paper?*

'Damn, damn, and damn.' *This makes me recollect that great novel I read, that while absorbing, proved a shocker when I realised the last, most important chapter was missing.*

As a girl who rarely voiced opinions, she recognised how Caroline's notes encouraged her to chatter aloud and, on this occasion, allowed it free rein. 'Must explore this. In the meantime, for even though unlikely, seems Catherine suspected they mixed up the babies.'

Dropped the book, stared at reflection in the mirror, and whispered. 'Worse still, did someone intentionally swap those children? Change mothers?' Agitated, she issued those comments loud enough to excite the three Jack Russells.

She determined to meet Angela and probe.

Given the two remained in touch, they never became real friends yet offered a useful platform to use as a sounding board. That stopped her as running into a brick wall does an out-of-control cyclist. 'No! If deceit occurred, is she involved? Angela, are you inadvertently mix in something serious? Or, and God forbid, did you play a part in some foul plot?'

Sharp, dropped book onto the table.

'Did you uncover the beginnings of a wicked example of child trafficking? Does that explain your sudden, dramatic exit from Overtoun? No!' A sudden expletive encouraged the dogs into action.

'Is that where your unexpected promotion came from? As it arrived directly from Matron's hands... Did she... Could she have offered that as a bribe to ensure your silence?'

An idea glimmered. *Must find and contact Celine for her memories, still poignant after horrid assault, will complete the package.*

Overall, enthralled by proposed investigations, the sensible woman stepped back, decided this matter potentially dangerous, damaging for her career, because she, as a staff member could find herself tainted with colour of deceit.

That said, took a break.

After she hobbled to the kitchen for tea, Elaine discussed her dilemma with the dogs. They listened with unparalleled patience; for Jack Russells and advised her to allow sleeping dogs to rest.

'So, friends. What about swapped children.' Mused again. 'If swapped, they are already grown, so only pain follows if retrospective investigation uncovers anything untoward.' *Irrespective of what went down, probably best to let sleeping dogs lie.*

Said that in a whisper then laughed and got the dogs going. 'Let sleeping dogs lie.' Dogs agreed.

80

ANGELA AND CELINE

Coincidence or not!

People shared interesting observations.

Once shared ten evening meetings with a well-educated, informed lady, an eminent psychologist with a haughty manner who informed the group she disregarded coincidence. Everything happened as part of a great plan.

But it was her attitude toward God that contributed an extra dimension to her character. 'While I disbelieve in God, accept there *must be something out there*[2].'

Explained God as her great inexplicable something and disagreed with her comments on chance. This meeting that took place in Dumbarton was the perfect example.

Elaine met with Celine and Angela.

Celine left Overtoun and medicine shortly after Sister Catherine Grant's attack. Moved away to recuperate with Sandra, a much-loved cousin in Denny near Stirling. In one of those fortunate accidents of life, she met, when almost convinced to capture the unsuspecting Henry, then entered marriage with the man who became her flawless life partner.

When Eileen tracked her down, she overjoyed to learn Celine prepared to visit Dumbarton for a family anniversary.

Thrilled at the prospect of meeting Eileen and Angela for lunch at Eileen's splendid home on Colquhoun Street, near its junction with Gibson Street in Dumbarton.

Satisfied with preparations for lunch, she looked around and gave hands a small clap.

---

[2] Found remarkable similarity in Jane Goodall's last interview. Released only after her death, she made a similar comment. But in a poignant moment, ended with *God bless*.

As Eileen finished putting everything into place, a noise made her glance through dining-room window. On seeing a car pull up, she walked down tarred driveway to greet her visitors.

Angela, let us be honest, never earned plaudits as world's best driver. By the time Eileen noticed her struggle to negotiate stone pillars that held apart already opened wrought-iron gates, she moved to intercept her on the pavement and instructed how best to enter the driveway.

With this almost accomplished, screeching brakes indicated a second vehicle had pulled up sharp by the kerb outside the house.

'Goodness me. A lovely surprise.' Angela pushed Francesca, driving her GTI, into an emergency stop when she spotted Elaine by the side of the road.

That promised an interesting meeting of five ladies.

To continue the event, Elaine instructed. 'Now ladies. All of you, I mean. Come inside and enjoy the loveliest, impromptu lunch party.'

Never brokered Holly's refusal. 'Nonsense. Sure, have enough food on hand for a dozen coal miners, never mind five genteel ladies. So, inside with you.'

Notwithstanding her confidence, as they followed Elaine, Angela, introduced her to a different possibility when she whispered to Francesca. 'Inspect the table and be prepared for FHB.'

Only later she educated the thoroughly confused Francesca. They used FHB, Family Hold Back, as an ancient warning on how to react when the host does not have enough food for everyone. Thus, family accepted their responsibility to delay helping themselves until after serving guests.

Two hours of their magnificent cold buffet flew past as everyone caught up with news of life and partners.

The situation changed for the inquisitive Francesca, as the new girl on the block, held centre of attraction.

With friendship bubbling, she turned the conversation along avenues where recent conversations raised interest. 'And as you can imagine, this talk of Overtoun, of Caroline's illness, of her dislike of the Cairns family. Well, as an intriguing subject, it attracts me.'

With Elaine more relaxed than in ages, the two glasses of wine worked magic. She joined the theme. 'Funny you should introduce that subject. For I only completed reading Aunt Caroline's diaries.'

'What!' At least three ladies exclaimed something similar.

Elaine, who rarely socialised, adored her party.

Aided by alcohol's lubrication, potent facts, better remaining silently hidden in diaries, nosedived across the table. Even allowing for unnecessary emphasis, revelations proved just that.

Revelations.

For, and inadvertently, she mentioned something about a situation that developed around the Stewart twins.

Although common sense exerted its necessary influence, helped her hold back the truly juicy bits, intricate neural pathways pushed her onwards.

But Francesca picked up on her important disclosure. 'Twins! They constantly jump into conversations. Common enough to convince me the incident holds truth and more intrigue than anyone ever uncovered.'

As she raced along, enthusiasm poured out in the form of questions, including who and what truths remained hidden. 'Twins, indeed.'

Elaine slipped up.

But we must allow some leeway.

As her acquaintance with Francesca's and Niall relationship, sat new with her and led into making what we accept as a mistake, a potentially party ending remark.

For Elaine released information she earlier determined to remain hidden. 'Sufficient evidence exists to suggest possibility of error around those twins births.'

Next, introduced a note of intrigue when she offered views on Caroline's conjecture on the basis her now recovering, hoped herself to release what she considered hard facts. In that case, expecting it to open, milked the story, and did so by firming tone with the tenor of a prosecution witness.

'Caroline intimated her positive belief Deirdre swapped out Fiona's natural birth son for one of the Stewart boys. Because only that can explain...'

Paused. That said, only when she caught on to how everyone stared at her did, she accept Angela's overt, determined effort to hush her.

The others homed in on Francesca.

The paleness of her face when associated with a marked slump into her chair, restored reality. Next, as the girl's face threatened to implode into surface of the smart Delft, recently cleared of excellent apple crumble with cream, Angela closed the meal. Smart.

Angela decided enough. Pointed at her watch, rose, and said, 'Goodness me girls. While lovely, we must get off.'

A bewildered Francesca delivered Angela to her home in Balloch.

But only as they arrived, she found courage to speak. 'Elaine offered me a frightening revelation. Overall, she suggests Niall may be Niall Stewart, not Niall Cairns. God. How do I mention this to his family? Should I be the one to break this news?' Amid a mind that vacillated with uncertainty, she wavered. 'Or should we?'

With them standing beside the car, Angela reached out with both hands, and as she shook her hard, pushed Francesca against the door. 'An impossible dilemma. For now, Elaine has resurrected suspicious facts, now released, the story may spread with the rush gossip always causes.'

Shook the now depressed and silent Francesca again. 'Like the Flying Scotsman, this will do the rounds and inevitably lead to shock, pain, and untruths.' With the girl unable to respond, she continued. 'Must now dig into this, research it. So, not a word on this until, we are sure. Insist you remain dumb.'

Francesca, as her head cleared gasped at a series of mind-boggling possibilities. 'Even worse than we imagined. Besides the horrors of the swap itself.'

Flung a hand over her mouth, then slapped it onto Angela's shoulder. 'That means the boy, Alroy Stewart, the one Niall's team hope to treat experimentally for his HIV infection, may be...'

Flooded both with tears. 'Niall's twin, his brother.'

As time unblocked her mind, she worried it time to visit the hospital. *For if Alroy has arrived and if Niall meets him, as an identical twin, he may suspect, even recognise him?'*

81

VETS PREPARE

Paulo never shared Leon's surprise.

Left his slaughtermen to stew in their deliberations.

As they finalised planning for the greatest equine insurance scam, and hopeful it was his last trip, Leon faced Paulo in his office.

The stealthy repositioning of enforcer Monty around the room added to his fearful state. For the man remained fixed in one spot, behind and to the side of his boss' left shoulder.

An odd variation in his pattern, it added further fuel to Leon's concerns, his desperate hope Paulo would allow him to leave. Already significant funds, when added to his reward for planning Senor Angel's death, assured everlasting wealth.

While living to embrace that luxury; fear I may disappear from the face of the earth.

No surprises there for Monti shared that hope.

Although as the savage man sank into his lowest level of depravity, he intended Leon's disappearance should take a different path.

For fear that he confuses the arrangements with lies, even white ones, Leon detailed his meeting with the vets, their sense of commitment and readiness to act on Paulo's instructions. When informed of the vet's restless nervousness, he detailed their state of mental readiness. 'Anxious, but keen to proceed, they satisfy me as to their willingness to act on your behalf.'

Paulo merely raised an eye as Leon looked at Monti who now draped himself against the door and received a flicker of a sneer, as Monti, in full view of Paulo, moved aside his coat and tapped belt mounted pistol.

Paulo, sensed Leon's emotional turmoil increased by the minute.

Concerned it might spiral into a Corryvreckan but remained satisfied enough to reassure Leon. 'It pleases me, my faithful friend to find the vets unfold this attitude, and do not try to fool you.'

In an exceptional display of energy, he rose, took his measured thinking pose from the window in his office, and allowed two minutes to pass then punched a palm against the wall.

When Leon jumped to attention, he said, 'We will achieve the success needed to eradicate all traces of horses from my empire. When the stallion dies, you then organise a dispersal sale. Everything goes.'

Now satisfied arrangements followed the desired pattern, he commended Leon.

If insufficient to calm fears that jigged inside his chest, his kind comment helped bridle the racing heart inside his chest as it sought to escape.

Still concerned, his boss asked. 'Come, friend, why so nervous? Consider our dealings, how your invaluable advice, detail, and eagerness to assist, always pay dividends.'

As the snaffle bit exerted control so too did Leon's heart slow from a gallop to a mere working canter as he continued. 'However, after removing horses from the equation, shall make changes. First, time for the Chinese who again express further interest in our... let's call them who medicines, to win the day.'

Thumped palms together. 'Next, time for me to grant Morgan her wish. We spotted the perfect Manor Farm in the South of England. So, yes. Deserves her place in English Royalty.'

Mind made up. After a glance through the window, he said, 'Last point is sad. For after sweeping away horses, you Leon must disappear, leave the US. With more than sufficient funds to support a decent lifestyle, suggest you slide gracefully away into exile for at least a year, even two.'

Because implications of that relocation made Leon step back and raise eyebrows, Paulo softened the blow. 'Granted, consider that as the extended holiday that will allow lingering doubts to dissipate.'

In an unusual move, he tapped Leon's shoulder. 'And then. When life continues at its normal trot, you should be able to return.'

A second tap, unfolded into the slight caress that caused a fleeting bolt of disgust and jealousy to race across Monti's face.

'With patience, as you test the waters, you could then to reclaim your place in your beloved horse society.'

Monti, whose face now again adopted its tough, non-reflective mask, even though still puzzled over his boss' reaction, continued in a manner out with his standard protective position when he moved things forward. 'Fear we consider the future before fully appreciating the stakes we face. For this horse's death to be a breeze.'

Gawked at Paulo, sharp enough to slice through butter. 'Anticipate, this being even tougher than you do, for we face significant hurdles with insurance, nosey parkers and others.'

Tapped his gun again. 'You have my guarantee. Any loose tongues, here or when these vets return to England, well... my task... to silence them.'

Leon gulped as he gave his revolver a tender stroking.

82

THE ENFORCER

The enforcer ignored Leon.

Accept threats and promises a fact.

While we encourage people with secrets to either release them, or in this case to bury them deep enough to make resurrection impossible, nothing claims effective focus as does a death threat.

In contrast to his earlier buoyant mood, Paulo, at last, realised the depth of Monti's concerns, but remained quiet, although his usually rigid pulse climbed.

For the first time, he worried for Leon's safety, made a mental note to discuss that fear with Monti when time permitted.

By the time various notions whipped through Paulo's brain as he tried to unravel Monti's ongoing and escalating behaviour, even he shivered as the man continued, uninvited to outline his backup plan. 'My job is to monitor the process. Concealed, shall hide in the shadows, discrete.'

With a display of faultless English, he rarely exhibited, explored the coming action. 'And... ensure we face no hitches.'

Patted his ever-present CZ-75 SP-01.

If the 9mm tucked into waist was not the most popular in use, awesome, terrifying stopping power at short range suited him. When faced with the threat, or promise of real action, he normally sported his Ruger LCR Revolver, the 38 Special model,

strapped to right ankle.

Only used it once.

Saved his life, ended two.

As the enormity of the slaughter unfolded Leon cringed at what they prepared to face. Backtracked, considered the Monti he thought he knew well, no longer faced him, and at once appreciated he plumbed depth of the man's psychopathy.

While he struggled to adapt to and fathom the different type of character in front of him, he replayed stories, half-truths of his early days with Paulo's father. Considered their abundant adventures, and now, Leon saw in the enforcer a ripe, yet nauseating example of primal mankind.

Now, seeing him in the raw, Paulo appreciated he had lost control over his man. As in some primitive fashion he generated the musky odour of a hunter whose superhuman awareness pushed him over the top, prepared him for battle.

Leon's sensitive nostrils closed, forced him to mouth breath, as the man's actions spoke tombs for the true animal instinct he exuded.

Also sensed Leon's critical situation.

Paulo held his tongue, but extraordinary and unanticipated thoughts floated to the surface. *Monti, fear you go too far. And I cannot intervene, for as you take control am powerless to interfere.*

Monti confirmed that wise decision when he gave Paulo a hint of his famous, malevolent stare then swung it full force over and through Leon.

The weak man felt his bowels loosen and release the powerful, noxious, foetid smell of fear. Stared as eyes flashed around the room, searched a bolt hole, where he might hide until they completed the slaughter.

With no hiding place, excused himself, raced to the bathroom where he emptied his colon in one flush of digested and still ripe material. Took three cistern flushes before he considered everything flooded out.

With him gone, Paulo dragged up a smile for Monti and tried to inject a touch of humour. "Come now, friend, you half scared the fool to death.

Triggered a mere glimpse of the man's desperate intentions but failed to raise a comment as Monti displaced him, took Paulo's privileged position by the window. *Fear my boss' nerves will not cope with this effort, so no prisoners.*

Leon's fear grew into something tangible enough to create a urine smell mixed with odorous gland excretions that poured from recently shaved armpits. *Could be the end of things.*

Sensed how this night set to play out as not just a watershed.

Convinced irrespective of a successful conclusion his life must end one way or the other, knew Monti intended for him to disappear, and not in the usual geographical manner.

Lodged hopelessly in the mire of despair he minced, almost crawled back to the room where Monti's final, withering stare almost caused guts to issue a repeat performance.

More concerned than ever, Paulo tried again to exert his authority, determined to win back control, and said, 'Our biggest effort ever. With our planning executed to perfection, and as everyone understands their parts, we do this. Let us go!'

As much as he tried to maintain some semblance of confidence even Leon spotted the tenor of weakness in his boss' voice worse than ever experienced and trembled to big toes.

Inasmuch as Monti now functioned as if the veil of terror that covered his face blew away, he acted his normal rational self when he stopped him. 'No boss! Need you to agree with me on this and go over the escape plan again until you nail it down as second nature.'

Monti grew in stature as they approached the killing act.

Now *Top Dog*, he emphasised when the possibility of their actions might involve violence, the scene demanded he take control. Although he addressed Paulo as *boss*, attitude left no room for doubt.

This commander led the way.

Paulo acceded to his control. 'You are probably right, so take us through it again.' Now affected by serious anxiety, he demonstrated a lack of control, subservience few guessed possible.

As Paulo understood how Monti's preparations affected Leon, his own nervousness increased. *Monti now reacts as any animal hunting for its life, in full protective killing mode. This must go well, for if caught up in any fracas, we are in danger of becoming the hunted.*

As though Monti, aware of their increasing mental disorder, decided it appropriate he take control, and acted out his best features. Drew from inner strength and numbered off the modus operandi on stubby fingers.

"These facts hold true.

Tick one. We have already prepared the horse with his overloaded, energy drink.

Tick two. Vet has examined him twice.

Tick three. The Greek vet, Georgiou, met him at the stables, and in busy mode, accepted his offer of support.

Tick four. The stallion's groom remains absent until summoned by Georgiou.

Tick five. Leon must now leave us to fetch him.'

Tick six. Checked his watch. 'Expect the second vet to arrive in exactly thirty-three minutes.'

Tick seven. Barked at Leon. "Go now! No slip ups, or' Patted his revolver.

Tick eight. 'When both vets are here, I will join them. They will administer the lethal injection in my presence.

Tick nine. Then Leon and the second vet shall disappear.

Tick ten. The first vet, concerned over the horse's deteriorating condition, will then summon his groom. For by then the horse will be ill enough to summon the vet.' Monti's deliberate choice of words heightened Paulo's fears.

Tick eleven. 'And then. We hide, and from a distance, sit around and watch the thing die.'

Monti explained how he would maintain his position as operations director and outlined the what-if scenario. 'When both vets arrive, I check them out. If they show any suspicion of a problem, any hesitation, I persuade them to get on with things.'

Repeated his favoured weapon tap, although he convinced Paulo his scowling face should prove sufficient in an emergency.

'Then the pattern follows as suggested.' Spoke with steady diction of authority and assurance which required no response.

Despite where earlier he threatened to submerge in darkness of nothing, it surprised Monti to find how Paulo's condition deteriorated. Always faithful, disturbed him to find his beloved boss plummeted into a state of anxiety the likes of which they never witnessed. *And this is my fault for should have insisted he left with his family.*

'But!' Monti also exhibited nervousness, when he suddenly lost his assured tone, outlined what happens if this goes seriously wrong. 'Witnesses disappear. Both vets and Leon will meet their maker.'

Peered hard at Paulo and patted his gun. 'You, boss, should now at once get away from here. Head for the Rose House, as agreed, and use the unmarked car concealed there for that purpose and join the family.'

Paulo nodded. 'We act to implement our escape.'

Monti swung back to Paulo, his request a statement. 'With Morgan as your alibi, confirm she understands the course of events?'

Paulo coughed, nervous. 'And from there while expecting to take a lot of flak, but will hopefully extract myself, somehow.'

Monti agreed. 'Good. Although you still have time to disappear now, for having changed my mind, please, get off this place now!'

He sorely tempted Paulo.

But having often analysed his escape route and convinced of success wished to complete the exercise and as he shook his head put on a brave face. 'No Monti. Cannot desert you, for faced with this fair plan, wish to be here when it goes down. Yes, I remain with you.'

In a touching moment Monti extended his hand, clasped Paulo's. 'To the end.' Took time but Leon's breathing, now settled from its earlier gale force, satisfied he, in the comfortable role of chauffeur, headed to fetch Calder, delighted the boss never instructed him to wait with them.

83

SOPHIA AT DINNER

They dined at 27 Mix.

Sophia arrived via an FBI chauffeured limousine.

To further enhance her credibility, the FBI insisted they transport a lady of Sophia's stature to the restaurant in a new, gleaming luxury Mercedes. And, to set the tone, her uniformed chauffer, an agent, also collected the vets.

Without delay, as she watched the limo rock up, Louise tucked a hand into Louis' arm. 'See dollar signs. Crispy notes will flood our coffers as though we cracked the casino jackpot.'

The restaurant, placed in Halsey Street's fashionable setting, serves a fusion of Asian and Italian dishes and reflects how US cuisine searches to uncover its identity. The nation has yet to establish a reputation for anything other than mimicking established worldwide kitchens.

Not a dreadful thing!

Sophia appreciated the meal and warmed by a single glass of decent Californian Burgundy, anticipated racing into the final bend of her chase. Despite her ability to remain distant, even cold, she slipped into a difficult, potentially weak phase where she enjoyed their company.

That said, were she fifteen years younger, such distraction may have proved problematic, but this seasoned officer, loaded with backup support, carried on with their effort.

As the evening unfolded, Sophia, reluctantly it seemed, steered conversation in an unexpected direction.

'Next, a confession.' Attractive eyes, enhanced by wine and lighting dilated and drew them into her mind.

'Since we share a table, eat as friends, may I explain niceties around my import business, that, having held back, mean I acted less than honest.'

Yvette's eyes, if they never matched Sophia's allure, flew wide and uncovered an overlarge portion of pure white sclera.

Sophia, while she concealed watchfulness, noticed Yvette gripped Louis' hand under the table as she continued. 'The parentage of your horses is not quite what you or anyone else considers as fact.'

Left that remark suspended over their heads, until Louis queried, 'You attract our interest. Fastened down our interest from the word go,' Beat out a series of drum notes as a lone finger tapped the desk. 'and must now clarify your intentions.'

Took three seconds, enough to raise alarm beats in Sophia's breast as she studied Yvette's face.

The vet, now en guard said, 'Enough now! No time for rubbish, explain yourself?'

By the time he unloaded his concern and sat back in his chair, Sophia wished to rise and dance as she dodged the winged shards of steel the vets in harmony winged her way.

A sense of the man's inner strength showed when he insisted on facts. 'Your tone smacks of dishonesty, suggests you wish to drag us into a dangerous arrangement.' Wrapped a knuckle on table. 'We are successful, professional people with a thriving practice.'

After he spent three long seconds to observe the still silent, tight-lipped Yvette, who aged five years in as many minutes Louis placed a protective hand on her thigh and as he offered her a reassuring caress, summoned a protective note.

Outlined his position. 'Cannot risk endangering our marital harmony by allowing you, or anyone, to introduce a note of corruption into our lives. Successful and content we need no dodgy practices to cause discord.'

Of course, the FBI never dumped Sophia into that charged environment without support. On the contrary, wired her with concealed equipment efficient enough to make even Bernard salivate.

A discrete earpiece matched the sophisticated and comfortable harness which supported the recording device that transmitted their conversation to a delivery van parked forty yards off.

It contained two technicians, Agents Waterman, and Blanchard.

From there, a superb sound system delivered everything back to base where Henry and Assistant Director Davidson listened.

Forty yards off lay two unmarked FBI cars loaded with field agents. Had Sophia seen them she must have shuddered at the degree of armament the vehicle supported.

The microphone that fitted snug in Sophia's left ear was protected by a sweep of well-styled hair, courtesy of an FBI makeup artist, to cover that side of her face and neck as fitting camouflage.

Excellent audio meant that when Henry whispered, his voice came through with such clarity and volume it made Sophia suspicious vets must detect them. 'Now, as it appears your approach has caused alarm, take care, for this may be difficult. Hold your patience and only when comfortable proceed.'

In the absence of any obvious lack of response from the target vets the surveillance set up confirmed test results obtained in the office before they set off on the mission.

Yvette's guarded responses, more passionate than expected, drew them out as Sophia hoped it should.

Amid the milieu of conflicting emotions that governed her responses Yvette's firm response bolstered Sophia's emotions to move on and introduce the second phase.

With artistry of a used car dealer who sells a vehicle with a dodgy engine, she smiled and followed that with the gentle chuckle which disarmed them. 'Respect your concern but ask for your patience, while you tuck into this magnificent seafood.'

As she leaned forward her confidence invited Louis' plethoric face to soften enough for her to go on. 'Shall explain how by following my scheme, you can make good, easy money.' Although both vets vibrated with tension, she continued. 'A consistent, regular and *safe* income will follow.' Highlighted, then repeated. '*Safe*.'

In fairness, although she played her part to perfection, a nervous Sophia looked around and guessed a couple at a table eight feet away were agents.

Needed a sip of wine.

Impressed Henry. 'Brilliant. You attract their attention. Slow, cunning.'

Again, sipped from her wine glass, until she realised it empty, an action that led to Louis half filling it before she could refuse.

Despite years of professional service in unusual situations, excitement of the chase threatened to derail her, and to improve her confidence, Sophia embraced the calming influence of something as mundane as sipping a glass of wine.

Propitious as desired, a server attended their table, enquired about the suitability of their meal, which allocated her and vets two necessary minutes to recover.

Appreciated where Henry's constant professional; even he at this stage never appreciated the attachment he felt for her support proved the expert backup required to bolster her through that stage.

Swirled her crystal glass. 'An excellent vintage, and now as I find you beginning to relax, please allow me to extrapolate, bring you to the winning post of our outrageous, masterful scheme.'

With the flair of Julie Roberts' portrayal of the Pretty Woman, she introduced them into unbelievable possibilities for duping the public and professionals. 'To make safe money.'

84

TRAPPED

'You now command the discussion.'

Sophia prepared to introduce her masterstroke.

Masterful, did so as Louis pulled out his wallet from an inside pocket.

Sophia's first thought was he set out to draw a weapon. The harsh pulling back of a chair over tiles indicated for her one of the nearby agents prepared to intercept.

Although only milliseconds passed, alarm settled as Louis opened the leather purse to draw money as he prepared to drop cash on the table.

Intended to guide his wife away from the table.

At once, appreciate the artist's magnificent portrayal of control as Sophia played her part, somehow managed to relax her demeanour.

Masterfully, sent him sufficient contented signals to make him change his tone.

Sophia built on that opening. 'Whereas I have caught your ear, listen while I explain how my system, soon to be ours, works.'

In contrast to Louis indignation of minutes earlier, he slipped under her spell and could not resist this different approach.

But compared to Louis, Yvette glowered, suspicious, her negativity issued warning signals for Sophia to first placate her. Fast. This encouraged Louis to stretch over and in a remarkably tender moment caused a fingertip to brush Yvette's wrist.

Did this as Sophia said, 'If not my intention to cause alarm, be fair.' Chuckled. 'Admit my opening caught your attention.'

Louis ignored Yvette's tough warning look and said, 'Got that for sure. Okay, as we are attentive, feed us your potent information.'

'Excellent.' Sophia settled into her well-constructed plan and reiterated they should make good, clean, *safe* money.'

Louis savoured how she stressed the safe word and appreciated how it encouraged Yvette to show more interest.

Sophia stuck to her detailed story.

Initiated that with the first inkling of how the simple fraud she introduced must prove undetectable and profitable.

Described how her company illegally bred the horses through AI and ovum transplantation from best quality international stock.

Guessed them hooked.

No matter their increasing interest, she excused herself. 'Best if you fine people share a moment, as I pop along to the powder room.'

When alone, Sophia took two minutes to admire spectacular the porcelain tiles in pink and gentle pastel colours, which brought extra dimensional life to the tasteful bathroom.

Toilet matters addressed; she closed off the microphone during that exercise.

In the meantime, as she left the vets space to stew, washed hands asked. 'So, boss, where do we go from here?'

Henry added to his already sound coaching. 'The crunch must come soon, for they can never resist this plan. Try to get them to unveil their past by exploring history. Find anything smoky in their background that smells dodgy? Get into insurance scams. Go, girl.'

In Sophia's absence, Yvette's nervousness increased, aggravated by what seemed merely an uneasy tummy. Despite them hoping to fall pregnant, it took days before the thought of *morning sickness* nagged, and as a palm caressed tummy, she outlined her concerns. 'What is this woman up to? I think we should get up and go. Slip away. Now.'

Louis, even though his thoughts drifted along similar lines, suggested patience. 'Match your sense of unease. But too early to bolt. Let us consider the rest of the story before jumping to conclusions.'

Before she returned, Henry's too tender warning, *take care my special friend*, issued with more that professional passion alerted not only Sophia to his growing interest in her as more than a colleague. *Gosh! Nothing for a decade and now two attractive men flirt with me. Gosh!*

On her return, Sophia enjoyed where two shining sets of eyes shimmered with expectation and even before she settled, Louis advised they deserved answers. 'Several things concern us.'

Sophia stroked palms together. 'Good. For your initial lack of response made me nervous. Cannot allow you to jump into this without asking me appropriate questions.' Henry liked that. 'Now, as you exert control, empower them to explore.'

She accepted validity of his prompt and satisfied them ready to gobble bait, said, 'I sense you may be the partners I need. But first, please, outline your concerns.'

In the office, Waterman said, 'This lady presents the perfect line to bring them out.'

'So, you constantly talk of money. But what money?' Notwithstanding her concerns, Yvette's hunger for wealth oozed, money aspect held most important.

Henry suggested she strike, lead with money.

Accepted that prompt, decided it sufficient stimulus to proceed, thus, Sophia said, 'Believe you may earn a consistent annual income of one hundred and fifty thousand fragrant dollars with fifty tax free cash.' Inclined head towards them, invited them to share her confidences. 'True, if not a fortune, remember you face no expenses. We pay all bills timeously.'

On balance, with Louis rivetted on her, he said, 'From your description, I sense we create nothing, no paper trail, nothing tying us down to anything other than a professional relationship.'

Assured in his approach, pinged a crystal wine glass with a nail. 'Do I follow the right track?'

'Theoretically you know nothing of the horse's origins, how we obtained them, or our plans. You act purely as agents on our behalf to facilitate their growth and juvenile training. For that, you bill us for professional services.'

Easily convinced, Louis said, 'We are in, for sure.'

'You have them, so milk this.'

Because Henry encouraged Sophia to explore, she said, 'Big bonuses follow when your stable agents introduce these horses to training. When they unfold as decent prospects, we sell them. We expect them to auction well and will reimburse you with a cash commission of twenty per cent.'

Because dollar signs landed Yvette, she forgot her queasy tummy and said, 'In synch with your understanding of the local situation, understand quality four-year-old imported European horses, with obvious potential are precious.'

Chuckle emulated Sophia's effort as she went on. 'But twenty percent.' Thought herself clever. 'Fear your offer sits low, unattractive.'

Because Sophia had prepared for that intervention, she haggled as well as any Romani scarf maker. Furthermore, after the normal to-and-fro of industry, she said, 'Twenty-two percent. Final offer.'

Sophia's stern statement as it threatened her overacting, forced frowns from both Henry and Waterman as when she laid her cards out, prepared to close. 'Time for decisions. In or out?'

Moreover, had Henry watched Sophia rise and pretend to leave, he may have choked. Need not worry, for Sophia engineered the process. Obvious when as she threatened to rise, Yvette, whose intentions swung to the stage where she appeared as he BFF, took her by the hand and asked her to please sit.

Having hooked them, but when she began to outline the plan's finer details, Sophia, when she sensed vestiges of initial barriers still in place from Yvette's side, buttered them up.

The ever-vigilant Henry sensed their timing right and suggested timing perfect for Sophia to take the step. 'Now, go softly, but dig.'

Also confident, Sophia explored their history. 'Own up to one last concern.'

As a hand ran through hair, she pulled it away, fast. *Almost exposed my ear plug.*

'To emphasise, while this project is cast iron safe for you, acting as mere, responsible agents, you appreciate our group of heavy investors, sail close to the wind.'

Patient, watched as puzzlement drenched eyes when she expressed concerns around security. 'As Go-Betweens, supplied with reams of correct, properly notarised paperwork, my people take the fall should we fail.'

Sophia mimicked an axe falling.

In conclusion, relaxed, watched a smug flicker run over Louis' face, as she gave her eyelids the merest, sexy flutter. Asked him to confirm them up to managing their

project. 'Must be sure? So, do tell.'

Gave the tiniest, cultured hand clap, 'Have you ever bent rules? Even a little? Can you uncover any slight discretions in your past that will give me confidence you will not fold on me? Any soupcon that might encourage me to take this forward?'

85

THE HIGH NOTE

The third bottle of wine worked its magic.

A smiling Yvette surprised Sophia.

To Louis' horror, and without consulting her, admitted they recently returned from Europe after being part of a profitable exercise involving...'

Before he could finish, Louis dug her in the ribs and called out *steady Yvette*. Voice insistent enough to make diners study them. Issued a tough question. 'Are you sure we are safe?'

While Henry and Waterman crossed fingers, she said, 'My dear we must join the Baroness in her venture, She must understand the calibre of her international partners.'

Then, stretched her hand out, touched Sophia's arm. 'Only when the Baroness is confident, she has sourced suitable partners, will she confirm us raring to go.

Yvette revealed her dissatisfaction at him for his ongoing urging to hold back when she prepared to divulge secrets. 'No! by taking this defensive approach too far and make us ladies uncomfortable.'

Henry whispered. 'Do not ease back. Tackle him now. Keep digging.'

Sophia rose. Masked her face with a disappointed stare and pretended to leave. 'Sorry, but if unsure.' Pulled out her phone. 'Shall summon my car.'

Louis, now that Yvette had convinced him to move forward, touched, almost grabbed her arm but released it as though red hot, apologised. 'Sorry Baroness, rude.'

Sophia responded to his rough treatment as must any lady. Haughty, displayed upper crust disdain at boorish treatment, and pretending cross, again pretended it time to exit. But when she almost reached the door, her overacting brought out a fear. *Have gone too far.*

Concerns proved groundless.

For Louis walked fast after her and offered the bow she as an aristocrat deserve and added further sincere apologies. 'No! Please stay. Let me explain an important development.'

Precious stones' involvement, throughout history reveal mankind's involvement with them have caused more sorrow than pleasure, and this relationship established that as factual when as they opened to her, vets could not stop talking. Complete and unabridged, Louis' version, compared to Yvette's more cautious approach, of their involvement in diamond smuggling operations tumbled. With Sophia genuinely enthralled by his disclosure, she exclaimed. 'Wow!'

Henry feared they suspected her situation, said, 'Quiet. Let him talk.'

Even Yvette, aware Louis loose tongue, opened them up to intrigue, joined his discourse in a rattling exhibition of how their pride in conducting themselves well in a quality crime, prevented them withholding any facts.

Ten minutes later, after Sophia drained their memories, Henry and Waterman shook hands and prepared to close off the investigation.

Sophia congratulated herself, offered them a most lady-like, soft clap of the hands, announced her confidence in having found new partners. 'Found the ideal match. What a story. Loaded with intrigue, appreciate the quality of my partners.'

Unlike Henry, Sophia carried on, intent on digging deep as any archaeologist, posed a finger heavenwards then coaxed it to drift into a lazy spiral to the tabletop. Louis decided her lost for words when she studied it against the pristine cotton tablecloth for a moment. Inasmuch as that pregnant pause permitted a gap for reflection until she continued. 'Perhaps, with us importing horses, we may develop a similar process.' Hesitated, disappointment to embrace her face, said, 'Although the money involved in dealing with quality stones, may well lie beyond even my partners.'

Still frowning, swirled ruby remnants in her wine glass carefully crafted from a recycled wine bottle, and when she went silent Henry said, 'Job done. Finish your desert while we plan to pick them up.'
Nevertheless, to everyone's surprise, her rambling vets, who now enjoyed themselves, continued to outline details of fantastically profitable trips. Because the information trail Sophia encouraged grew longer, deeper than her backup crew supposed.

Waterman, as excitement grew, said, 'Precious. Are they about to divulge something even bigger than hoped for, and...'

Henry shooshed him to listen as Yvette, tongue now loose enough to reach the table, raced on. 'In truth, because we collaborated with experts, their flair for planning meant they set up the deals to perfection. When approached by Chao and Gregor, the vast resources they commanded established them as major international players.'

Louis broadened her theme. 'And although names meant nothing to us, they took pride in being Chinese when they expound their great wealth.'

Waterman's excitement overflowed, and as he gripped Henry's arm suggested Sophia continue to probe into the Chinese connection.

Sophia developed that theme as instructed. When she poured dregs of their third bottle of wine she queried. 'The Chinese, you say. Never guessed them interested in horses. Odd.'

Yvette agreed with her. 'They also surprised us.'

Sophia extemporised. 'If talking drugs, I understand, for their established involvement in narcotics makes sense, but diamonds.' Brain raced at notion of how this fresh evidence could link with their important investigation, and how they might reach for the moon.

Whereas Louis, loaded with confidence, said, 'We spent so much time with our agents, considered them friends and they explained how their situation changed, dramatically so, by the involvement of a powerful family called Zhāng. That admission made us appreciate where they had found their big money players.'

At that point, Waterman almost choked.

But a call from his Assistant Director floored even him.

Henry, voice now urgent, instructed their arrest and commanded they rescue Sophia. 'Get her out. Enough. Close this down now. Get out.'

Issued Sophia with a similar instruction and pride in her professionalism ensured she never shocked at the intensity of Henry's instructions, but as Sophia brought the discussion to a close, promised their final preparatory meeting to follow in two days. 'Wonderful. The start of something big. Superb.'

She moved her chair back from the table.

Agents at the nearby table erupted into action as doors crashed, heralded intervention of the task team's takedown force.

Later, she wondered who paid the bill.

86

FBI TOP BRASS

Sophia's chauffeur disappeared.

In his place Agent Blanchard pulled up beside her.

Played part of a passing New York taxi driver.

Reached her as Sophia exited the restaurant. As she climbed in beside her, a swift glance caught where an additional agent, revolver already in hand lay stretched out partly covered by a blanket on the rear seat.

Her timing perfect, mind you, taking nothing to chance, they blocked off all taxi cabs in the vicinity.

When safely ensconced in the yellow cab, Blanchard's congratulations were most effusive. 'Well done, DI Sophia. Your skill exposed something bigger than we ever imagined, so back to HQ for gallons of coffee for we face an intense, demanding night.'

The investigation moved up another notch.

By the time they extracted then delivered Sophia to HQ, she faced their largest operations room where a powerful air of expectancy embraced fifteen agents.

Waterman introduced Director Zaleski, who as he assumed control said, 'Your magnificent team uncovered unexpected information of immense value.'

Saw the Director's enthusiasm mirrored in sparkling eyes of all participants. Nothing thrills law enforcement officers as the thrill of a hot chase.

Zaleski greeted, smiled at Henry.

But and noticed by everyone, proffered Sophia a slight bow. 'The Baroness deserves our compliments on how she expertly infiltrated the suspects confidence. Why nailing them for insurance fraud and smuggling is quite wonderful.'

Although Sophia enjoyed those compliments, she was aware more must follow and as he continued to speak the Director laid out other areas for the team to investigate.

'But and thankyou Special Agent Waterman for your excellent effort means as well as immediate promotion I appoint you as task commander, instruct you to develop these other leads.'

He embraced the entire staff. 'This is now a top priority issue. Commission you to research this complex areas where we hope to take down tougher targets.'

As the FBI team continued to expand, Waterman outlined how Sophia's investigation created interest. 'When they introduced the Chinese Zhāng family bells sounded, for that raised this investigation to the highest level.'

After he accepted a further confirmatory nod from Zaleski, Waterman, as he tried not to show excitement at his unexpected promotion, updated Met officers on the Zhāng family enterprises. 'From drugs, human trafficking and diamond smuggling, this family always attracted us as five-star targets.'

Spread arms wide to encourage the room. 'Now, because of the efforts of our British colleagues, we move forward in a positive manner.' Enthusiastic praise triggered off a another, even more passionate round of applause.

Next, Henry took centre stage.

His turn to introduce FBI agents to Alroy's teams investigations. 'Remarkable how separate exploration on both sides of the Atlantic exhibit a serendipitous channel which includes corruption in senior personnel in both forces.'

Although Director appointed Waterman to lead the team, he continued to add his ten cents worth. 'Also declare our recent conundrums in that area and expect to find this corruption extends to one of our assistant directors. Also like to explore that with your team, to either rule out, or firm a connection with your research.'

'In that case,' Henry got them going when he handed Waterman, a memo. 'Declare this officer may be involved with your corrupt agents. You may be able to cross reference something with your man.'

'Great. And as we share, ask you to check out our Assistant Director Rhodes with your people.'

Handed Henry a similar memo. 'Thanks. And excuse me, need to get this off to our boffins at once. For we face an incredible chain of events which should expose significant crime.'

87

BERNARD'S WEAKNESS

Bernard never settled into sleep.

Struggled to cope with insecurity.

Family and friends found coping with him difficult, always considered the man a nerdy loner. He grew with his relationship with team members, especially their obvious enjoyment of and appreciation for his company and skill. They opened his personality out as effectively as any cheap can opener dismembers a tin of HP baked beans.

But with his team dispersed, two days with minimal contact, he allowed the devastating news of Alroy's horrid debilitating illness to hit hard. Depression followed when last evening receiving news of Alroy's deteriorating condition, that doctors feared for his life.

Also, as they flung his confident Pauline into investigative searches distant from him, this contributed to that sense of loss and began restoring ancient inadequacies, fuelled from his own senseless, undeserved impressions.

Few slammed themselves as he did when faced with what he termed his *kit bag of inadequacies.*

To worsen matters, he, when in need of a decent rest, awakened after a restless sleep that lasted a boiling kettle over three hours, which made him affected by two successive, disturbed nights.

Plagued by insomnia for two reasons. First, as we may expect, shared the team's anxiety, their hyped nervous systems because mounting evidence from superb investigations ensured teamwork drew loose straws into solid bundles fit for thatching roofs.

Without team support, anticipated scenarios where failure to offer deserved support disappointed, and meant they faced disorder, defeat. The thought he may not be up to the task constantly chewed at psyche.

Worried over how they embraced him, a relative youngster, idolised his skill. Feared their brilliant team demanded he fashion noose after noose to finish their prey. Admiration they showered over him, their hopes, desires he alone could unravel almost magical evidence weighed heavily on slim shoulders.

Another reason for his uncomfortable nights lay in a heap on floor after he struggled out of his ancient, thin; could spit peas through it, sleeping bag. The formless structure crumpled on tiled floor beside his beloved equipment may have been bright orange at one time.

Now a miserable mixture of brown shades past its sell by date.

Poured coffee. 'Nice, helpful.' Slurped over well dunked muesli rusks a friend gifted him from Johannesburg.

Given the stimulatory effects of Pauline's exceptional blend of *Coffea arabica*, mien improved, until as imagined reality once again nagged, Bernard moaned. 'Still, I am missing something here. Where are these vets, my vets?'

Because he spent hours researching, sneaking around personal matters, brain instructed an unexpected change of direction.

Bernard sank into a dank, flavourless place.

Criticised himself, deciding he paid the vets disservice for leaving them alone, unprotected in the same big cruel world disinfecting his police brain.

With disappointment came distress.

Alarmed at perception he neglected them, apologised for not offering them needed support which might have changed their pathways from death and destruction. *If only I could have picked them up before something terrible happens.*

It happens hunters feel sympathy for their prey.

Robin Hoods of this world often earn ill-deserved empathy, for crime. Guardians of the law must ignore the easy euphemisms and half-hearted explanations for disorder.

A crime is a crime.

A woman is either pregnant or not.

A horse is lame or not.

No half measures exist in the minds of investigating officers. Only courts dish justice.

So, it transpired Bernard, inadvertently threatened to remove himself from the hunter role and went soft on them. Faced an unexpected danger wherein lay possibility he might flip his role, assume responsibility of protector.

Insidious notions led him to an incorrect impasse.

Aware his vets were on a par with himself, he could stop them digging themselves into deeper holes, rescue them from each other and from his team.

Hope flared that prompt intervention on his part may result in them facing shorter sentences and thus, after workings of the judicial system had its way, they may still face a reasonable future.

Debate raced through a brain tormented with confused neural synapses which distorted decision making pathways. *If I allow them to get into serious trouble, they may remain incarcerated for ever, and that fault may rest with me. Any delay or error during my inadequate investigative work must distort their impossible futures?*

Brilliant people often criticise themselves, assume character of their worst enemy. Although not a fundamental problem for Bernard, who held his place in the top half a-dozen people in the world at his speciality.

On occasions, when weak brain dopamine levels depleted, dangerous talons of lack of worth, snared him in vice-like fingers. Such a dangerous tendency places its victims in danger, and canny, because his team appreciated that weakness, they worked hard in the background to protect Bernard from himself.

Astute, Alroy alongside Pauline, unnoticed, managed, mothered his team.

Recognised Bernard's defect, arranged for fortnightly counselling sessions alongside safe homoeopathic remedies to bolster weakness neurotransmitter levels.

Helpful, but immediate urgency of their investigations, coupled with major overseas complications meant he missed three appointments.

Which left him alone and insecure during a time when Bernard's amazing brain demanded interaction, support.

A written mantra offered sustenance.

A business card sized piece of embossed paper.

Prepared for him by his counsellor, a fellow Christian and graduate of the Alpha movement, it held a single sentence.

If Jesus loves me,

I must consider myself unique,

Must accept my role in life.

Bernard read this four times.

Meditated using his favoured version of a breathing technique for five minutes.

Until during a third cup of coffee, as contacts and messages from team members raced across his computer, these shook him back into the saddle, resurrected him as a changed man.

At last. Here we go, my friends, back in the saddle, encourage me to face the world.

Reached underneath his desk to where the main cables extended away from him to the units computing processors.

Caressed the cable, blew his screen a kiss. *Meanwhile, no prevarication. Forthwith, forget the rubbish. Hunt them down.*

88

LONDON AND LEXINGTON

Bernard plunged into work mode.

Brain back in working order.

Throughout the tough, brutal, and often seemingly wasteful process of evolution, environmental factors played their part, developed resilience factors necessary to create the *Top Dog*.

Inherent flexibility of human mind as it harmonised with nature instilled the remarkable buoyancy which enables people to rise above themselves and achieve greatness deserved of our blessing as *Imago Dei*.

Seen at its best during the confessions of the great Saint Augustine.

Bernard appreciated his human frailty implanted through Original Sin imperfect, but we, with God's help, can overcome weakness.

If not yet saint-like, although Pauline raised him to that lofty pedestal, this power, as he worked for common good, inculcated desire to act in synch with the acceptable moral standards which aided Bernard's recovery.

After a struggle, intense as any giraffe that shakes off attentions of a lioness as it clings to a thigh, he, and he alone, righted mental balance.

Next, while he stared into the bathroom mirror, demanded shaking off what he termed senseless juvenile irrationality. 'Go Bernie, better than this, back into fighting mode.'

Overall, surprised at how much and how fast he accumulated reams of information on Georgiou and Calder.

Pulse elevated when it appeared his wobbly information ball, firmed.

Rolled both palms around each other as if he tried to encourage them into a solid, spherical shape of efficiency.

Late at night, thrived on regular pinging of incoming facts and left them to self-analyse and coordinate.

Fed enough facts into his computer to build an algorithm which, when combined with sneaky bits-and-bobs, filched from clandestine sources, encouraged his system to run a similar facial recognition programme to the one the Newark chaps used on Yvette and Louis.

Even his smart program took time, and incomplete data prevented him following that to a conclusion the previous night.

After which Bernard flopped onto the floor, pulled his disreputable sleeping bag over himself, and crashed into a useful, if inadequate three-hour hiatus from work.

Take cognisance of how the man worked like a Clydesdale gelding; did as much as four of the researchers in Kentucky for three days and nights, and how that resulted in sleep being necessary and irresistible.

With synchronicity of neonatal breaths providing oxygen after birthing process, which bring life, so too as Bernard delivered his mantra to the mirror, his beeping computer advised it coughed out important news.

Yes! Ignored coffee.

Tapped a single key to bring now dormant screen into action, and at once gasped, 'Got them. And different airports.'

With Bernard back in proper cop-mode, he clapped hands, issued a stream of instructions to his friend, now voice activated to clarify, and homed in on their whereabouts.

Established departures from Athens and London.

Confirmed both vets active, headed for JFK on the same day, three hours apart, which made him slap a fist against temple. Too hard. 'Ouch! Today!'

Flipped to fourth screen of his five-wall mounted information centre.

Cogitated on fresh streams of information, drained the coffee pot, grabbed two rusks, and almost choked on a rough-edged chunk as he gulped when eating. 'Confirmed. Different flights from different countries. Now! Both headed from JFK to Kentucky, Lexington.'

Never considered the range of clocks installed on his screens as he placed a call to Pauline.

She sprang from bed, shared instant awareness of all fired up officers, and began pulling on clothes as she listened to his excited, but logical update. 'With both our horse vets headed to Kentucky, guess them commissioned to commit fraud.'

Because Pauline agreed that meant they must escalate their investigation, she contacted Henry. 'Besides your superb news with Sophia, our chance to add a twist. Our two vets, Houdalakis, and Stewart,' Bad taste left in her mouth from last night's unwelcome news caused a slight pause, 'head for Lexington.'

Outlined Bernard's diligent research established them travelling on false passports. 'Is it possible someone shipped them in to kill something.'

Deputy Director Lomond made the correct conclusions. 'Too much for coincidence. These stories merge for solid reasons.' A pen tapped a prominent canine tooth. 'DI Higgins, ask you to please slow down your side. Inasmuch as you wish to take them down, please, pause all planned searches and arrests on the Met's bent officers.'

In synch, eager for the hunt, Henry, appreciated his point, said, 'Correct. By working together, that may enable us to undertake a full sweep.'

Clenched both fists and as he surveyed Sophia's beaming face, said, 'Must plan to pick up all of them, yours, and ours, together.

Looked in turn at all of the information screens. 'In the meantime, must ask if your team focuses on tracing our two vets?'

When Davidson agreed, Sophia noticed how, for the first time, even that fifty something, seasoned agent's lips quivered with anticipation as Henry continued, 'Doubtless these chaps are here to kill a horse or horses. Need to conduct intensive search for their recent movements, so, please FBI agents, find them.'

'Sir,' 'O'Malley, the agent who worked earlier with Bernard, said, 'I am in contact with the met officer in London. With us combining resources, expect an update soon, but already suggest the name Paulo Grizelli is important.'

'Grizelli. At last.'

Updated Henry. 'Fabulous work. Taste the icing on this enormous cake.'

Palpably savoured the moment then continued. 'We recorded suspicious circumstances around Grizelli's connection with heroine.' Frowned. 'At this stage, circumstantial, without solid evidence. But as well.' Eyes embraced flashing screens, searching for information. 'Have positive evidence his wife spent time with the Zhāng twins. Bang and bang again.'

Agent Blanchard, while aware of her junior position, had remained inconspicuous in the background. Now, wrapped up in everyone's enthusiasm she made an obvious, unnecessary suggestion. 'Sorry sir if I may?' When he nodded at her, she continued. 'Time for prompt action. For then we could catch them in the act.'

Director jumped at that. 'Also, on my mind. Because of fresh information, I escalate our investigation by two notches.'

With barely a pause in thought processes, he moved on and while he tapped a tooth again, pointed at agents. 'Special Agent Waterman. Organise transport to Lexington. You, Agent Blanchard coordinate circulation of vet's pictures. Hotels, so on.' Made one younger agent wither as his got tough.

'Now, top priority, need feet on the ground. Where do they stay? Whom do they meet? Where are they now and find a link with the Chinese?'

Slowed, showed a rarely evidenced humane touch. 'Feel this in my water. Find a connection.' Hesitated. 'Furthermore, get a local agent's task force tooled up, headed in their direction. Ready to fire on my command. But first, catch them doing something.' Held his hand up to indicate silence. 'However, we can trap them when they target horses, as soon as they kill.'

Blanchard dared interrupt. 'Sorry sir, I know we need hard evidence, but surely not at the expense of taking the life of a valuable horse.'

Despite acceding to her fair request, he remained untroubled by that possibility when, after listening to Waterman, issued further instructions. 'To begin with, establish the terrain. Can we land a helicopter on or near the property?'

'Affirmative, sir. We have two suitable landing sites. Large, grass paddocks close to house and buildings.' O'Malley impressed by finding information fast. Since modern day technology, including investigative satellites and drones, resulted in maps detailed enough to identify a tick in a horse's ear.

'Get to that farm. Fast, Where is my helicopter?'

89

LEXINGTON

Team arrived in Lexington.

Waterman barked out a series of orders.

Blanchard instructed a swat team.

Had them up and running with admirable speed then phoned Director Lomond back within fifteen minutes after receiving instructions. 'Confirm subjects' arrival in Lexington.'

Before he completed his report, Davidson asked. 'Are they together?'

'Negative. Drivers convey them in separate vehicles. While following the same route, they head towards horse country. The one identified as subject A, Georgiou Houdalakis, left two hours before the other. We monitor them. Discrete, will not contact until you command.'

'Good. Calibrate their route. Any chance they head for Roxio Stud?'

'Affirmative Sir. One hundred per cent.'

Excused himself for a seven second update, then advised subject A already on Roxio. In situ for,' glanced at the wall mounted clock. 'ninety-eight minutes.' Turned to the director. 'Moreover, with subject B, Calder Stewart, moving in that direction, extrapolate they arrange his journey to join them.'

Director explained. 'Paulo Grizelli again. That slippery customer owns Roxio. Our suspicions of heroin hold up, but taking no risks, absence of error makes his involvement difficult to confirm.'

Furthermore, considered how well Agent Blanchard blended with and constantly received information from O'Malley who manipulated two keyboards with the upper body dexterity of *Alondra de la Para* conducting *Ravel's Bolero*.

Seized a moment to comment.

Waited for his nod, then said, 'Sir. In Senor Angelo, he owns one of the country's most valuable horses.'

Thereafter, Henry, privy to this update, phoned Anderson. 'Check out Roxio Stud in Kentucky. Ask officers Collins and Anderson to establish if anything significant happens with their bloodstock, with one horse Senor Angelo, in particular.'

As they buckled up to land, Bernard phoned back and confirmed. 'Interesting facts. Roxio Stud owns the precious Senor Angelo. They recently insured him for tons of money.'

Anderson joined in. Her role to update team with real time information as it arrived on her monitor. 'Story takes an interesting twist when we consider his breeding record.' Perceptive, her knowledge of the thoroughbred industry allowed her to reach a significant conclusion faster than the less-informed agents.

She contextualised incoming information and released facts around the horse's disappointing stud performance. 'Established his first batch of progeny cause marked disappointment.'

Paused, asked for two seconds. Next, unfolded a positive report and explained. 'As the horse, initially, will be a failure, an unsuccessful sire, they stand to lose fortunes in covering fees. With enormous value of insurance cover, confirm it likely they target that stallion.'

Bernard again. 'My ongoing research on the horse uncovers relevant data. Concur with Sgt Anderson. Convinced Grizelli organises a fraud aimed at killing Senor Angelo for he has spent millions buying back shares in the horse at reduced prices.'

A *whoosh* slipped as the dollar's money involved reached his monitor. 'They insured him to the hilt. A fortune.'

Henry said, 'Fits in well with these vets and previous killings.' Broadcast to his team via a secure form of Facetime. 'As we approach our big pay day, owe this to DS Stewart to get it right.'

90

MONTI PREPARES

Paulo secreted family on their holiday home.

Planned slaughter during children's school holidays.

He and enforcer remained on Roxio.

When Paulo monitored Monti's actions he decided never was his nickname so apt.

They hid in a first-floor flat, his secretary's usual residence. She thrilled when her kind boss, appreciating he had overworked her and insisted she take two days off. For them, the flat proved the absolute observation spot as three curtained windows directly faced the barn that housed the stallion stables and adequately covered the yard.

Monti never revealed his growing sense of awareness, although an expert student of human behaviour must have spotted flared nostrils and increased respiration. Designed to absorb maximum oxygen, these physiological changes prepared his body for battle.

In complete control, deadly.

Checked weapons and moved with searching action of a fidgeting rabbit hunting, Red-tailed hawk. Restless eyes moved constantly as he monitored barns and yards bathed under maximum volume of the target areas splendid flood lights.

Paulo, while he appreciated Monti's competence, now, wished he had left the farm, and as he recognised Monti's professionalism, hung back, slunk into the background.

Still and quiet.

Earlier discussions with Leon, led by Monti convinced him to bow to the man, accept his leadership.

Doubtless, action as it prepared to unfold fitted Monti's job description.

Even Paulo carried a weapon.

Nervous fingers tapped the Beretta M9A3; modern equivalent of the famous ninety-two. Although proficient in basic training, firearms never appealed. Besides, notion of adverse factors that might force him to use it threatened to induce vomiting. Knees weak as jelly threatened collapse.

Monti, from vantage of a window seat, tried to dissuade him from carrying, but checked Paulo's Beretta twice during the previous hour.

Monti settled into killing mode.

Dissected every movement with dedication of a special force's sniper determined not to miss this, his one kill shot.

Despite understanding the man like a brother, Paulo appreciated he never witnessed the look of calm certainty that embraced Monti's face, nor anticipated his complete plan which included murder. *If I find opportunity, that ponce Leon gets it tonight.*

Paulo wished he could fathom the man's mind as he watched him peer through the window with intensity of a peregrine falcon swooping on a hapless feral pigeon. *Seen nothing like him adopt this pose before. Does he hope for proper action?*

In unstoppable mode, Monti continued to muse, *should anything go wrong, my pleasure to drop him alongside the horse. Preparations on hand for how and where to dispose of hi, perhaps their bodies. Lake again.*

91

ROXIO'S STALLION

Nine pm, as agreed.

Monti's contact had already tubed the horse with starch.

Four hours before he entered a scene well-prepared by Monty. Devoid of personnel for he had created a diversion. Called all staff together and informed them of a need to update security which meant all must remain inside.

Kept them distant, occupied for forty minutes, far enough from stables to ensure the killers practiced evil in peace.

The ex-jockey: always tight for cash, as are his compatriots, constantly worked dodgy jobs for Monti. Substantial pay outs for services rendered, ensured silence.

Easy money got him there.

The death threat that caused him to rejoice in a fast departure down the driveway, ensured tight lips.

Content for the preliminary part of their plan, the administration of the starch, slotted in with perfection.

As intended, Flannery, Senor Angelo's groom summoned Ozzie Thomson, the yard's usual vet, when the horse developed a mild colic at around six that afternoon.

Both pleased to find the horse showed initial and expected response to treatment for mild discomfort, although when Ozzie visited two hours later, he disappointed to find him still uncomfortable.

Ozzie advised his groom. 'Still not right. Shall inject flunixin again, then swing past later, around ten.'

Said that as the decent man showed his fondness for horses when he patted Senor's the horse's neck and added. 'Good chap. Let's hope that injection softens your pain.' After a final pat, turned to Flannery. 'Must check out another case but will not be far away, should you need me before then.'

Georgiou arrived early as planned and disguised his visit under cover of him taking a late stroll before he had to prepare for the bogus upcoming coffee marketing conference.

But careful, he spent thirty minutes on a sneaky tour of the premises, where he snooped around empty yards and peaked into open doors.

On cue, arrived in the stable block while Ozzie was busy treating the horse and when he peered into Senor Angel's stable, said, 'Hi chaps. Can I help?'

Curious and suspicious at the stranger presence, Ozzie challenged him. 'Who are you? Why are you here?' As the stable vet's possessive nature surfaced it uncovered his his normal abruptness with two-legged animals as distinct from his empathy for four-legged ones.

'Sorry man. Never meant to interrupt.'

Ozzie accepted that response and permitted Georgiou to explain in logical format his presence. Finished with. 'Know nothing about thoroughbred stallions, although rode and worked regularly with pleasure horses.' He declared sympathy for Senor when he ran fingers through his mane. 'And yes. Seen lots of colic cases. Find it easy to dislike the condition.'

As horsemen do, while they awaited the horse's response to pain killers, they shared experiences. Ozzie enjoyed Georgiou's experiences of Trail Riding in Greece. 'We consider it the finest in the world.'

As kindred spirits, Georgiou's equine knowledge impressed Ozzie as they continued to chat while they monitored the horse's condition and despite intensity of the situation,

Georgiou acted not merely as his created character.

Under the circumstances, bizarre for he conducted himself as any vet should in the presence of a wounded animal. Thus, despite true reason for being on the farm centred on him killing this horse, he felt the horse's pain. Genuine sympathy seeped as he said, 'His condition worries me.'

Five minutes later, Ozzie now comfortable with Georgiou's company and satisfied with the horse's improved condition, he and Flannery discussed the stud's apparent shortage of staff.

As a man cognisant of the industry, Ozzie enlisted Georgiou's help. 'With this horse giving cause for concern, I am on the brink of admitting to him to our hospital but will first check out these blood sample for basic parameters.'

Excused himself to study a short *WhatsApp* message then frowned, 'Although I must make another quick visit, and as you are obviously familiar with horses, and here may I assume you do nor race of on other business?'

Georgiou admitted as few of the other conference's attendees arrived, he was content to offer his assistance.

Ozzie appreciated that offer. 'In that case I may delay a decision to hospitalise him for an hour.'

For fear of upsetting Flanner, he turned to the Irishman, put an arm around his shoulder and said, 'Sorry, friend. While I have complete faith in you, but as they have worked you hard, this man may prove helpful.'

Flanner's reply, bathed in fast flowing words and his Cork accent, meant Georgiou concentrated to understand him.

Meanwhile, as the vet shook Georgiou's hand, Ozzie's parting remark brought relief. 'Shall visit later but bell me if he worsens.' Made the standard telephone sign by putting two fingers to ear.

Relished how Ozzie gave the handsome colt a firm slap on his sweat drenched neck and left the scene.

Georgiou worried stiff when the vet threatened to hospitalise the colt for fear, he might take the horse away before they did the business. Which hit hard.

Now relieved he focused on how to deal with the groom.

Flanner talked nonstop and Georgiou battled to catchup with his fast, broad, Irish brogue.

Until *Irish*, as Georgiou christened him, yawned hard and flopped onto a smart bench outside the stable. A propitious move for it permitted Georgiou a chance to introduce the next stake.

He took it. 'Now then, friend. You are useless to anyone at present. Get your head down for an hour. Leave him to me to relax, sit here, read a book on my Kindle app, while acting nursemaid for a couple of hours.'

As one might expect, the conscientious groom expressed reluctance to desert his horse.

Patient and positive, Georgiou exerted considerable people skills. 'Go on, man, be sensible.'

Dug firm fingers into the fossa below his neck and massaged a tense spot.

Landed the big one. 'If the vet decides to hospitalise your horse, you shall travel with him. A decent bit of shut eye now, might be all you will manage during a tough night.'

Fair comment, which convinced the man.

Soon Georgiou trailed Flanner to his apartment. 'Now I know where you rest, easy to find. First-rate.'

Pushed the exhausted, middle-aged man into his house.

92

GET THIS DONE

Monti checked the time.

Again.

And worried. 'Come. Now, any minute and we can swing into action.'

Paced the floor again and as he reached the window on the fourth revolution, welcomed the sight of car headlights as they drifted gently up the driveway as if to reward him for his vigilance. 'Yes! Here comes the second player. Now we move.'

Glanced at Paulo, barked at him for drawing his gun. 'No Paulo. Expected this, must be the second vet, and I warned you to keep away.'

Eyes darted between Paulo, the driveway, and the gun. 'To begin with, make sure the safety is on. This is my job, and if you must use your gun, well we will already be in trouble. Finished. So, put it away.'

Leon, as Calder's driver allowed the vehicle to trundle up the blacktop, pleased to find stable area bathed in super troopers of powerful floodlights. Oddly enough, remained calm, resigned to what should follow. Satisfied with his remarkable level of self-control.

Also relieved when Georgiou popped out to meet.

Never waited for driver to bring the car to a stop before he directed him to where to park for a quick getaway. 'Closer, and now swing around, point down the driveway. You never know.'

As the younger vet joined him, Georgiou held Calder by his jacket sleeve, and when he pulled him into the stable block, said, 'Right! Let us get this done.'

Pointed out Senor Angelo's box as first on the left.

Only three extra-large stables filled the north side of a magnificent structure built in native hardwood and wheelbarrow sized blocks of local stone. A horse palace, an equine residence better than most people could ever dream.

Calder, despite intensity of the moment enthralled in spectacular surroundings. 'Take a gander at this place. Doubtless this is six-star accommodation.' Said that as he ignored the second stallion to check Senor's ID against an A3 copy of his passport.

Anxious, Georgiou took control and instructed. 'Now Calder, prepare the injection, as discussed.' Nervousness showed and was picked up by the horse as his overloud hard voiced bounced off the high vaulted ceiling.

Leon, who had accompanied Calder into the yard, stepped back from the stable, left the barn and surprised himself with the power he put into the effort when he gave a confident thumbs-up sign to Monti twenty feet away, although partly obscured by stable's north wall.

Monti, already headed towards the scene, turned, looked up at a window where he expected to find Paulo. Gave him an obvious, similar thumbs-up sign and grunted. 'Everything is set. We can finish this job in ten minutes.'

Until, on full alert, headed into a panic attack.

'No! What is this? What happens here?'

Monti reacted first, left shadows, ran towards the flat and ascended half of the steps as his boss opened a door, and shouted. 'What is happening? Are we in trouble?'

Monti also barked instructions as urgency in his voice escalated to fearful levels. 'Paulo, we are in trouble, get out now as planned. Go.'

Turned away from him on soundless feet.

Flashed downstairs as he moved faster than anyone imagined possible.

Ran towards the stables, and initially hidden from approaching officers, on reaching the vets called out, 'No. Abort. Get out of here. Cops!'

93

WELL, DONE SENOR

Enter a big noisy bird.

Massive engines roared through still air.

Sleek, appeared bigger than it was, the helicopter whirred onto the scene.

In a whirlwind of grass and leaves, blades rotated for three revolutions then landed a mere thirty yards from the stables.

An excellent set of headphones ensured agents talked even over the noisy whirlybird. 'This is positive. We face definite action. Over.' Waterman's voice trilled when he called his director.

In synch, FBI ground reinforcements transported in two bulky black cars roared into view.

Absence of running lights kept them shrouded in darkness as they zoomed up the driveway, and when they cruised up to the stable block, switched on their portfolio of augmented, powerful lights.

They, when combined with the helicopter's formidable super troupers and yards floodlights left no hiding places.

A loudspeaker instructed. 'FBI. Everyone on the ground.' Blanchard's commanding voice rang out as she constantly repeated instructions.

Meanwhile, Georgiou, rooted to the spot, stared at the needle he held in his hand.

Calder held the horse by the head collar as Leon interfered, when he inexplicably countermanded Monti's instruction. 'No. Do this. The injection takes only take twenty seconds. We can kill the horse and be off and away. My escape plan will work.'

Monti exhibited inherent terrible savagery.

Attended to his primary aim.

Without warning or fuss, dropped Leon with a close range shot to the head.

As brain and blood spilled over Calder, he screamed. 'Out now. Run to the rear of the stables.'

Calder and Georgiou dropped everything and lost the plot.

In a scene reminiscent of comic cops featured in the *Thin Blue Line*, they collided.

In their haste to escape, knocked each down into the stable's thick straw.

Waterman acted out his role as leader.

Pistol drawn, reached them first. While running towards the stables, roared. 'FBI stand down!'

Bedlam ensued!

Monti spun around and fired two shots at the agent but narrowly missed him.

Caught the fleeing Calder in the chest.

As Monti darted away from the second FBI agent who followed tight and on the left side of Waterman, he got in the line of fire.

Three agents discharged eight shots.

Despite chaos and confusion, their calculated, well-focused firing appeared to Georgiou and Monti haphazard, delivered from everywhere.

As horses screamed their fear, they contributed to cacophony.

Hoping to avoid the agents Monti ducked into Senor Angelo's stable.

But the big, rough, noisy man slipped, and as he bounced off the stallion's hindquarters, roared at him. 'Move out of my road you stupid thing.'

Fired off half a magazine of bullets.

In the melee, one bullet grazed the panicking horse along his rump.

As he must, Senor Angelo reacted by squealing and lashing out.

Monti took the full force of a flashing hoof on the left temple.

Crashed unconscious to the floor.

Georgiou surrendered.

Threw himself face down to the floor in the passageway outside the third stable.

As an agent fastened him in handcuffs, Paulo still could have used their escape route.

But with nervousness gripping, became irrational.

Next, and unintentionally, instead of at once implementing his exit by fleeing the scene, he drew his gun.

On reaching the barn, Agent Blanchard, spotted the weapon and challenged Paulo.

But panic forces people into mistakes and so it was with Paulo when, forgetting he held the gun, waved arms in her direction.

Blameless, she never guessed his lack of intent, nor could she appreciate intention to discharge the weapon. Functioned as her training demanded.

Two sharp cracks.

Saw a man drop to the floor as Paulo took two shots in right arm and shoulder.

Blanchard continued to impress.

Acted the utter professional, holstered her weapon then handcuffed him.

Raced to the stable.

Gasped at the sight of the berserk Senor Angelo as he trampled Monti and ignored where two agents dragged Calder's prone form from the stable.

Brave, she grabbed the horse's head collar.

Director Davidson joined her, determined to be part of the action but when he took a sharp glancing blow from Senor Angelo's leg, he screamed through his pain for someone to *shoot the thing.*

Regardless of her director's instructions, Blanchard placed herself between armed agents who pointed weapons at the horse. Amid surrealist scenes from movie fantasies, holstered her weapon and approached the bucking animal.

Hand outstretched, moved towards him then she without taking up eye contact, used a firm, strong and confident voice to encourage calm. Called out the well-known single word. "Foot.'

As she repeated this, moved towards the horse and as many anxious specimens do, when faced with the single command foot, he relaxed sufficiently for her to stroke him. Creatures of habit familiar with people cleaning their feet, he settled into an almost normal state.

Impressed the FBI agents who ignored captive criminals to stand open-mouthed as the slim, athletic woman controlled the stallion.

Even if she needed eight minutes with the horse the agent's her seemingly unflappable technique surprised herself and everyone else when she constrained him.

Then again, her partner Waterman approached her in the stable, and as his left arm went around Blanchard's shoulders the other stroked the horse's neck.

Amid that mutual admiration society he said, 'Well done Senor Angelo. And our director called for someone to shoot you!'

Her boss heard this.

Walked away with a huge grin. *Lucky to work with such superbly trained agents.*

Helicopter disgorged two passengers.

Henry and Sophia joined the scene.

As unarmed and foreign officers, the director followed protocol when he instructed them to remain inside the helicopter until they rendered the scene safe.

On seeing Agent Blanchard twenty yards from the barn, Sophia guessed she arrested a prone man.

Despite being a proficient shot, gun ranges never hold the same influence as the real thing.

Thus, excited, and shaking from noise of a terse, deadly gun fight, remained aghast when she faced carnage.

So much so, Henry gave her a most unprofessional embrace.

Lingered for three seconds longer than required, then pushed her away. 'Stiff upper lip, my dear. Show no weakness.'

Sophia, in curious detached manner, never shared his enthusiasm for success, and a thought, even if brewing in its infancy, jumped to the fore. *Now, dear lady, after this a trip to York. Time for retirement, and well, suspect a place in the Faith family awaits.*

Henry who had experienced two armed interventions, fared better and his calm, detached mien absorbed sight of the arrested Georgiou and three prone figures. While satisfaction at a job well done flowed, he as did the others, regretted loss of life.

Death immersed the barn and despite this, Sophia hugged Blanchard, kissed Senor Santa's black muzzle, and shared self-satisfied grins of horse lovers pleased to find their charge well.

Apart from an obvious, bleeding eight cm nick over one hindquarter.

Straightaway, the stallion's vet and groom arrived.

The initially mesmerised Ozzie revelled in the extraordinary event of his armed escort to the stables.

Professional to the end he placed five stitches in the gunshot wound.

Thereafter, during the horse's breeding career, never failed to run fingertips over his scar.

Newspaper articles featured him and his charge.

After going viral, new owners mounted one superbly silver mounted headline opposite his stable door.

FBI AGENT AND HORSE FULL AROUND.

Agents Blanchard and Waterman revelled in promotion.

When they visited the horse three weeks later found Senor Angelo, fully recovered and busy breeding his ladies.

When he greeted them, the Senor nipped her arm.

Caught off guard, Blanchard said, 'Ouch!'

Rubbed the spot and continued. 'Nice one Senor, so you remember me?'

Waterman buttered her up. 'Swear he winked at you.'

94

WRAP UP

Started with six days intensive debriefing.

Evidence collected initiated months of deeper, widespread research.

Georgiou's sweet song rang out like the proverbial bird when he helped lay down a detailed trail that protected him from manslaughter charges over Sean's death and reduced his jail sentence to eight years.

Trainers he implicated, included Saunders and Humphrey permanently lost licences, home bases and after prison terms, never again got within twenty yards of a horse.

Inasmuch as three countries argued over which country deserved Georgiou; the Greeks, fingers burned from Alroy's team's investigation, won in the end.

Forthwith, when Yvette implicated Louis as mastermind behind their effort, she received a shorter sentence than him.

Louis only saw his child eight years later and never understood the diatribe Yvette spat his way, always blamed him for allowing Sophia to trap them.

Altogether, after being at the top of the pile their flop hit hard.

Paulo faced the most marked lifestyle changes.

Remained hospitalised in intensive care for three days before fit for FBI interviews.

Despite hoping to protect his sources, the promise of them sanctioning Morgan to retain their holiday home and coffee-based business, meant he exposed his drug network from farming to distribution.

Because his evidence against Assistant Director Rhodes of the FBI led to a conviction, and when he disclosed his Chinese dealings, plea bargaining resulted in a significantly reduced nine-year sentence.

Financial assets, including properties and horses forfeit to the state.

Worse followed when eight months later a warden found him dead in the shower room. Shanked by a sharpened toothbrush. The Chinese gained their revenge.

Morgan escaped prosecution.

After a name change, and a slinky relocation to darkest Texas, never attained the desired state of royalty.

Senor Angelo came out on top.

One of the rare horses to recover from a massive starch intake and a bullet wound.

Nature works wonders and thus, his system kicked into gear as onrush of circulatory benefits from excitement and focused treatment saved his life after Georgiou, with an odd show of humanity, advised vet Ozzie and Blanchard how they drenched him with starch.

Confessed this before FBI took him away.

With this unexpected, welcome turnaround, Senor Angelo's crop, sired after this adventure won everything.

That set the horse out on a successful stud career as leading stallion for sixteen seasons which earned shareholders fortunes and glory.

The Chinese empire took a hammering.

Inasmuch as their ancient cultural practices held sway, five members of the Zhāng family disappeared. Callous, vengeful masters engineered in-house execution style deaths, which included the twins, with synchronised efficiency.

As louis outlined the routes of the diamond smuggling chain this resulted in multiple arrests.

If Gregor and Chung resisted arrest, they barely survived.

Although their Mongolian postings which included herding feral ponies amid the great sweeping grassland never held flavour of earlier campaigns.

The Chinese empire took an enormous knock.

Required almost fourteen years of tentative probing before they induced a follow up team of a Special Agent FBI and a DCI in the Met to begin building their sordid empire, as a minor player on the world's corruption stage.

95

WOLF COMMANDS

Henry telephoned Wolf on his special number.

Delighted to respond to his instruction they meet.

'Damn bad news about DS Stewart, damn bad.'

Henry agreed. 'Indeed sir, most unfortunate.'

Straightaway, after he laid out facts, the Commissioner instructed. 'In the absence of Superintendent Stewart need you, Superintendent, and the full team at HQ. Time to take down these bastards and your team deserve the honour.'

When they met with the Commissioner, he bathed in the success he hoped for and now relished.

Clasped Henry's hand. 'Remarkable, quite remarkable. Anticipate studying your team's in-depth report on this superb investigation.'

Continued in that vein, satisfied their secret meeting in a North London park secure. 'This becomes a case study for students. Brilliant work. Award winning as well. A lovely thought.'

As he rose from the modern composite bench, he took a final fond glance over a colourful bed of flavourful annuals that burst into blossom. When he turned to leave, stared at Henry. 'Not a word to anyone in the team, but the FBI also prepare to give you chaps a decent send off.'

As that worked out as promised the teams jet flight to New York and their *three-day conference* went better than anyone dreamed.

Henry, even though famous for his hard, impregnable manner, could not help smiling as Wolf continued. 'Need your team in conference room four. Ten forty-five sharp tomorrow morning; conference room four.'

Outlined how they should sneak in as individuals, filter in throughout the morning, separate. 'The business will follow at eleven in room five. Timing critical, for in synch, FBI will nail Rhodes.'

Repeated. 'But first. Gather in conference room four. Got that?'

Henry saluted. 'Got it, sir.'

'Of course, intend we arrest all three bastards with impeccable synchronicity. With you as arresting officer. An honour Superintendent Stewart deserves. Sadly, as he cannot attend, your well-deserved honour.'

Later that afternoon. Wolf, confident and in command, thoughts of her misinterpreting actions never even entering his head, buzzed PA. 'Inspector Pastor. Organise our best lunch ever. Spare no expense, champagne the lot, in conference room five at 11.15am tomorrow.

Plan on around twenty, no make that thirty people, including,' Rhymed off names, 'ACs Flynn, Meakins, and Proudley if available. Also, three or four of the CS's. Whoever, is available, although Gordon and Milroy are in for starters.'

While they constructed the event, could not resist an outpouring of deceitful magnanimity. 'Of course, yourself. After years of faithful service, could not neglect you for this important event.'

Excitement contagious, she almost dropped the phone. 'Yes sir.'

'That will be all.'

Hung up, permitted himself a big smile. That should throw the bitch off the scent.

Placed a call to Assistant Commissioner Proudley. 'Need you here. Imperative. Use helicopter, if necessary, but be here tomorrow at eleven.' Take no excuses. 'Just be here.'

Wolf tapped desk, and when he looked at the photograph of HM, chuckled. 'Got them Mam. Hooked the bastards.'

Pastor popped her head around the door. 'Sorry Sir. Your instruction disturbs CS Fletcher. With something important going on, he queries necessity of his attendance. Indeed, as do the others. On balance, they request information, your meeting's agenda. Time involved.'

'Damn them.'

Considered options for a moment. 'Not a word to anyone else.'

Fingered side of nose and distributed a generous smile. 'Tomorrow promises to be a memorable day... For I shall announce my retirement and indicate those I recommend succeeding me.'

'Gosh! Mean, thank you, sir.'

As an obviously flustered Pastor left, he smiled to himself. *Notwithstanding my instruction to secrecy, bet she takes less than two minutes to leak my news.*

Without delay or complaints, he expected them to come at the gallop, joyful school children at their graduation. Spoke aloud. 'Then. Chop, chop and then firm, a most pleasant third chop.'

But because he associated that with firm hand thumps against the top of his desk, they were hard enough to cause Pastor to run in without knocking and ask. 'Sorry sir, is there a problem?'

No matter her concerns, pleased with his effort, he pretended to whisk a dead fly from desk. As grins danced over face, he chuckled. 'Not at all, but it took me three goes to get the rubbish thing.'

Three minutes later, strolled from the office, forced a grin at his still stunned PA as he passed her desk. Thirty yards into corridors of power found AC Meakins, still rushed after a hectic rush in one of the boardrooms with officers and civilians.

Wrapped on the window, held up a finger, and mouthed. 'Give me a minute.' Motioned him away from prying eyes. 'Got them. Our big takedown. Conference room five, tomorrow at eleven.'

To emphasise seriousness of the effort instructed him to arrange for two armed officers and Internal Affairs top brass. 'Drag them up from the bowels of this place if you must.'

When he gave his friend a most unprofessional hug that raised eyebrows. 'The decisive moment. Need everyone here at exactly ten minutes past eleven.'

Smiled, turned to leave, and continued. 'Shall grin like a Cheshire cat until then.'

AC Meakins' cover held up. The only officer Alroy never sussed as being knowledgeable of his investigation.

DI Pastor's call to Flynn, indicated high hopes. 'Okay, Geraldine, here we go.'

'Fantastic news my darling.' Thought for a moment. 'Mind you. If they offer me the post of commissioner, consider the money we could make.'

'No! Geraldine, do not do this to me.'

Flynn's greedy mind did cartwheels at the thought as she dropped the call.

96

ALROY'S SUCCESS

Ten forty-five am.

Wolf briefed Henry and his team in conference room four.

Adjacent to the larger number five where they prepared to make the arrests.

When he addressed the team, they appreciated genuine dissatisfaction in the Commissioner's voice. 'Disappointed our DS cannot be with us.'

After that brief soft moment, he changed, became the competent leader they expected. 'Besides that, are my officers prepared for this showdown?'

All eight snapped off a quick fire. Yes sir.

Harmony impressed Wolf who approved how Henry coached them for the event.

Three passing senior officers, unable to recognise anyone in the discussion group, wondered why the Commissioner spent time with lower ranks. Luckily, whispered questions never raised sufficient notice to interfere with the business.

Only AC Meakins was privy to the commissioner's intentions.

As Bernard stood closest to the window, he anxiously peeked through the almost closed venetian blind, intent on spotting their prey arrive. Warned the others. 'And here come the lambs.'

Flynn and Gordon arrived together with Pastor five minutes later.

Because they approached the conference room from the blind side, they spotted nothing untoward.

'Not lambs. Sheep ready to face the wolves, I mean Wolf. Appropriate.' Pauline shared her disgust, although although others relished her smart play on the Commissioner's code name.

Sophia said, 'And now. Look at them, wreathed in smiles. Unaware of what they face. Lovely.'

'Yes friends. If we remain in the force for forty years, our part in this takedown will still hold interest. Without doubt, the pinnacle of our police careers.' As DI Mandy rose to peek, she performed her posing trick.

Staff had suitably prepared the conference room. The Met's biggest and best furnished conference room, as *guests*; nice word, arrived they admired the magnificent lunch. The best Pastor's special expense account ever managed.

After six senior officers arrived within five minutes, sparkling eyes and noisy chatter created a jolly scene.

Magnanimous, as he acted the complete host, the Commissioner encouraged the three marked officers, including his PA, to dig in and enjoy themselves. 'As we share this, our final, intimate meeting together, let us enjoy ourselves.'

Laughed, a powerful ringing tone which encouraged everyone to settle. 'Because, I intend having a splendid day.'

Flynn, beside herself with joy at the news Pastor earlier delivered, whispered to her behind a bubbling glass of decent champagne. 'Wonderful news for us. Only joked about working on. Now, propitious, we can time our departure to his. As an excuse or turnaround, no one will give us a thought. Fantastic.'

Wolf noticed their sniggering and barely resisted temptation to crack heads. Only just. *Enjoy your bubbly ladies. Final glass for years.*

At ten minutes past eleven, Wolf winked at Meakins.

Excused himself from the group, popped around the corner, wrapped the glass window, and clicked fingers at Henry. His signal summoned them from the adjacent room.

Five minutes before, Henry had prepared the armed officers and those from Internal Affairs on upcoming arrests. So, Henry reminded the armed guards. 'After I make the arrests, the Commissioner demands you parade the handcuffed guilty slowly, with lots of fanfare through each floor to the cells.'

Admired how they, as seasoned officers, accepted their role without question.

Henry, in full uniform, as were his team, acted model of police correctness when he ordered armed officers to stand guard outside the door.

Used an extravagant flourish to open both doors, invited his team and the officers from Internal Affairs to join the others in the vibrant conference room.

The sight of this dramatic change of affairs caused much flapping tongues and forced temperature of the meeting to plummet from plenty to zero.

The commissioner snapped. 'Attention, everyone.'

Crowd sprang into gear as he pointed out Henry, said, 'Meet CI Higgins, now formally Superintendent Higgins.' He will introduce his team and take us into the morning's true business.

There was a deathly silence as each of Henry's officers responded to their name and new ranks, with a smart salute and a strong, *yes sir*.

Without delay, a final nod from the commissioner allowed Henry to switch on the video projector. His succinct presentation, audio, and visual disgorged damning, solid evidence in less than five minutes.

With the room speechless, Wolf's livid face spat into three guilty faces. 'DS Henry. Arrest this scum.'

Armed guards were unnecessary.

Neither Flynn nor Gordon commented or offered resistance.

Only Pastor reacted, did so in the manner of a sixteen-year-old dumped by first ever boyfriend. Her constant wailing when guards escorted them along corridors, ensured many aghast colleagues witnessed the parade of the guilty.

Wolf shook hands all around. 'And now you wonderful officers can party as never before.'

The Commissioner enjoyed himself.

His best day in years.

While he handed out compliments and promotions to the team, Henry's flashing phone alerted him to take a call. 'Sorry sir. The one we await.'

Listened and reported on that brief communication. 'All gone to plan on the other side. Arrests made. Thet thank us. Invite the team to join them in New York and together we will debrief.'

Henry's face, awash with news further advised on the gathering of the overseas successful sting. 'The FBI picked up two of their people, an Assistant Director and a Deputy Director, already linked to AC Flynn.'

'Thank you, Superintendent, and team. For now, our project ends on the highest note ever.'

THE END

A TASTER

FINAL VOLUME

OVERTOUN FIVE

OVERTOUN RHINO
SUBTITLE: PRINCESS GUGU

1

YOUR BROTHER

Entombed in her flashy car, Francesca phoned her mother.

Evan decided the Golf GTI never matched the driver's personality.

Declared a Discovery Sport suited to her robust temperament.

However, amid this tricky situation, she embraced its manoeuvrability and speed.

With her tearful daughter in full flow, Clarice, through the car's speaker phone, winced as the girl mistreated even its competitive gears.

Missed the connotation for barely a second, and then as her mind displayed perambulations of an indecisive flock of Red-billed queleas, shared her shock. 'No! You cannot be right. This news astounds me.'

Francesca disregarded the following hint of indecision and insecurity as her mum sought conformation. 'Are you sure?'

As brain headed heavenwards it made her as careless of traffic as a bolting horse gallops after it dumps jockey in the starting pens. Raced on, reckless of her mother's reaction, when hurrying through evidence without thinking.

'Whereas they have no facts set in stone.' Struggled to unfold the heady information garnered during the girl's lunch with Elaine. Hurried through the careless, stabbing manner with which Elaine introduced the subject of Sister Catherine's dislike for the Cairns family.

Clarice gasped on understanding how that information related to criminal activity around Niall's birth. Turbulent mind sensed her daughter's pain.

The notion that had already hammered Francesca's psyche, now pounded Clarice's already revved mind. Daughter's overloud modern music, Bruno Mars, and drummer Anderson proved too much.

In the meantime, she, keen, yet unsure about discussing the saga with Niall, her mum, as her best friend, remained her choice of confident.

A necessary wait because of her carelessness when she overtook a truck made her drift the car and pause the conversation. Nevertheless, hectic noise of squealing brakes through her phone increased Clarice's anxiety and demanded an extra-large dose of willpower to remain silent until her daughter continued.

Francesca forced herself to explain. 'Yes. The evidence mounts. Unbelievable, for people suggest my Niall and Alroy Stewart are twins.' Her tone climbed. 'People suggest someone at Overtown may have separated them at birth.' Shouted above the din of motorists peeping horns in response to her wayward, agitated progress.

Clarice headed into panic mode. *Likewise, if some mix up at the hospital means those boys are the real Stewart twins, my daughter's future lays in tatters.*

Pictured the girl's agitated hands as her breathing escalated into the effort of an in-labour first timer as she grunted her next statement. 'Will fill you in as information seeps out.'

With Francesca, taking a necessary and sensible step, the control of her law trained mind asserted her actions to improve necessary control. While she forced tense, sweaty hands to soften their grip on the steering wheel, she peered through the increasing drizzle.

Until she found a gap that allowed her to tuck her car into a lay bye, when she even killed the music. Regardless of her intense news, when she settled sufficient to phone her mum back, disappointed followed when Clarice cried off from their conversation. Pleaded she must take an urgent, international call.

Thus, Francesca barely gained time to discuss her significant concerns, before her mum offered a quick, love you, and dropped the call.

Clarice worked two phones.

Hot from activity, she contacted her second-in-command. 'So, Janice, I do not care how difficult you perceive the situation. A family emergency demands I head off at once for Dumbarton.'

In response to the competent Janice's initial attempt to complain her unprepared for a top-level meeting, she broke one of her cardinal rules by shouting at a staff member. 'Spent too much time training you to assume command. Do not waste this marvellous opportunity to demonstrate your value to me, the company. You are ready to take this meeting, so I need you to get on with this.'

Given the circumstances, no traveller ever packed a bag as fast as Clarice. Agitated as never since birthing her daughter, she pushed her five series BMW through three speed traps up the A1.

Now, mantra-like, repeated the same impossible to imagine, possibility. Because I seduced Angus Stewart, that resulted in him fathering Francesca. And as for Niall Cairns. If true, that makes my daughter's fiancé her half-brother.

Because she left within thirty minutes of ending her conversation with Francesca, her rush when packing released an omission.

'Oops. No knickers must buy six pairs.'

DR ALEX NIVEN

Website: dralexniven.com

THE MEMOIR STORIES

As one would expect Dr Alex' VETERINARY MEMOIRS written during forty years of veterinary practice where he treated various animals is an absorbing, five volume series.

The stories reflect on cases that touched Dr Alex' life and his family, during adventures with animals as diverse as cattle, dogs and horses to elephant, rhino, and lions.

His career took him through Scotland and England to South Africa.

In Volume One: **THE BENT BULL**, gasp at the charging lion.

Thrill with him as he rejoiced over Hansie's cancer cure.

Gulp as he did when Lady Nordic; his much-loved SAAB saved his life.

Laugh with him as Charlie, the nutcase Jack Russell Charlie found himself trapped when he assaulted a newspaper. While it left Charlie embarrassed it always draws laughter. Mind you... that is the nature of the breed.

Come on man! Did he in 1978 really use superglue to repair a dogs fractured leg? And it healed well.

Then there was the tale of the bossy police officers mentally disturbed and baldy bird which he only cured after she dumped her boyfriend. Soon content, her tale of naughty goings-on with what we must term a *gentleman's club* got local tongues wagging.

When a trainer rejected the chestnut gelding Red Heaven the owner consulted Dr Alex. When given appropriate treatment under a fresh trainer they won a group one race, another case which illustrated the value of homoeopathy.

Consider a dangerously ill patient who benefitted from his often-employed mantra. Never give up. *They are only dead when the heart stops!*

In Vol Two: **OUR CALF TESSA** share Dr Alex' hysterical tale of the lollipop which stuck to Chang's...... and made him lame.

Not all cases are soft, cuddly happy ones.

Rachael's death is a tearjerker that illustrates vets do more than wrap bandages on puppies' paws. From disaster came *Lady Tess*, one their favourite animals.

When teaching **Simon** how to unblock a cat's penis jampacked full of crystals, flighty urine illustrated how young vets can learn if they accept advice.

An **abused lady** is a human-interest story. One which illustrates vets always have at least two patients to consider. The human guardian deserves respect.

Theresa's **bed warmer** illustrates Alex's dedication to saving lives. Accept how the exercising of his vocation depended on the fabulous girl who shares his life.

GOATS AND GIRLS highlights Slug Bait poisoning in Vol Three. A story that illustrates Niven's concern for the environment when he discusses two dangers.

Associated the first with the careless use of poisonous chemicals.

Second reflects on desirability of teamwork.

For him, a sad story reflects on how the tractor destroyed the romance of the heavy horse, the fabulously strong **Clydesdales** who made Scotland famous.

The impossible **Grumble Guts** was not so difficult when Dr Alex diagnosed his behavioural problem was due to partial sight. A simple management change set him off on the road to showjumping success.

In **TURKEY TALES:** Vol four introduces a remarkable animal lover who funded her hobby from jewellery theft. Her bird's egg-bound plight first created interest.

The extraordinary truth of the British government's approach to **anthrax** as a weapon in the second world war came to the surface when he diagnosed it killed a cow. No! He never brought it back to life!

An **overturned horsebox** not only describes the plight of the injured horses, but also the attitude of the owner which declared he deserved the same fate. Horrid human greed illustrates why not all people should never own animals.

In a similar theme, when the American vet described his farmer client's method of catching a wild **pregnant cow**, while successful proved unbelievable.

His first experience of **dehorning** an adult cow led to plastic surgery.

Ever wondered at where the expression **SHIT** came from? Dr Alex describes its derivation. Does so amid another absorbing tale of the link between human and animal distress, and how he involved social services to help Mrs Woods, who as she threatened to die from neglect, triggered powerful.

As a youngster, the family's adventures with a collection of wild things from frogs to **hedgehogs** kept them entertained in days before TV and computers.

FAMILY MATTERS in Vol five, illustrates happy moments including the best day of his life when his gorgeous Dumbarton girl, **Theresa;** the catch of Dumbarton married him. The **vet's first day** almost never made it into print as it still evokes powerful, unpleasant memories. Everything went wrong on what he hoped must be a fabulous introduction to his longed-for career. Yes! Perhaps engineering might have suited him better.

Theresa's first visit to a **calving cow** gave her an exceptional insight into farming, including how to reflect on a bull's massive equipment when deciding... male or female. But her experience birthing a calf got her hormones flowing.

Juliet, a silly **fantailed pigeon** added a different dimension to animal welfare.

When he knelt beside a sick pony and used his ears to listen for signs of pneumonia, were the connections entitled to believe **Christianity** cured its bronchitis?

A case of **Siamese twins** began as an extraordinarily difficult birthing, but not only did he save the cow's life but also, she continued to breed normal calves.

***

DR ALEX NIVEN

WORKS OF FICTION

OVERTOUN

A five volume novel.

OVERTOUN

VOLUME ONE

OVERTOUN

Story line. August 1982. Begins when Henderson attends a road traffic accident. As this medic treats Gerry discovers him as an old nemesis, he fought with over a girl. Concussed, Henderson's aberrant personality unfolds when to get his revenge, he kills Gerry by blocking his oxygen tube.

Celine, a trainee medic under his wing, witnesses enough of Henderson's malpractice to make her suspicious Gerry's death is needless, possibly criminal. Unable to cope, she leaves the Vale Hospital and joins Overtoun Maternity Hospital.

Haunted by unpleasant memories, she, encouraged by colleagues digs into the case until convinced Gerry died due to murder.

June 1981. Fiona, rejoicing at the success of her engagement party, drives her fiancée Tom to a special layby on Loch Lomond where they first consummated their relationship.

Reckless after drink, she crashes the car and kills Tom. Maurice and Alice witness the accident. She supports Fiona while he attends to Tom. Finding him dead; he removes the body from the passenger seat and lays him out on the beach beside the driver's door.

Does this to prevent Fiona from a drunk driving charge. Persuades his girlfriend to lie to the police, convince them Tom drove the car.

Medic Henderson captivates Fiona when he transports her to the hospital. Later, she enters an abusive marriage with him. Treating her as a surrogate mother, she delivers a weak infant.

Matron, fearful of him dying and how that must have desperate consequences for Fiona's life, swaps him for one of the Stewart's twin boys born at the same time.

When both boys become ill, we meet Sr Holly, a neonatal ICU specialist, and her determination to romance and later marry the brilliant, perfect but hopelessly shy specimen, Dr Patrick Cairns.

His concern for Fiona results in him suggesting they swap twins, although Deirdre changes his opinion. She, to protect her brother from repercussions, convinces him it a bad idea, then orchestrates the swap by herself.

Sr Angela, as Matron Cairn's deputy, develops increasing concerns around matron's management of the infants. When on the point of uncovering this, Deirdre in a masterstroke of perfect timing, promotes her to assistant matron. A move that suppresses further investigation.

Nurse Ingrid is well paid for collecting tissue samples from newborn infant girls. Does this on behalf of a North Korean company. Unknown to her they hope to develop a biological weapon against Caucasian women. The volume ends when this goes wrong.

OVERTOUN

VOLUME TWO

OVERTOUN TWINS

Story line. Overtoun's Matron Deirdre Cairns earlier swapped her sisters infant, believing him dying for a Stewart infant, one of twins. Swaps to protect her sister Fiona from her increasingly difficult husband, Henderson.

Oldest of the three siblings. Matron of Overtoun Hospital. Intrigue and innuendo floods the hospital. She despairs authorities must uncover her crime.

Her only solution, as she sees it, is to prepares for suicide.

Until news of Nurse Ingrid's death brings hope, but her mental instability worsens.

Deirdre hates Henderson. Rejoices when Celine divulges how other medics intend to mount an investigation around Gerry's death and reveal fresh information.

Midwife Sister Catherine's investigations increase tension throughout the hospital. After establishing twins have birthmarks, she uncovers the swap. Before she can unmask the crime, a road accident results in her sustaining a debilitating, chronic, head injury.

Her diary uncovers the truth around her dislike of the Cairns family.

While enraptured with her stolen child, the swapped Stewart twin, Fiona's remarkable sense of smell, alerts Deirdre to the possibility she recognises the child as not hers.

The infant becomes ill.

Henderson's distorted personality worsens when he appreciates the medics may uncover, he murdered Gerry. Tremendous mood swings lead to impotence and increasing dependence on Mirror Man, his alter ego who decides Henderson must murder Deirdre to prevent her uncovering their crime.

Patrick Cairns, middle of the siblings is a doctor at Overtoun Hospital. His medical skill saves lives of both infants.

Patrick and Henderson fight, during which the latter sustains a head injury. In time, this leads to serious altercation between him and Mirror Man.

The massive fight between him and Henderson results in them breaking the mirror.

Henderson slashes at Mirror Man with a piece of broken glass.

Henderson collapses from a severed jugular vein.

In danger of dying Deirdre arrives to convince him not to divulge her secret.

But finds him lying in a bloody pool. Although she summons ambulance, does she work hard enough to save his life?

Their black Labrador, Afrika, continues to support Patrick.

Sr Holly is midwife and ICU specialist. An effervescent, dedicated character, she works hard with Patrick to save infants. At last, she wears down his resistance and under the best imaginable romantic circumstances he proposes.

Margaret Stewart, the twins mother copes with the swap until one child, her true child, takes ill.

Husband Angus' support helps her through a tough time.

Francesca Cormie is born at Overtoun at same time as the subject children.

Clarice, her mother, disguised her pregnancy, maintaining she adopted the girl.

With no intention of having a permanent man, but wishing to get pregnant, she selected Angus Stewart as her sperm donor and seduced him for that purpose.

Three infants play significant parts in later volumes.

Sr Samantha from the Vale Hospital plays a role when during an emergency power failure at that hospital, she leads a team of staff and pregnant mums to Overtoun.

Tiredness causes her to make a significant medical error. This opens the way for Deidre to promote Angela to matron, thereby allaying her interest in the crime.

Ends with Deirdre, convinced her crime exposed by Sr Catherine, secludes herself at home and awaits police.

OVERTOUN

VOLUME THREE

OVERTOUN: HORSES

Story line. Police visit Deirdre's home and ask her to accompany them. At first, relieved for she expected their visit.

Great surprise followed when they advised they were taking her to Overtoun hospital.

A massive train crash in Dumbarton Central Station meant they drafted in all available medical personnel to assist with disaster management.

Eight years later. Holly and Patrick, now married with two children host a Cairn's family lunch. Still ravaged by guilt and loss, Deirdre, her mental health regularly deteriorating she almost reveals how she swapped the infants.

Life progresses to the children as teenagers then adults as we follow their careers into vet medicine and the police force.

Vet and twin Niall's involvement with best friend Evan when they research homoeopathy in HIV research at Glasgow University promises wonderful things.

Niall becomes engaged with Francesca; unknown to both, they share a father.

Twin Calder meets bogus vet, Georgiou Houdalakis, and together enter the hideous life of killing horses to claim insurance payouts.

In parallel, the Commissioner of Police instructs Calder's brother Alroy to run a secret investigation into that business.

We follow this through twists and turns between Britain and Kentucky, where it involves Paulo Grizelli, horse breeder, and drug distributor.

Overtoun

Volume four

OVERTOUN: KENTUCKY

Story line. Niall and Evan's research on HIV promises success.

As his first patient he treats Alroy; not yet introduced as his twin, and on death's door from HIV.

Only after saving his life does, he learns of their happy relationship.

Introduce Yvette and Louis, American horse vets who engage in fraud in parallel with Calder and Georgiou. They link up with Chinese agents to create a novel method for diamond smuggling by transporting gems inside horses which leads to Europe.

Patrick Cairns establishes Deirdre had swapped the twins, that Calder is Fiona's natural son, while Niall and Alroy are true twins.

Corrupt racehorse trainers collaborate with bogus vet Georgiou and Calder to kill horses.

Alroy and the FBI sniff the prospect of a major takedown, including American and Chinese drug dealers.

The vets travel to Kentucky to kill Senor Angelo, a fabulously successful racehorse, now a stallion at stud.

In a smart takedown, the FBI rescue the horse and conduct arrests.

Senor Angelo has the last laugh.

OVERTOUN

Volume five

OVERTOUN: RHINO

Story line. When Glasgow University sells off Niall and Evan's HIV project to a multinational company, they horrify to learn how they mothball what should have been a fabulous effort proving homoeopathy is real, lifesaving medicine.

They sacrifice it for a less effective but more lucrative product. This leads to Niall and Evan leaving the world of research and while undecided about their future, Niall received the potentially fatal hammer blow which leads to his split from fiancé Francesca.

Her mother Clarice reveals devastating truth around her parentage and how she selected a sperm donor.

After a disastrous attempt to enter farming practice in Dumfries, Niall heads off to join Gugu on her family farm in South Africa. He, hoping for an extended holiday to recharge his sagging mental state lands in a situation where Gugu and her family have other intentions.

While they work hard to ensure she captures the man of her dreams, animals bring her intentions to fruition.

Introduce Sarah Kelly, a Dumbarton girl, and another vet. Her tempestuous life with a would-be suitor which never gets beyond a simple kiss, leads to her visiting South Africa to work on Gugu's second then Ipulazi their main family farm.

There, amid a gun battle she saves Evan's life from a deranged poacher and killer which by awakening deep seated neurochemicals controlling love, confirms it time for Sarah to involve herself in affairs of the heart.

Rhino poaching takes centre stage where the hideous reality of a Nigerian and Chinese partnership threatens to wreaking havoc on Ipulazi.

In a masterly stroke, they invite the recovering Alroy to visit the farm to continue convalescing from his near-death experience with HIV, but in practical terms, they ask him to lead the investigation against the poachers.

Gugu's aunt leads the team who interrogate two Nigerian embassy workers. Via a brutal but effective session of intense questioning, a scalpel opens tongues.

A fitting finale finds poacher and their informants receiving suitable, tribal punishment with Gugu at last claiming her man.

DR ALEX NIVEN

NON-FICTION

HOMOEOPATHY TEXTBOOKS

Volume One

REPERTORY AND MATERIA MEDICA

The Repertory includes a detailed discourse on four hundred and eighty remedies and their interactions. This includes detailed clinical indications and the signs of disease and the conditions to which they relate.

The Materia Medica illustrates various disease parameters, their signs and offers pointers towards selecting appropriate remedies.

As an example, consider the remedy *Berberis aquifolium* (Berb-a) of proven value in the management of lameness conditions in horses.

The indications alongside the various organ implicated, help in confirming clinical conditions where this remedy may assist.

The role that aggravating conditions play in mediating disease are reflected.

By way of example consider the following as an illustration of how the remedies are setup in the volume.

Berb-a

BERBERIS AQUIFOLIUM

Mahonia aquifolium Plant

MODALITIES Agg; evening and night.

Amel; cold washing.

Also significant is it relationship and similarity with other remedies including Aloe Ars Berb Psor Sulph which offer alternative selections.

UROGENITAL Azoturia. Lithiasis with proteinuria and tenesmus. PU.

LAMENESS Azoturia; profound muscle pain and stiffness.

SKIN Widespread blisters and papules.

COMPETITION Azoturia and high muscle enzymes in sport horses.

MODALITIES Agg; evening and night. Amel; cold washing.

COMPARE Aloe Ars Berb Psor Sulph.

CONSIDER

- Acute allergic eczemas including flea bite and veld mange.
- Azoturia; better than Berb

- Cystitis and lithiasis.

POTENCY 6X. 30CH.

Worth pointing out where the author emphasises Berberis aquifolium as being more useful than the similar Berberis vulgaris. An indication of where his extensive clinical experience and willingness to experiment allow him to make such a confident claim.

Volume two

THEORY AND CLINICAL APPLICATION

While other authors have written extensively and well on the theory of homoeopathy, Niven's basic introduction accents the main points with a twist.

For here he regularly discusses a detailed approach to an individual case, and how various animal species in his experience show different cure rates and reaction responses to homoeopathy.

His introduction to the management of cancer with nosodes because it includes cure in field cases offer groundbreaking research for the future.

His collection of samples using specialised PRP syringes, and their further preparation under the NIVEN KORSAKOVIAN system is a first, as it recognises the necessity of succussing samples one thousand times during nosode and sarcode preparation. Far more than standard practice, by reporting clinical success, this must offer hope for future workers to refine and achieve success.

Because space prevents the description of an extensive number of conditions, the author picks out this nuisance of a disease which causes marked distress in animals and owners.

Also, as this is one which responds especially well to homoeopathy, it illustrates where cure is possible. Thus, he includes secondary, and concomitant conditions, with the ever-present threat of serious, chronic gastric ulceration.

Understand how homoeopathy restored desperate conditions to full function.

IBD - INFLAMMATORY BOWEL DISORDER.

May be related to or worsened by food sensitivities.

IBD Is associated with chronic diarrhoea, flatus, and colic.

Individuals may develop secondary liver disease and often is associated with skin problems.

Gastric ulceration possible.

Treatment considers toxaemia from standard drug therapy.

Widespread use of cortisone results in a partial improvement but is toxic.

Reduce such treatments slow. Aim for complete resolution.

Remedies: APIS BELL CORTISO LACH MERC RHUS-T THUJ Acid-oxal Carb-v Gaert-b Mag-s Op Urt-u.

Treatment:

Chronic; Cortiso Gaert-b or Merc 30CH. Hydr or Acid-oxal 12X. Apis Bry or Urt-u 6X. TD. Months. SD.

Eco-Vet management with the following medicines often brings success.

ECO-HEAL for first aid relief.

ECO-DIARRHO for the control of gastroenteritis.

ECO-ULCER for controlling damage to the lining of stomach and intestines.

Volume three

EQUINE HOMOEOPATHY

Practicalities of training horses, irrespective of which disciplines, is dependent on the attitude of the horse and the owner. While it does not fall within the author's remit to treat people... well, he presents situations where a slight modification in the trainer's approach has resulted in excellent in the horse's behaviour.

A sad fact is obvious. In the author's practice he often faced difficult horses, either because they are either inherently problematic or have reached a state whereby faulty or imperfect human interaction creates barriers.

It was because cases became terminal, they drove Niven into researching the topic to establish which if any might respond to adjustment with homoeopathic medication.

Important to state this, although it can be spectacularly successful, this can at best be only likely with good owner management. Remembering always that horse, rider, and trainer work best when as a team they act in synch.

Niven's skill becomes apparent when considering his management and where he describes case reports which engender confidence.

Volume Four

MATERIA MEDICA

A stand-alone collection of the homoeopathic remedies.

Does not include a repertory.

Volume Five

COMPANION ANIMAL HOMOEOPATHY

The focus in this volume is mainly animals which are linked to people as pets.

Dogs and cats form the bulk of the work.

As many vets lack the necessary tools to deal with birds, this volume should help.

Small furry creatures from guinea pigs to rabbits are important.

Touches of reptiles and amphibians.